Advances in Hemophilia Treatment

E. Carlos Rodríguez-Merchán
Editor

Advances in Hemophilia Treatment

From Genetics to Joint Health

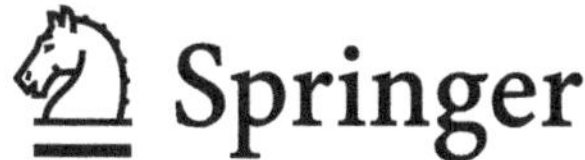

Editor
E. Carlos Rodríguez-Merchán
Department of Orthopedic Surgery
La Paz University Hospital
Madrid, Spain

ISBN 978-3-030-93992-2 ISBN 978-3-030-93990-8 (eBook)
https://doi.org/10.1007/978-3-030-93990-8

This Springer imprint is published by the registered company Springer Nature Switzerland AG
The registered company address is: Gewerbestrasse 11, 6330 Cham, Switzerland

Preface

Recent advances in treatment allow many people with hemophilia to live a life which is similar to that of the rest of the population. The basic treatment of hemophilia consists of intravenous infusion of coagulation factor concentrates (CFCs), factor VIII in hemophilia A and factor IX in hemophilia B, throughout the patient's life (so-called primary prophylaxis). The objective is to avoid the repeated bleeding that patients present with when their hemostasis is not controlled: the goal is to have zero bleeding in any anatomical area, but especially in the joints (elbows, knees, ankles). A major problem is that some hemophilia patients develop antibodies against CFCs (called inhibitors) and then need another type of hematological treatment, such as immune tolerance induction (ITI) and by-passing agents [recombinant factor VII activated (rFVIIa) and activated prothrombin complex concentrates (aPCCs)].

In practice, hemophilia is considered a hematologic disease that mainly affects joints (elbows, knees, ankles) and muscles (iliopsoas, muscles of the volar aspect of the forearm, gastrocnemius). Without hemostasis control, repeated hemarthroses will soon lead to complications in the joints (initially synovitis, progressing to chondral degeneration, contractures, and deformities), and in the muscles (hematomas that may lead to acute compartment syndromes, pseudotumors, and compression of peripheral nerves).

The most important hematologic advances in recent years are the CFCs with extended half-life (which allow intravenous infusions to be more infrequent than was previously necessary) and some drugs that are administered subcutaneously (emicizumab, concizumab, etc.), which can even be used in patients with inhibitors. Another important advance has been in Genetics, i.e., gene therapy applied to hemophilia. Although it is in its early stages, it opens a new way to raise, with a single therapeutic action, the level of deficient factor sufficiently so that the patient does not need lifelong primary hematologic prophylaxis.

Although hematologic treatment is the basis of hemophilia management, we should not underestimate the importance of Physical and Rehabilitation Medicine (PRM) to maintain a good musculoskeletal condition in these patients, and of Orthopedic Surgery for those patients in whom nonsurgical treatment [hematologic treatment, PRM, intraarticular injections of corticosteroids, hyaluronic acid or platelet-rich plasma (PRP), analgesics, and cyclooxygenase-2 (COX-2) inhibitors] fails, leaving the patient with severe, polyarticular joint pain due to polyarthropathy. On the other hand, it is important to emphasize the importance of the correct management of hemophilia carriers and the great value of pharmacoeconomic studies (given the great economic burden that hemophilia treatment places on health systems).

In this book, expert authors in the management of hemophilia have presented their knowledge and reviewed the recent literature on all of these aspects, which are absolutely necessary for a comprehensive management of the patient with hemophilia. I must recall the great importance of constant coordination among all the specialists who treat these patients. Also, taking into account the rarity of hemophilia, I recommend that this disease be treated only in large centers specialized in it, but always in constant coordination with the physicians (hematologists, orthopedic surgeons, rehabilitation specialists) of hospitals that, due to their size, cannot specialize in its treatment.

As editor and author of several chapters of the book, my objective has been to concentrate in a single volume the most important topics related to the current treatment of hemophilia from the only possible point of view: the multidisciplinary one.

Madrid, Spain E. Carlos Rodríguez-Merchán

Contents

Pathophysiology of Hemophilia

1

E. Carlos Rodríguez-Merchán
and Víctor Jiménez-Yuste

1.1 Introduction

Classic hemophilia is caused by mutations in either the factor VIII (FVIII) or factor IX (FIX) genes, classified as hemophilia A and hemophilia B, apiece. Both genes are located on the X chromosome, causing the classic X-linked inheritance of these conditions. Defects in other coagulation factors produce very analogous clinical phenotypes, although these conditions are by far less frequent than the hemophilias and easily recognized by laboratory testing for specific coagulation factors [1].

1.2 Pathophysiology of Hemophilia

The comprehensive incidence of hemophilia is commonly estimated at between 1:5000 and 1:10,000 males [2]. Hemophilia A is due to missing or diminished FVIII procoagulant function, caused by mutations in the FVIII gene. Other congenital coagulation factor deficiencies can exhibit an analogous picture of mild to severe clinical bleeding. Nonetheless, the diagnosis of hemophilia A is usually easily confirmed by the detection of an isolated scarcity of plasma FVIII activity [3, 4]. Hemophilia A accounts for approximately 75–80% of all hemophilia cases. The severity of bleeding related to hemophilia A can be precisely foreseen by the level of residual FVIII or FIX activity in plasma. Factor levels of <1% of normal are associated with severe hemophilia, 1–5% levels with moderate hemophilia, and levels of 5–25% with only mild condition. Around 70% of people with hemophilia are classified as severe [2].

Clinical symptoms of hemophilia B are almost indistinguishable from that of hemophilia A, although the two conditions can readily be distinguished by means of routine laboratory testing and the determination of FVIII and FIX activity [4, 5]. Hemophilia B accounts for around 20–25% of all hemophilia cases [2]. As for hemophilia A, the severity of condition is intimately correlated with the residual level of FIX activity.

Von Willebrand disease (VWD) is an extremely usual inherited bleeding disorder with incidence calculated to be as high as 1% in various populations [6, 7]. As a consequence of the dependence of FVIII stability in the circulation on its association with VWF the diminished levels of von Willebrand factor (VWF) in the majority of VWD patients are also associated with a decrease in plasma FVIII activity. Indeed, parallel decrease of VWF [measured as either ristocetin co-factor activity or VWF antigen ("FVIII

E. C. Rodríguez-Merchán (✉)
Department of Orthopedic Surgery, La Paz University Hospital, Madrid, Spain

V. Jiménez-Yuste
Department of Hematology, La Paz University Hospital, Madrid, Spain

E. C. Rodríguez-Merchán (ed.), *Advances in Hemophilia Treatment*,
https://doi.org/10.1007/978-3-030-93990-8_1

related antigen")] and FVIII activity to the range of 20–50% of normal is the distinctive characteristic of type 1 VWD [8, 9]. The type 2 N variant of VWD can cause isolated deficiency of FVIII activity in the presence of otherwise normal VWF. Type 2 N VWD is due to mutations within the FVIII binding domain of VWF, causing selective loss of this relevant function [10]. Type 2 N VWF otherwise shows normal platelet adhesive function and bleeding in these patients seems to be due solely to the diminished FVIII procoagulant activity. Type 2 N VWD should be specifically considered in families with uncommon patterns of hemophilia inheritance, including affected females.

1.3 Pathophysiology of Hemophilic Arthropathy

1.3.1 Joint Bleeding

Articular bleeding is the characteristic manifestation of hemophilia, but can also happen in the context of VWD [11], as an adverse event of anticoagulant therapy [12], upon trauma [13] or major joint surgery [14]. Irrespective the intrinsic reason, joint bleeding can cause significant articular damage and further major morbidity. In hemophilia, hemorrhages in the locomotive apparatus account for 80% of all bleeds and most usually the elbow, knee, and ankle are affected [15]. Synovial joints are prone to unprovoked hemorrhages because the synovial membrane is well-vascularized. Mechanical stress is a relevant factor as suggested by the beginning of articular hemorrhage with weight bearing. Furthermore, local hemostasis in an articulation differs from other tissues [16, 17]. Commencement of the coagulation cascade in articulations is restrained and this lack of balance is even more reflected in articular tissue of hemophilia patients [18]. Besides, there is a notable activation of the synovial fibrinolytic system after joint bleeding [19]. It has been reported that articular hemorrhage in hemophilic mice induces the expression of synovial urokinase-type plasminogen activator (uPA); besides, the levels of active uPA and plasmin are augmented compared to healthy controls [20]. This hyperfibrinolysis causes a rapid degradation of blood clots in a zone very vulnerable to mechanical stress.

Basically, development of hemophilic arthropathy is characterized by the following main processes: synovitis, cartilage degeneration, bone damage, and vascular development and angiogenesis [21–23].

1.3.2 Synovitis

After an acute articular hemorrhage, it takes around a week prior to the blood is eliminated from the articular cavity by the synovial lining cells [24]. Macrophages and other inflammatory cells migrating to the articulation participate in this elimination process. In case of recurrent extravasations or ongoing hemorrhage, the quantity of blood surpasses the synovial elimination capacity. Erythrocyte-derived iron accumulates as synovial hemosiderin deposits [25–27]. It has been shown that macroscopically hemosiderotic synovial membrane contains considerably more inflammatory cytokines than normal tissue [25]. Nuclear factor kappa β (NF-kβ)-associated signaling pathways are essential in inflammation, and also in a murine hemophilia model its upregulation has been shown. An articular hemorrhage led to upregulation of several genes of the NF-kβ pathway and the irresponsive pro-inflammatory cytokines like interleukin (IL)-1b, IL-6, interferon-gamma (IFNγ), and tumor necrosis factor-alpha (TNFα) [28]. This is in line with findings of the role of NF-kβ in synovitis [29] and cartilage degeneration in osteoarthritis [30] and rheumatoid arthritis [31]. Besides, patients with hemophilic arthropathy show high expression of synovial levels of Receptor Activator of NF-kB (RANK) [32]. The existence of iron turns the thin synovium into a hypertrophic, villous membrane, by means of induction of DNA-synthesis and cell proliferation. Iron stimulates the amplification of c-myc, a proto-oncogene associated with cell proliferation [33], and mdm2, a protein that targets the p53 tumor suppressor gene, by that means inhibiting synovial cell apoptosis [34].

The inflamed and hypertrophic synovial membrane has an augmented oxygen demand stimulating the liberation of growth factors like vascular-derived endothelial growth factor (VEGF). VEGF causes neoangiogenesis, both locally and systemically [35, 36]. Systemic angiogenic factors liberated in response to articular hemorrhage can also cause hypervascularity in otherwise unaffected articulations [37].The combination of iron, inflammation, hypertrophy, and neo-vascularization can cause a vicious cycle. Articular hemorrhage causes synovitis (hypertrophy of the synovial membrane), making it more prone to mechanical damage and by means of vascular remodeling more vulnerable to subsequent hemorrhage. In this manner a so-called target articulation can develop, which happens in around 25% of patients with severe hemophilia. A target articulation is clinically defined as a joint in which three or more unprovoked articular hemorrhages happen within a consecutive 6-month period [38]. Over time, repetitive articular hemorrhages cause chronic synovitis and eventually the synovial membrane turns into fibrotic.

1.3.3 Cartilage Degeneration

Cartilage degeneration after an articular hemorrhage is due to both synovial dependent and independent mechanisms. First, synovitis creates an invasive and destructive stratum (pannus) over the cartilage surface [39]. Pannus tissue contains aggressive macrophage- and fibroblast-like mesenchymal cells and other inflammatory cells that liberate collagenolytic enzymes [40]. Additional degradation of the cartilage matrix is caused by synovial derived pro-inflammatory cytokines, plasmin and matrix metalloproteinases (MMPs) [41]. Pro-inflammatory cytokines produces cartilage degradation by means of MMPs and aggrecanases. Plasmin makes a contribution to cartilage degradation directly by causing proteoglycan liberation in human cartilage [42], or indirectly by means of activation of pro-MMPs [43]. MMPs are endopeptidases implicated in the degradation of extracellular matrix components, like collagen and proteoglycans [44]. Besides, plasmin is able to have an influence over cell signaling by means of proteinase activated receptors (PARs) resulting in synovitis and cartilage degradation [45]. Upon articular hemorrhage an augmented expression of PARs is encountered in chondrocytes and synovial membrane. In addition to this synovial membrane-dependent mechanism, blood also has a direct detrimental effect on cartilage. Cartilage is a rather inert tissue that is made up of chondrocytes and extracellular matrix. Chondrocytes synthesize cartilage matrix, synovial fluid contributes nutrients as cartilage has not blood supply. Blood exposure produces both extracellular matrix degradation and chondrocyte apoptosis. Brief exposure to a small amount of blood already causes lengthy and unchangeable disturbances in matrix turnover [46, 47], still present 10 weeks after initial blood exposure [48]. These persistent disturbances in matrix turnover are due to chondrocyte apoptosis caused by oxidative stress. Synovial and blood derived pro-inflammatory cytokines provoke the creation of hydrogen peroxide by chondrocytes. In the presence of erythrocyte-derived iron, hydrogen peroxide is able to react according to the Fenton reaction, producing very toxic hydroxyl radicals and subsequent apoptosis of chondrocytes [49].

1.3.4 Bone Damage

As the development of synovitis and cartilage degeneration advances, the underlying bone becomes damaged. Osseous changes are due to a disturbed equilibrium in bone resorption and bone formation, causing a reduction in bone mineral density (BMD) and osteoporosis [50, 51]. A diminished BMD is encountered both in children [52–54] and older hemophilic patients [55–57], and local osteoporosis is also a characteristic of hemophilic arthropathy. Other osseous changes in hemophilic patients are cyst formation, subchondral sclerosis, osteophyte formation, and epiphyseal enlargement [58]. While osseous damage in hemophilic patients is considered a late fact, both in hemophilic rats and mice excessive bone remodeling has been found as early as 2 weeks after induced articular hemorrhages [59, 60]. These severe osseous changes in animal models might be an augmented reflection of the human situation, caused by discrepancies in matrix turnover rate, cartilage thickness, and articular biomechanics [61]. The precise mechanism by which articular hemorrhages cause osseous damage is mostly unknown. It is not clear whether osseous damage is an indirect or direct consequence of articular hemorrhage. Acute hemarthrosis and chronic hemophilic arthropathy cause local disuse and generalized decrease in physical activity. As such, it may negatively affect BMD by reducing peak bone mass and augmenting bone resorption [62]. Furthermore, infection with hepatitis C virus (HCV) or human immunodeficiency virus (HIV) and their therapies may affect BMD negatively [63–65]. Local changes in osseous turnover upon articular hemorrhage are hypothesized to be due to changes in the RANK-Ligand (RANK-L)/RANK/osteoprotegerin (OPG)-pathway, a crucial pathway in osseous resorption induced by swelling [66–69]. RANK-L is chiefly expressed on osteoblasts/stromal cells and is synthesized by reactive lymphocytes and synovial cells [66]. By binding to its receptor RANK, it stimulates osseous resorption by osteoclasts [23]. OPG acts as a decoy receptor and competes with RANK for the binding to RANK-L. By averting the interaction between RANK-L and RANK, OPG protects bones from excessive resorption. In synovial tissue of hemophilic patients with severe arthropathy an augmented expression of RANK and RANK-L and a reduced expression of OPG is shown, which favors osteoclastic differentiation and thus osseous resorption [32]. The doubt remains whether articular injury is the primary cause of osseous loss in hemophilia or a contributing factor. In FVIII deficient mice a reduction in BMD was shown in spite of having experienced articular hemorrhages [70]. Several molecular mechanisms are hypothesized to directly affect bone density in FVIII deficiency. A reduced thrombin production [71] causes less thrombin induced PAR-1-mediated proliferation of osteoblasts [72]. Furthermore, FVIII deficient mice were more likely to have undetectable levels of two crucial bone regulating cytokines, IL-1a and interferon-b, thereby theoretically inducing osseous resorption [73]. To sum up, articular hemorrhage causes iron deposition, swelling, synovial proliferation, cartilage degradation, neoangiogenesis, and fibrinolysis, making the articulation prone to recurrent hemorrhages and as such inducing a vicious cycle. Additionally, osseous damage is due to a multifactorial process, of which articular hemorrhage, amongst others, is a major contributor.

1.3.5 Vascular Development and Angiogenesis

Vascular development and angiogenesis are paramount to both physiologic [74] and pathologic processes [75, 76]. Just as angiogenesis is needed for tumor growth, angiogenesis is also likely to be needed for the synovial membrane to expand beyond several millimeters in size [77]. The novel capillaries created throughout angiogenesis are composed of endothelial cells and pericytes, which are formed from differentiated intimal/subintimal smooth muscle cells [78]. The influence of iron on blood vessels may be deduced from experiments in which the intravenous administration of iron at a concentration sufficient to saturate transferrin causes hypervascularity and subsequent expansion of the synovial lining and subsynovial tissue [79]. Two hours after administration, a four-fold increase in synovial cell mitotic activity and pinocytosis by endothelial cells was found. After 8–24 h, mature collagen appeared between endothelial cells, pericytes, and pericyte layers, and iron-containing mononuclear cells. Evidence of the direct impact of blood, particularly platelets, on vascular permeability was observed in an experiment in which blood was directly injected into the articulations of rats [80]. A remarkable augmentation in the permeability of synovial venules was found that persisted for up to 16 h.

Figure 1.1 summarizes the pathophysiology of hemophilic arthropathy. Figure 1.2 shows the blood constituents potentially responsible for

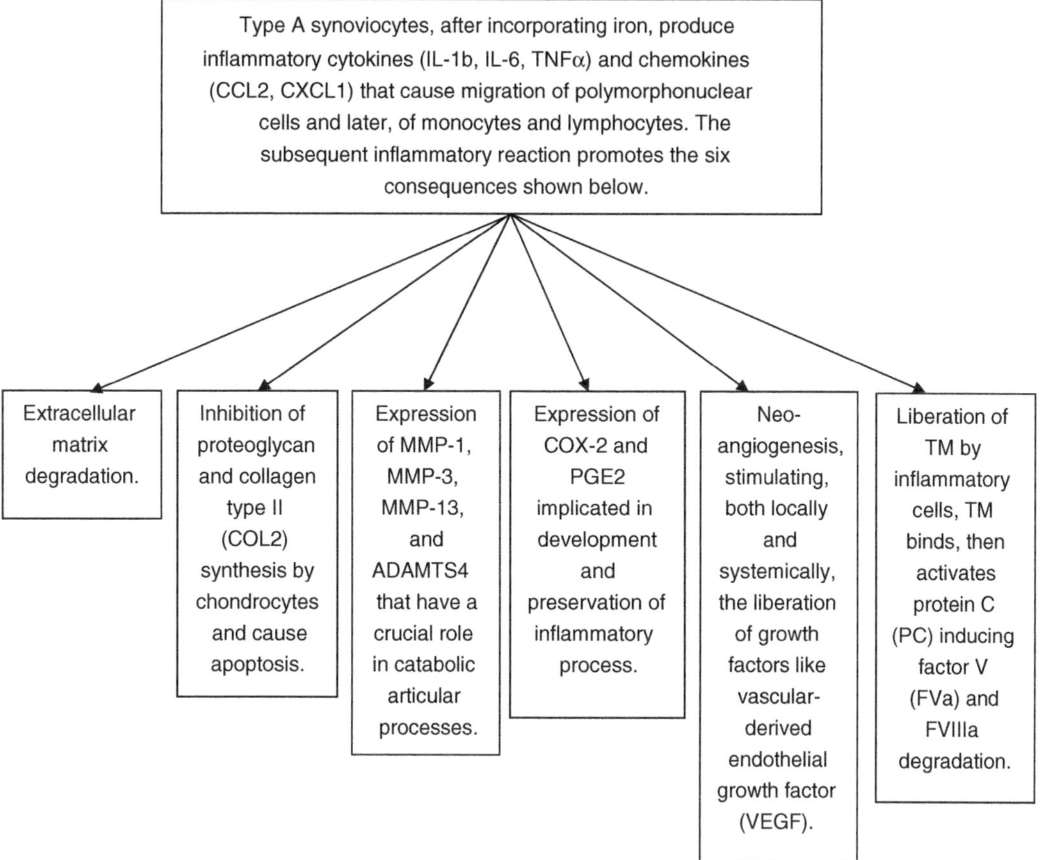

Fig. 1.1 Pathophysiology of hemophilic arthropathy (IL = interleukin; TNF = tumor necrosis factor-alpha; MMPs = matrix metalloproteinases; COX-2 = cyclooxygenase 2; PGE2 = prostaglandin E2; TM = thrombomodulin)

Fig. 1.2 Blood constituents potentially responsible for hemophilic arthropathy (MMPs = matrix metalloproteinases; PG = proteoglycan; IL = interleukin; TNF = tumor necrosis factor alpha; MCP-1 = monocyte chemoattractant protein-1; VEGF = vascular endothelial growth factor; PDGF = platelet derived growth factor; TIMP-1 = tissue inhibitor of metalloproteinase-1)

PLASMA COMPONENTS

* **Enzymes** (MMP-1, MMP-3, MMP-13, Thrombin, Tryptase/chymase, Elastase, Cathepsin, PG-degrading activity).

* **Cytokines and chemokines** (IL-1, IL-6, TNFα, MCP-1).

* **Growth factors** (VEGF, PDGF).

CELLULAR COMPONENTS

* **Erythrocytes** (hemoglobin, iron).

* **Leukocytes.**

* **Monocytes/macrophage** (TIMP-1).

* **CD3+ T cells, platelets** (growth factors).

ARTICULAR CARTILAGE	BONE CELLS	SYNOVIAL MEMBRANE	BLOOD VESSELS
*Chondrocytes *Matrix	*Osteoblasts * Osteoclasts	*Fibroblasts *Synovial macrophages	*Endothelial cells *Smooth muscle cells *Pericytes

Fig. 1.3 Joint components that are potential targets in the development of hemophilic arthropathy

hemophilic arthropathy. Figure 1.3 shows the joint components that are potential targets in the development of hemophilic arthropathy.

1.4 Conclusions

Albeit the complex molecular mechanisms underlying the abnormal synovial hypertrophy in hemophilic arthropathy are still poorly comprehended, some studies have shown that a variety of mediators may play a significant role in blood-induced articular damage. Collectively, such mediators are thought to trigger a synovial over-reaction which, once commenced, may act independently of the intra-articular hemorrhage. Hemarthrosis causes intra-articular iron deposition, synovial proliferation and neoangiogenesis, and cartilage and subchondral bone damage, triggering a vicious cycle that causes severe arthropathy. Albeit osseous damage may arise from a multifactorial process in hemophilic patients, articular hemorrhage appears to be an important contributor. This complex scenario eventually causes clinical manifestation of hemophilic arthropathy.

Spontaneous articular hemorrhage and recurrent hemarthroses cause hemophilic arthropathy—a debilitating condition with a significant negative effect on mobility and quality of life. Iron, cytokines, and angiogenic growth factors play a crucial role in the beginning of the inflammatory process that implies the synovial tissue, articular cartilage, and subchondral bone, with early damages and molecular changes determining the maintenance of a chronic inflammatory condition. Synovitis is one of the earliest adverse events of intra-articular hemorrhage and is characterized by synovial hypertrophy, migration of inflammatory cells, and a high degree of neoangiogenesis with subsequent bleeding.

The pathogenic mechanisms and molecular pathways by which blood in the articular cavity produces articular cartilage and subchondral bone destruction have yet to be fully clarified. Both cytokines and matrix metalloproteinases and hydroxyl radicals may cause chondrocyte apoptosis. Members of the tumor necrosis factor receptor superfamily (such as the molecular triad: osteoprotegerin—OPG; receptor activator of nuclear factor kB-RANK; RANK-Ligand—RANKL) appear instead to play an important role in the inflammatory process. These pathogenic processes interact with each other and eventually cause a fibrotic articulation and the disabling condition typical of hemophilic arthropathy.

References

1. Hedner U, Ginsburg D, Lusher JM, High KA. Congenital hemorrhagic disorders: new insights into the pathophysiology and treatment of hemophilia. Hematology Am Soc Hematol Educ Program. 2000;2000:241–65.
2. Soucie JM, Evatt B, Jackson D. Occurrence of hemophilia in the United States. The Hemophilia surveillance system project investigators. Am J Hematol. 1998;59:288–94.
3. Hoyer LW, Hemophilia A. N Engl J Med. 1994;330:38–47.
4. Furie B, Limentani SA, Rosenfield CG. A practical guide to the evaluation and treatment of hemophilia. Blood. 1994;84:3–9.
5. Ginsburg D. Hemophilia and other inherited disorders of hemostasis and thrombosis. In: Rimoin DL,

Connor JM, Pyeritz RE, Emery AEH, editors. Emery and Rimoin's principles and practice of medical generics, vol. II. New York: Churchill Livingstone; 1997. p. 1651–76.
6. Werner EJ, Broxson EH, Tucker EL, Giroux DS, Shults J, Abshire TC. Prevalence of von Willebrand disease in children: a multiethnic study. J Pediatr. 1993;123:893–8.
7. Rodeghiero F, Castaman G, Dini E. Epidemiological investigation of the prevalence of von Willebrand's disease. Blood. 1987;69:454–9.
8. Nichols WC, Cooney KA, Ginsburg D, Ruggeri ZM. Von Willebrand disease. In: Loscalzo J, Schafer AI, editors. Thrombosis and hemorrhage. Baltimore: Williams & Wilkins; 1998. p. 729–55.
9. Nichols WS, Ginsburg D. Von Willebrand disease. Medicine. 1997;76:1–20.
10. von Mazurier C. Willebrand disease masquerading as haemophilia A. Thromb Haemost. 1992;67:391–6.
11. van Galen KP, Mauser-Bunschoten EP, Leebeek FW. Hemophilic arthropathy in patients with von Willebrand disease. Blood Rev. 2012;26:261–6.
12. Andes WA, Edmunds JO. Hemarthroses and warfarin: joint destruction with anticoagulation. Thromb Haemost. 1983;49:187–9.
13. Shaerf D, Banerjee A. Assessment and management of posttraumatic haemarthrosis of the knee. Br J Hosp Med (Lond). 2008;69:462–3.
14. Saksena J, Platts AD, Dowd GS. Recurrent haemarthrosis following total knee replacement. Knee. 2010;17:7–14.
15. Aronstam A, Rainsford SG, Painter MJ. Patterns of bleeding in adolescents with severe haemophilia a. Br Med J. 1979;1:469–70.
16. Drake TA, Morrissey JH, Edgington TS. Selective cellular expression of tissue factor in human tissues: implications for disorders of hemostasis and thrombosis. Am J Pathol. 1989;134:1087–97.
17. Brinkmann T, Kahnert H, Prohaska W, Nordfang O, Kleesiek K. Synthesis of tissue factor pathway inhibitor in human synovial cells and chondrocytes makes joints the predilected site of bleeding in haemophiliacs. Eur J Clin Chem Clin Biochem. 1994;32:313–7.
18. Dargaud Y, Simpson H, Chevalier Y, Scoazec JY, Hot A, Guyen O, et al. The potential role of synovial thrombomodulin in the pathophysiology of joint bleeds in haemophilia. Haemophilia. 2012;18:818–23.
19. Storti E, Magrini U, Ascari E. Synovial fibrinolysis and haemophilic haemarthrosis. Br Med J. 1971;4:812.
20. Nieuwenhuizen I, Roosendaal G, Coeleveld K, Lubberts E, Biesma DH, Lafeber FP, et al. Haemarthrosis stimulates the synovial fibrinolytic system in haemophilic mice. Thromb Haemost. 2013;110:173–83.
21. Pulles AP, Mastbergen SC, Schutgens REG, Lafeber FPJG, van Vulpen LFD. Pathophysiology of hemophilic arthropathy and potential targets for therapy. Pharmacol Res. 2017;115:192–9.
22. Lafeber FP, Miossec P, Valentino LA. Physiopathology of haemophilic arthropathy. Haemophilia. 2008;14(Suppl 4):3–9.
23. Valentino LA, Hakobyan N, Enockson C, Simpson ML, Kakodkar NC, Cong L, et al. Exploring the biological basis of haemophilic joint disease: experimental studies. Haemophilia. 2012;18:310–8.
24. Letizia G, Piccione F, Ridola C, Zummo G. Ultrastructural appearance of human synovial membrane in the reabsorption phase of acute haemarthrosis. Ital J Orthop Traumatol. 1980;6:275–7.
25. Roosendaal G, Vianen ME, Wenting MJ, van Rinsum AC, van denBerg HM, Lafeber FP, et al. Iron deposits and catabolic properties of synovial tissue from patients with haemophilia. J Bone Joint Surg Br. 1998;80:540–5.
26. Wood DD, Ihrie EJ, Hamerman D. Release of interleukin-1 from human synovial tissue in vitro. Arthritis Rheum. 1985;28:853–62.
27. Brennan FM, Chantry D, Jackson AM, Maini RN, Feldmann M. Cytokine production in culture by cells isolated from the synovial membrane. J Autoimmun. 1989;Suppl 2:177–86.
28. Sen D, Chapla A, Walter N, Daniel V, Srivastava A, Jayandharan GR. Nuclear factor (NF)-kappa B and its associated pathways are majormolecular regulators of blood-induced joint damage in a murine model of hemophilia. J Thromb Haemost. 2013;11:293–306.
29. Muller-Ladner U, Gay RE, Gay S. Role of nuclear factor kappa B in synovial inflammation. Curr Rheumatol Rep. 2002;4:201–7.
30. Ma B, Zhong L, van Blitterswijk CA, Post JN, Karperien M. T cell factor 4 is a pro-catabolic and apoptotic factor in human articular chondrocytes by potentiating nuclear factor kappa B signaling. J Biol Chem. 2013;288:17552–8.
31. Min S-Y, Yan M, Du Y, Wu T, Khobahy E, Kwon S-R, Taneja V, et al. Intra-articular nuclear factor-kappa B blockade ameliorates collagen-induced arthritis in mice by eliciting regulatory T cells and macrophages. Clin Exp Immunol. 2013;172:217–27.
32. Melchiorre D, Manetti M, Matucci-Cerinic M. Pathophysiology of hemophilic arthropathy. J Clin Med. 2017;6:63.
33. Wen FQ, Jabbar AA, Chen YX, Kazarian T, Patel DA, Valentino LA. C-mycProto-oncogene expression in hemophilic synovitis: in vitro studies of the effects of iron and ceramide. Blood. 2002;100:912–6.
34. Hakobyan N, Kazarian T, Jabbar AA, Jabbar KJ, Valentino LA. Pathobiology of hemophilic synovitis I: overexpression of mdm2 oncogene. Blood. 2004;104:2060–4.
35. Acharya SS, Kaplan RN, Macdonald D, Fabiyi OT, DiMichele D, Lyden D. Neoangiogenesis contributes to the development of hemophilic synovitis. Blood. 2011;117:2484–93.
36. Zetterberg E, Palmblad J, Wallensten R, Morfini M, Melchiorre M, Holmstrom M. Angiogenesis is increased in advanced haemophilic joint disease and

characterised by normal pericyte coverage. Eur J Haematol. 2014;92:256–62.
37. Bhat V, Olmer M, Joshi S, Durden DL, Cramer TJ, Barnes RF, et al. Vascular remodeling underlies rebleeding in hemophilic arthropathy. Am J Hematol. 2015;90:1027–35.
38. Donadel-Claeyssens D. European Paediatric network for Haemophilia. Current co-ordinated activities of the PEDNET (European paediatric networkfor haemophilia management). Haemophilia. 2006;12:124–7.
39. Hoots WK. Pathogenesis of hemophilic arthropathy. Semin Hematol. 2006;43(Suppl. 1):S18–22.
40. Furuzawa-Carballeda J, Macip-Rodriguez PM, Cabral AR. Osteoarthritis and rheumatoid arthritis pannus have similar qualitative metabolic characteristics and pro-inflammatory cytokine response. Clin Exp Rheumatol. 2008;26:554–60.
41. Rippey JJ, Hill RR, Lurie A, Sweet MB, Thonar EJ, Handelsman JE. Articular cartilage degradation and the pathology of haemophilic arthropathy. S Afr Med J. 1978;54:345–51.
42. Furmaniak-Kazmierczak E, Cooke TD, Manuel R, Scudamore A, Hoogendorn H, Giles AR, et al. Studies of thrombin-induced proteoglycan release in the degradation of human and bovine cartilage. J Clin Invest. 1994;94:472–80.
43. Cawston TE, Young DA. Proteinases involved in matrix turnover during cartilage and bone breakdown. Cell Tissue Res. 2010;339:221–35.
44. Nagase H, Visse R, Murphy G. Structure and function of matrix metalloproteinases and TIMPs. Cardiovasc Res. 2006;69:562–73.
45. Nieuwenhuizen L, Schutgens RE, Coeleveld K, Mastbergen SC, Schiffelers RM, Roosendaal G, et al. Silencing of protease-activated receptors attenuates synovitis and cartilage damage following a joint bleed in haemophilic mice. Haemophilia. 2016;22:152–9.
46. Hooiveld MJ, Roosendaal G, van den Berg HM, Bijlsma JW, Lafeber FP. Haemoglobin-derived iron-dependent hydroxyl radical formation in blood-induced joint damage: an in vitro study. Rheumatology (Oxford). 2003;42:784–90.
47. Roosendaal G, Vianen ME, Marx JJ, van den Berg HM, Lafeber FP, Bijlsma JW. Blood-induced joint damage: a human in vitro study. Arthritis Rheum. 1999;42:1025–32.
48. Hooiveld M, Roosendaal G, Vianen M, van den Berg M, Bijlsma J, Lafeber F. Blood-induced joint damage: long term effects in vitro and in vivo. J Rheumatol. 2003;30:339–44.
49. Hooiveld M, Roosendaal G, Wenting M, van den Berg M, Bijlsma J, Lafeber F. Short-term exposure of cartilage to blood results in chondrocyte apoptosis. Am J Pathol. 2003;162:943–51.
50. Katsarou O, Terpos E, Chatzismalis P, Provelengios S, Adraktas T, Hadjidakis D, et al. Increased bone resorption is implicated in the pathogenesis of bone loss in hemophiliacs: correlations with hemophilic arthropathy and HIV infection. Ann Hematol. 2010;89:67–74.
51. Kovacs CS. Hemophilia: low bone mass, and osteopenia/osteoporosis. Transfus Apher Sci. 2008;38:33–40.
52. Tlacuilo-Parra A, Morales-Zambrano R, Tostado-Rabago N, Esparza-Flores MA, Lopez-Guido B, Orozco-Alcala J. Inactivity is a risk factor forlow bone mineral density among haemophilic children. Br J Haematol. 2008;140:562–7.
53. Barnes C, Wong P, Egan B, Speller T, Cameron F, Jones G, et al. Reduced bone density among children with severe hemophilia. Pediatrics. 2004;114:e177–81.
54. Abdelrazik N, Reda M, El-Ziny M, Rabea H. Evaluation of bone mineral density in children with hemophilia: Mansoura University children hospital (MUCH) experience, Mansoura, Egypt. Hematology. 2007;12:431–7.
55. Nair P, Jijina F, Ghosh K, Madkaikar M, Shrikhande M, Nema M. Osteoporosis in young haemophiliacs from western India. Am J Hematol. 2007;82:453–7.
56. Wallny TA, Scholz DT, Oldenburg J, Nicolay C, Ezziddin S, Pennekamp PH, et al. Osteoporosis in haemophilia-an underestimated comorbidity? Haemophilia. 2007;13:79–84.
57. Gerstner G, Damiano ML, Tom A, Worman C, Schultz W, Recht M, et al. Prevalence and risk factors associated with decreased bone mineral density in patients with haemophilia. Haemophilia. 2009;15:559–65.
58. Pettersson H, Ahlberg A, Nilsson IM. A radiologic classification of hemophilic arthropathy. Clin Orthop Relat Res. 1980;149:153–9.
59. Sorensen R, Roepstorff K, Wiinberg B, Hansen AK, Tranholm M, Nielsen LN, et al. The F8(−/−) rat as a model of hemophilic arthropathy. J Thromb Haemost. 2016;14:1216–25.
60. Lau AG, Sun J, Hannah WB, Livingston EW, Heymann D, Bateman TA, et al. Joint bleeding in factor VIII deficient mice causes an acute loss of trabecular bone and calcification of joint soft tissues which is prevented with aggressive factor replacement. Haemophilia. 2014;20:716–22.
61. Stockwell RA. The interrelationship of cell density and cartilage thickness in mammalian articular cartilage. J Anat. 1971;109:411–21.
62. Zehnder Y, Luthi M, Michel D, Knecht H, Perrelet R, Neto I, et al. Long-term changes in bone metabolism, bone mineral density, quantitative ultrasound parameters, and fracture incidence after spinal cord injury: a cross-sectional observational study in 100 paraplegic men. Osteoporos Int. 2004;15:180–9.
63. Brown TT, McComsey GA. Osteopenia and osteoporosis in patients with HIV: a review of current concepts. Curr Infect Dis Rep. 2006;8:162–70.
64. Brown TT, Qaqish RB. Antiretroviral therapy and the prevalence of osteopenia and osteoporosis: a meta-analytic review. AIDS. 2006;20:2165–74.
65. Schiefke I, Fach A, Wiedmann M, Aretin AV, Schenker E, Borte G, et al. Reduced bone mineral density and altered bone turnover markers in patients with non-cirrhotic chronic hepatitis B or C infection. World J Gastroenterol. 2005;11:1843–7.

66. Boyce BF, Xing L. The RANKL/RANK/OPG pathway. Curr Osteoporos Rep. 2007;5:98–104.
67. Anandarajah AP, Schwarz EM. Bone loss in the spondyloarthropathies: role of osteoclast, RANKL, RANK and OPG in the spondyloarthropathies. Adv Exp Med Biol. 2009;649:85–99.
68. Gibellini D, Borderi M, De Crignis E, Cicola R, Vescini F, Caudarella R, et al. RANKL/OPG/TRAIL plasma levels and bone mass loss evaluation in antiretroviral naive HIV-1-positive men. J Med Virol. 2007;79:1446–54.
69. Moschen AR, Kaser A, Stadlmann S, Millonig G, Kaser S, Muhllechner P, et al. The RANKL/OPG system and bone mineral density in patients with chronic liver disease. J Hepatol. 2005;43:973–83.
70. Liel MS, Greenberg DL, Recht M, Vanek C, Klein RF, Taylor JA. Decreased bone density and bone strength in a mouse model of severe factor VIII deficiency. Br J Haematol. 2012;158:140–3.
71. Dargaud Y, Beguin S, Lienhart A, Al Dieri R, Trzeciak C, Bordet JC, et al. Evaluation of thrombin generating capacity in plasma from patients with haemophilia a and B. Thromb Haemost. 2005;93:475–80.
72. Mackie EJ, Loh LH, Sivagurunathan S, Uaesoontrachoon K, Yoo HJ, Wong D, et al. Protease-activated receptors in the musculoskeletal system. Int J Biochem Cell Biol. 2008;40:1169–84.
73. Recht M, Liel MS, Turner RT, Klein RF, Taylor JA. The bone disease associated with factor VIII deficiency in mice is secondary to increased bone resorption. Haemophilia. 2013;19:908–12.
74. Semenza GL. Therapeutic angiogenesis: another passing phase? Circ Res. 2006;98:1115–6.
75. Sosman JA, Puzanov I. Molecular targets in melanoma from angiogenesis to apoptosis. Clin Cancer Res. 2006;12:2376s–83s.
76. Valentino LA. Blood-induced joint disease: the pathophysiology of hemophilic arthropathy. J Thromb Haemost. 2010;8:1895–902.
77. Paleolog EM, Miotla JM. Angiogenesis in arthritis: role in disease pathogenesis and as a potential therapeutic target. Angiogenesis. 1998;2:295–307.
78. Nicosia RF, Villaschi S. Rat aortic smooth muscle cells become pericytes during angiogenesis in vitro. Lab Investig. 1995;73:658–66.
79. de Sousa M, Dynesius-Trentham R, Mota-Garcia F, da Silva MT, Trentham DE. Activation of rat synovium by iron. Arthritis Rheum. 1988;31:653–61.
80. Bignold LP. Importance of platelets in increased vascular permeability evoked by experimental haemarthrosis in synovium of the rat. Pathology. 1980;12:169–79.

Genetics of Hemophilia A and B

2

Pedro A. Sanchez-Lara and Leonard A. Valentino

2.1 Introduction

Hemophilia is a rare inherited bleeding disorder caused by a deficiency of coagulation factor (F) VIII (FVIII) or factor IX (FIX), known as hemophilia A or B, respectively [1]. The prevalence (per 100,000 males) is 17.1 cases for all severities of hemophilia A, and 3.8 for hemophilia B [2]. Bleeding occurs most commonly in joints, soft tissues, and muscles; it can be serious, causing debilitating pain and musculoskeletal complications, resulting in morbidity, chronic disability, or even death [3]. Acute and chronic complications result in a major impact on health-related quality of life (HRQoL) for people with hemophilia (PWH) [4]. The mainstay of treatment in PWH is intravenous factor replacement therapy, for either prevention of bleeding (prophylaxis) or its treatment on demand [5]. Prophylaxis has been proven to maintain joint status and function, but requires maintenance therapy over a lifetime [6–9].

P. A. Sanchez-Lara
Genetics, Cedars-Sinai Medical Center, David Geffen School of Medicine, UCLA, Los Angeles, CA, USA

L. A. Valentino (✉)
National Hemophilia Foundation, New York, NY, USA

Rush University, Chicago, IL, USA
e-mail: lvalentino@hemophilia.org

2.2 History of Hemophilia

Instances of excessive or abnormal bleeding were first recorded thousands of years ago, including referred to in The Talmud dating back to the second century AD [10]. It was written that if first two boys of a mother died due to bleeding following circumcision, then the third boy shall not undergo the procedure [11]. Abu Khasim, a tenth-century Arabian physician, described families whose male children died from uncontrolled bleeding after trauma, while a modern description of hemophilia appeared only at the beginning of the nineteenth century [12–14]. In 1803, John Conrad Otto was the first North American to publish an article describing a recurrent bleeding disorder primarily affecting males in certain families (tracing it back three generations) [15]. The impact of X-linked recessive conditions on female carriers wasn't apparent until 1930, when Schloessman was able to definitively show protracted coagulation time in the blood from carrier females [16]. Hemophilia is often called the "Royal Disease" due to descendants of Queen Victoria of England and Empress of the Indies being affected by the disease [17, 18]. Among her descendants, possibly no one more infamous than Tsarevich Alexi of Russia and heir to the Russian crown until the Bolshevik Revolution was affected by hemophilia [18]. Later, it was determined that the form of hemophilia affecting the descendants of Queen Victoria including Alexi was hemophilia

E. C. Rodríguez-Merchán (ed.), *Advances in Hemophilia Treatment*,
https://doi.org/10.1007/978-3-030-93990-8_2

B [19, 20] Unfortunately, because of the association with a recurrence within royal families (and potential for consanguinity), many within the public and lay media naively mistake hemophilia as an autosomal recessive condition, rather than an X-linked recessive condition, perpetuating sensationalized misinformation [21].

2.3 Types of Hemophilia

There are two major forms of hemophilia [1]: hemophilia A, also known as classic hemophilia [22] which is due to the deficiency of the activity of FVIII and hemophilia B, due to the deficiency of coagulation FIX, also known as Christmas disease, named after the first individual identified with this form of the disease (5-year-old Stephan Christmas [23, 24]). The two forms of hemophilia have very similar clinical manifestations with frequent signs of bruising and bleeding including bleeding into the joints [5] and symptoms including pain at the site of bleeding [25]. Despite these similarities, they are caused by mutations in different genes, *F8* in classic hemophilia and *F9* in hemophilia B [26]. Hemophilia A is six times more common than hemophilia B with a prevalence of 1 in 5000 male live births compared to 1 in 30,000, respectively [27]. Although both types of hemophilia are usually considered clinically indistinguishable with negligible differences in severity and outcomes, several studies challenge this concept, regarding severity of bleeding tendency and risk of inhibitor development.

2.4 Inheritance of Hemophilia

Hemophilia A and B are inherited in an X-linked recessive pattern since the *F8* and *F9* genes are both located on long arm of the X chromosome. In males, who have only one X chromosome, one mutated copy of the gene is sufficient to cause the disease. Females, having two X chromosomes, are often silent carriers of a mutation, but can present with a spectrum of clinical symptoms when they have sufficiently reduced levels of FVIII or FIX to result in bleeding manifestations. This occurs in instances of extreme skewed inactivation of the X chromosome, in females with Turner Syndrome (45X) who carry a mutation on the remaining single X chromosome, or when both the maternal and paternal copies of the gene carry a pathogenic mutation. Nonetheless, females who carry one X chromosome with the mutated *F8* or *F9* gene can transmit the mutated gene copy to half their children with a 1 in 2 chance (50%) of a male offspring being affected with the disease and half of the females or 1 in 2 chance of being carriers of the disease-causing mutation [28]. Affected males will pass the mutation to all of their daughters and none of their sons. Although many de novo mutations occur in families, clues in the family history of an X-linked recessive bleeding disorder will show primarily affected males who do not transmit the trait to their sons, but their daughters may have affected sons.

2.5 Molecular Genetics of Hemophilia A

The molecular location of the *F8* gene was identified in 1986 and found to be located in the distal part of chromosome Xq28 [29]. Its relative close location (within 500 kb) to the glucose-6 phosphate dehydrogenase (G6PD) gene facilitated its early physical mapping [30]. *F8* is an extremely large and complex gene (consisting of 180 kb and 26 exons) in comparison to *F9* which is only 34 kb and 8 exons.

There are a wide spectrum of *F8* mutations identified in individuals with Hemophilia A, with almost half of the severe cases found to carry the intro 22 inversion (Fig. 2.1). Up to 30% newly diagnosed simplex cases have no family history. As many as 15% of probands with a single nucleotide variant and no known family history of hemophilia A have somatic mosaicism for an F8 pathogenic variant [31]. A review of the CHAMP Mutation Project database (available at CDC Hemophilia Mutation Project (CHAMP & CHBMP) https://www.cdc.gov/ncbddd/hemophilia/champs.html, accessed 27 June 2021 [32])

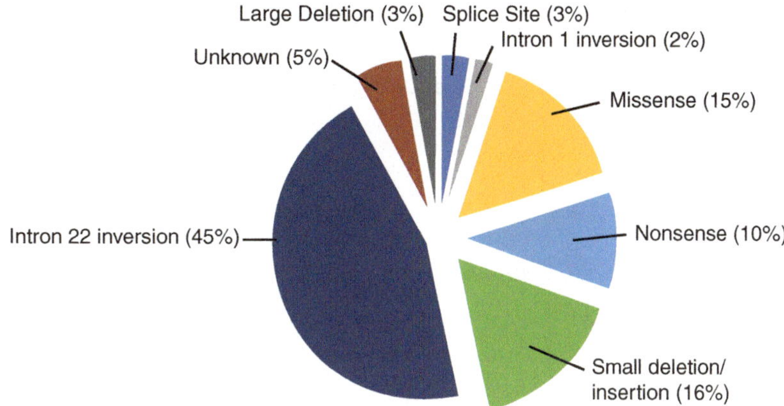

Fig. 2.1 Characteristics of hemophilia A (adapted from Castaman and Matino [27])

Table 2.1 Mutation types causing hemophilia A

Variant type	No.	%
Missense	1745	46.5%
Nonsense	416	11.1%
Frameshift	908	24.2%
Splice site change	320	8.5%
Large structural change	210	5.6%
Small structural change	86	2.3%

identified 3756 unique mutations of which 46.5% were due to a missense mutation and 24.5% due to a frameshift mutation (Table 2.1). Many of these mutations resulted in the absence of FVIII activity and severe hemophilia A. In approximately half of hemophilia A patients, there is no detectable FVIII activity and roughly 5% have normal levels of dysfunctional FVIII protein and are termed CRM-positive (for Cross-Reacting Material-Positive). The majority of genetic alterations that result in CRM-positive hemophilia A are missense mutations within the A2-domain [33]. The remaining 45% have a commensurate reduction of the FVIII antigen and coagulant activity of the protein in the plasma and are designated CRM-reduced. It was found that almost all CRM±/reduced mutations (24/26) were due to missense events [34]. In a 1995 review [35] of more than 1000 people with hemophilia, the disease-causing mutations included point mutations (46%), inversions (42%), deletions (8%), and unidentified mutations (4%) among those individuals with severe disease and 91%, 0%, 0%, and 9%, respectively, of those with non-severe disease.

Among individuals with hemophilia A without a family history of the disease, so-called sporadic mutations, point mutations occurred at a rate five to tenfold-higher and inversions at a rate more than tenfold-higher in male germ cells, whereas deletions showed a more than fivefold-higher mutation rate in female germ cells [36].

The *F8* gene (https://www.ncbi.nlm.nih.gov/gene/2157) is large, consisting of 26 exons that code for a signal peptide and a 2332 amino acid polypeptide with three different domains. Intron 22 of the human *F8* gene is hypomethylated on the active X and methylated on the inactive X. Mutations involving regions of intron 22 resulting in defective joining of exons 22 and 23 in the mRNA were identified as a cause of severe hemophilia A [37]. These same investigators then showed that exons 1–22 of the *F8* mRNA had become part of a hybrid mRNA, which were due to inversions involving intron 22 repeated sequences [38]. The mutation rate was very high (approximately 4×10^6 per gene per gamete per generation) and occurred 300 times more frequently in male germ cells than females. Inversions of introns 22 and 1 of the *F8* gene are common and lead to severe hemophilia A [39–42]. Although deletions and nonsense mutations have been well characterized as having an increased risk of developing inhibitors, it is important to note that some individuals with mild hemophilia A (secondary to a missense mutation) have gone on to develop inhibitors, while this has never been reported in patients with mild hemophilia B [43].

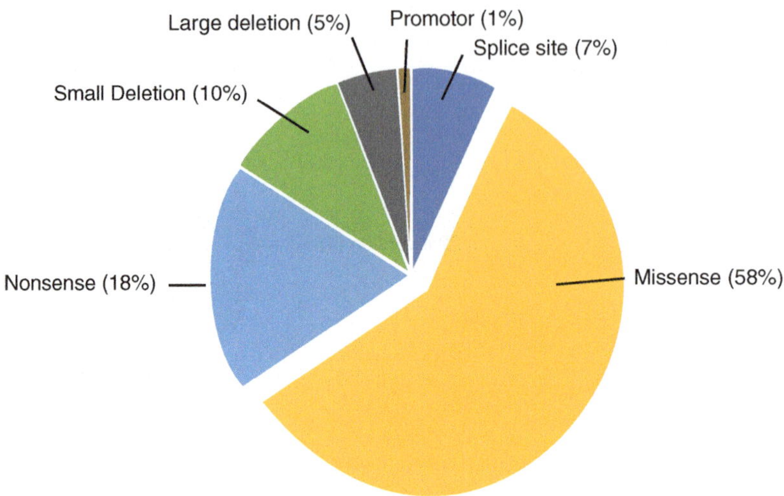

Fig. 2.2 Characteristics of hemophilia B (adapted from Castaman and Matino [27])

2.6 Molecular Genetics of Hemophilia B

The molecular location of the *F9* gene was identified in 1982, and found to be located in the proximal part (toward the centromere) of chromosome Xq27.1 [44]. The cDNA consists of 1466 base pairs coding for human FIX, and includes 11 and 18 base pairs at the 5′ and 3′ ends, 138 base pairs coding for an amino-terminal leader sequence, a stop codon, 48 base pairs of noncoding sequence at the 3′ end and 1248 base pairs that codes for the mature polypeptide chain composed of 416 amino acids [44].

There are a wide spectrum of *F9* mutations identified in individuals with Hemophilia B including gross genomic alterations (which accounting for ~15% of cases) (Fig. 2.2). Approximately, half of all affected males have no family history of hemophilia B. Somatic variant has been reported in less than 11% of families [31]. A review of the CHAMP Mutation Project database (available at CDC Hemophilia Mutation Project (CHAMP & CHBMP) https://www.cdc.gov/ncbddd/hemophilia/champs.html, accessed 27 June 2021 [32]) identified over 1000 unique mutations in the *F9* gene (Table 2.2). Nearly 60% of all disease-causing mutations in the *F9* gene are missense mutations followed by frameshift (16.1%) and splice site change (9.4%) mutations. Almost one-third of patients with hemophilia B are classified as CRM+ and can produce variable amounts of the FIX protein. There is a reduced prevalence of inhibitors in individuals with hemophilia B possibly due to the smaller protein size (less antigenic epitopes) and higher prevalence of less severe mutations (less stop codon or partial/whole gene deletions). The relative contribution of the various mutation types to hemophilia B disease severity is shown in Table 2.3.

Table 2.2 Mutation types causing hemophilia B

Mutation type	%
Frameshift	16.1
Large structure change (>50 bp)	2.9
Missense	58.1
Nonsense	8
Promoter	2.2
Small structural change (in-frame, <50 bp)	2
Splice site change	9.4
Synonymous	0.9

The FIX coagulant protein is a vitamin K dependent serine protease, which belongs to peptidase family S1. The mature protein is composed of four domains: the Gla domain, two tandem copies of the EGF domain, and a C-terminal trypsin-like peptidase domain, which contains the catalytic activity. It is synthesized as a zymogen which is processed to remove the signal peptide, glycosylated and then cleaved by FXIa or FVIIa to produce a two-chain form, where the chains are linked by a disulfide bridge [45, 46]. When activated into FIXa, in the presence of calcium ions, membrane phospholipids, and FVIII,

Table 2.3 Mutation types and hemophilia B severity

Mutation Type	Total	Severe *N* (%)	Moderate *N* (%)	Mild *N* (%)	Various severity *N* (%)
3'UTR	4	2 (0.3)	3 (0.9)	2 (1)	2 (1.1)
Frameshift	138	115 (18.4)	25 (7.6)	3 (1.5)	5 (2.7)
Large structure change (>50 bp)	10	9 (1.4)	1 (0.3)	0 (0)	0 (0)
Missense	568	342 (54.7)	229 (69.6)	169 (83.3)	129 (70.1)
Nonsense	77	74 (11.8)	17 (5.2)	3 (1.5)	16 (8.7)
Promoter	18	7 (1.1)	10 (3)	10 (4.9)	7 (3.8)
Small structural change (in-frame, <50 bp)	18	13 (2.1)	5 (1.5)	1 (0.5)	2 (1.1)
Splice site change	87	60 (9.6)	35 (10.6)	10 (4.9)	18 (9.8)
Synonymous	7	3 (0.5)	4 (1.2)	5 (2.5)	5 (2.7)

it hydrolyzes one arginine-isoleucine bond in FX to form FXa. Analysis of the structure–function relationships of FIX with cofactors and substrates have been reviewed [47] and provide much information on the molecular and biochemical basis of hemophilia B. Amino acid substitutions at or near the activation site lead to inactive FIX or to a FIX protein with decreased enzymatic activity. Release of the activation peptide is necessary for optimal interaction of FIX with its cofactors and substrates. Abnormalities in the calcium binding region, whether Gla independent or dependent, also decrease enzymatic activity. Other mutations may affect the FIX heavy chain, probably at or near the active site. Amino acid substitutions may cause conformational changes in FIX protein that interfere with other interactions, such as with antithrombin, its natural inhibitor and FVIII.

2.7 Conclusions

Hemophilia is a rare inherited, bleeding disorder caused by a deficiency of coagulation FVIII or FIX. The deficient protein activity is due to a mutation in the *F8* or *F9* genes, resulting in hemophilia A or B, respectively. These genes are present on the short arm of the X chromosome and follow an X-linked recessive pattern of inheritance. There are many different mutations that cause hemophilia, but most commonly due to inversion of intron 22 in hemophilia A and missense mutations in hemophilia B; however, there are multiple genetic mechanisms leading to different types of mutations. Genetic testing and characterization of the causative mutation testing will not usually result in a change in treatment, but does have implications for genetic counseling and prenatal testing, family counseling, and in the prediction of alloantibody formation (inhibitor). In the future, the introduction of precision medicine principles may make it possible to use this information to help guide clinical care. For example, defining the specific underlying genetic mutation may eventually have a role in determining eligibility of future novel therapies that are on the horizon [48, 49].

References

1. Zimmerman B, Valentino LA. Hemophilia: in review. Pediatr Rev. 2013;34:289–94. quiz 295
2. Iorio A, Stonebraker JS, Chambost H, Makris M, Coffin D, Herr C, et al. Establishing the prevalence and prevalence at birth of hemophilia in males: a meta-analytic approach using national registries. Ann Intern Med. 2019;171:540–6.
3. Booth J, Oladapo A, Walsh S, O'Hara J, Carroll L, Garcia-Diego DA, et al. Real-world comparative analysis of bleeding complications and health-related quality of life in patients with haemophilia A and haemophilia B. Haemophilia. 2018;24:e322–7.
4. von Mackensen S, Gringeri A. Quality of life in hemophilia. In: Preedy VR, Watson RR, editors. *Handbook of disease burdens and quality of life measures*. Heidelberg: Springer; 2010.

5. Simpson ML, Valentino LA. Management of joint bleeding in hemophilia. Expert Rev Hematol. 2012;5:459–68.
6. Pipe SW. New therapies for hemophilia. Hematology Am Soc Hematol Educ Program. 2016(1):650–56.
7. Manco-Johnson MJ, Abshire TC, Shapiro AD, Riske B, Hacker MR, Kilcoyne R, et al. Prophylaxis versus episodic treatment to prevent joint disease in boys with severe hemophilia. N Engl J Med. 2007;357:535–44.
8. Manco-Johnson MJ, Kempton CL, Reding MT, Lissitchkov T, Goranov S, Gercheva L, et al. Randomized, controlled, parallel-group trial of routine prophylaxis vs. on-demand treatment with sucrose-formulated recombinant factor VIII in adults with severe hemophilia A (SPINART). J Thromb Haemost. 2013;11:1119–27.
9. Manco-Johnson MJ, Lundin B, Funk S, Peterfy C, Raunig D, Werk M, et al. Effect of late prophylaxis in hemophilia on joint status: a randomized trial. J Thromb Haemost. 2017;15:2115–24.
10. Bernstein A, Bernstein HC. Medicine in the Talmud. Calif Med. 1951;74:267–8.
11. Rosner F. Hemophilia in the Talmud and rabbinic writings. Ann Intern Med. 1969;70:833–7.
12. Franchini M, Mannucci PM. The history of hemophilia. Semin Thromb Hemost. 2014;40:571–6.
13. Ingram GI. The history of haemophilia. J Clin Pathol. 1976;29:469–79.
14. Aledort LM. Hemophilia. N Engl J Med. 2001;345:1066. author reply 1067
15. Otto JC. (1774-1844) Kindly physician. JAMA. 1968;204:1139.
16. Kemp T. The rise of human genetics. Hereditas. 1949;35(Suppl 1):298–306.
17. Grobler SA. Hemophilia - a royal disease. S Afr Med J. 1981;60:143–4.
18. Lannoy N, Hermans C. The 'royal disease'--haemophilia A or B? A haematological mystery is finally solved. Haemophilia. 2010;16:843–7.
19. Rogaev EI, Grigorenko AP, Faskhutdinova G, Kittler ELW, Moliaka Y. Genotype analysis identifies the cause of the "royal disease". Science. 2009;326:817.
20. Rogaev EI, Grigorenko AP, Moliaka Y, Faskhutdinova G, Goltsov A, Lahti A, et al. Genomic identification in the historical case of the Nicholas II royal family. Proc Natl Acad Sci U S A. 2009;106:5258–63.
21. Bildirici M, Kökdener M, Ersin O. An empirical analysis of the effects of consanguineous marriages on economic development. J Fam Hist. 2010;35:368–94.
22. Pavlovsky A. Contribution to the pathogenesis of hemophilia. Blood. 1947;2:185–91.
23. Biggs R, Douglas AS, Mcfarlane RG, Dacie JV, Pitney WR, Merskey C, et al. Christmas disease: a condition previously mistaken for haemophilia. Br Med J. 1952;2:1378–82.
24. Merskey C. The laboratory diagnosis of haemophilia. J Clin Pathol. 1950;3:301–20.
25. Rodriguez-Merchan EC. Musculoskeletal complications of hemophilia. HSS J. 2010;6:37–42.
26. Antonarakis SE. The molecular genetics of hemophilia A and B in man. Factor VIII and factor IX deficiency. Adv Hum Genet. 1988;17:27–59.
27. Castaman G, Matino D. Hemophilia A and B: molecular and clinical similarities and differences. Haematologica. 2019;104:1702–9.
28. Ratnoff OD, Bennett B. The genetics of hereditary disorders of blood coagulation. Science. 1973;179:1291–8.
29. Tantravahi U, Murty VV, Jhanwar SC, Toole JJ, Woozney JM, Chaganti RS, et al. Physical mapping of the factor VIII gene proximal to two polymorphic DNA probes in human chromosome band Xq28: implications for factor VIII gene segregation analysis. Cytogenet Cell Genet. 1986;42:75–9.
30. Patterson M, Schwartz C, Bell M, Sauer S, Hofker M, Trask B, et al. Physical mapping studies on the human X chromosome in the region Xq27-Xqter. Genomics. 1987;1:297–306.
31. Konkle BA, Huston H, Nakaya Fletcher S. Hemophilia A. In: GeneReviews(®), Adam MP, et al, eds. 1993, University of Washington, Seattle. Copyright © 1993–2021, University of Washington, Seattle. GeneReviews is a registered trademark of the University of Washington, Seattle. All rights reserved.: Seattle (WA)
32. Payne AB, Miller CH, Kelly FM, Soucie JM, Craig HW. The CDC hemophilia A mutation project (CHAMP) mutation list: a new online resource. Hum Mutat. 2013;34:E2382–91.
33. Amano K, Sarkar R, Pemberton S, Kemball-Cook G, Kazazian HH Jr, Kaufman RJ. The molecular basis for cross-reacting material-positive hemophilia A due to missense mutations within the A2-domain of factor VIII. Blood. 1998;91:538–48.
34. McGinniss MJ, Kazazian HH Jr, Hoyer LW, Bi L, Inaba H, Antonarakis SE. Spectrum of mutations in CRM-positive and CRM-reduced hemophilia A. Genomics. 1993;15:392–8.
35. Antonarakis SE, Kazazian HH, Tuddenham EG. Molecular etiology of factor VIII deficiency in hemophilia A. Hum Mutat. 1995;5:1–22.
36. Becker J, Schwaab R, Möller-Taube A, Schwaab U, Schmidt W, Brackmann HH, et al. Characterization of the factor VIII defect in 147 patients with sporadic hemophilia A: family studies indicate a mutation type-dependent sex ratio of mutation frequencies. Am J Hum Genet. 1996;58:657–70.
37. Naylor JA, Green PM, Rizza CR, Giannelli F. Factor VIII gene explains all cases of haemophilia A. Lancet. 1992;340:1066–7.
38. Naylor JA, Green PM, Rizza CR, Giannelli F. Analysis of factor VIII mRNA reveals defects in everyone of 28 haemophilia A patients. Hum Mol Genet. 1993;2:11–7.

39. Kilian NL, Pospisil V, Hanrahan V. Haemophilia A, factor VIII intron 22 inversion screening using subcycling-PCR. Thromb Haemost. 2006;95:746–7.
40. Mahmoud Abu Arra C, Samarah F, Sudqi Abu Hasan N. Factor VIII intron 22 inversion in severe hemophilia A patients in Palestine. Scientifica (Cairo). 2020;2020:3428648.
41. Rastegar Lari G, Enayat MS, Arjang Z, Lavergne JM, Ala F. Identification of intron 1 and 22 inversion mutations in the factor VIII gene of 124 Iranian families with severe haemophilia A. Haemophilia. 2004;10:410–1.
42. Sawecka J, Skulimowska J, Windyga J, Lopaciuk S, Kościelak J. Prevalence of the intron 22 inversion of the factor VIII gene and inhibitor development in polish patients with severe hemophilia A. Arch Immunol Ther Exp. 2005;53:352–6.
43. Castaman G, Fijnvandraat K. Molecular and clinical predictors of inhibitor risk and its prevention and treatment in mild hemophilia A. Blood. 2014;124:2333–6.
44. Kurachi K, Davie EW. Isolation and characterization of a cDNA coding for human factor IX. Proc Natl Acad Sci U S A. 1982;79:6461–4.
45. Di Scipio RG, Kurachi K, Davie EW. Activation of human factor IX (Christmas factor). J Clin Invest. 1978;61:1528–38.
46. Taran LD. Factor IX of the blood coagulation system: a review. Biochemistry (Mosc). 1997;62:685–93.
47. McGraw RA, Davis LM, Lundblad RL, Stafford DW, Roberts HR. Structure and function of factor IX: defects in haemophilia B. Clin Haematol. 1985;14:359–83.
48. Pipe SW, Selvaraj SR. Gene editing in hemophilia: a "CRISPR" choice? Blood. 2019;133:2733–4.
49. Morishige S, Mizuno S, Ozawa H, Nakamura T, Mazahery A, Nomura K, et al. CRISPR/Cas9-mediated gene correction in hemophilia B patient-derived iPSCs. Int J Hematol. 2020;111:225–33.

Inhibitors in Hemophilia A

3

Víctor Jiménez-Yuste

3.1 Introduction

The development of inhibitory antibodies to factor VIII (FVIII) or factor IX (FIX) is currently the most serious and important complication of replacement therapy with clotting factor concentrates and is the biggest challenge in the management of hemophilia patients [1]. Prospective studies in previously untreated patients with severe hemophilia A indicate that the cumulative incidence is generally estimated at 25–44%, although the prevalence is around 12% due to the transient nature of these antibodies in some patients [2–5]. Development of inhibitory antibodies leads not only to a decrease in the quality of life of patients, but also has important socio-economic consequences due to the increased cost of treatment [6].

3.2 Concept of Inhibitor

An inhibitor is generally defined as a high-affinity immune globulin G (IgG) antibody of polyclonal nature to the coagulation FVIII or FIX. They are usually detected by laboratory techniques in the follow-up of patients using screening techniques or inhibitor-specific quantitative tests. An inhibitor may also be suspected in the event of an unexpected poor clinical response to replacement therapy for a hemorrhagic episode.

Inhibitors are classified as high or low responders based on their titer and demonstration of anamnestic response after factor administration. The International Society on Thrombosis and Hemostasis (ISTH) defines a high-responder inhibitor as one with inhibitor levels greater than 5 Bethesda units and a rapid anamnestic response after factor administration as opposed to a low-responder inhibitor with less than 5 Bethesda units and no anamnestic response, a definition that has been maintained and ratified over time [7, 8].

3.3 Etiopathogenesis of Inhibitors

In relation to etiopathogenesis, there has been much speculation as to what causes the development of inhibitory antibodies. Factors related to the ethnic origin of patients [9, 10], family history of inhibitor development [10–12] and mainly related to the type of genetic alteration that conditions hemophilia [13, 14] have been implicated.

Molecular alterations at the FVIII gene level have been shown to be the most important risk factor for inhibitor development [13, 15–17]. It is now possible to stratify the different types of mutation at

V. Jiménez-Yuste (✉)
Department of Hematology, La Paz University Hospital, Madrid, Spain
e-mail: vjimenezy@salud.madrid.org

E. C. Rodríguez-Merchán (ed.), *Advances in Hemophilia Treatment*,
https://doi.org/10.1007/978-3-030-93990-8_3

the FVIII gene level and their prevalence of inhibitor development. Thus patients with large deletions affecting more than one domain have a high risk of inhibitor development (approximately 88%) which is three times higher than the prevalence when only a single domain is affected [18].

Nonsense mutations affecting the light chain coding region have twice the risk of inhibitor development as those affecting the heavy chain. Intron 22 inversion represents a high-risk mutation with a prevalence of inhibitor presence of 21%. This mutation is the most prevalent mutation in patients who develop inhibitor, being found in more than 60% of cases [18].

Small deletions or insertions differ in their inhibitory risk. Those within the poly-A region (exon 14, codons 1191–1194 and 1439–1441) present a low risk due to gene sequence correction mechanisms. Other types of small deletions or insertions that generally lead to stop codons have a risk of approximately 20%.

Point mutations represent 15% of those found in severe hemophilia and account for the majority of mild-moderate cases. Being able to produce non-functioning protein, but capable of producing immune tolerance, the prevalence of inhibitor in this group is low (around 5%). Within this group it is interesting to note that point mutations at the level of the C1 and C2 domains present a risk of inhibitor development of 10% compared to 3% in mutations in other regions. This is because these domains are crucially involved in the binding of FVIII to von Willebrand factor (vWF) and phospholipids and any changes in these critical regions affect the immunogenicity of the molecule. Finally, so-called splice-site mutations represent a type of mutation with a low risk of inhibitor development [18, 19].

The possible involvement of the HLA (human leukocyte antigen) system has been known for some time [20, 21], but more recently it has become known what its relationship with genetic alterations may be [22]. Other molecular alterations described with a possible role in the development of inhibitors include polymorphisms in the promoter region of the gene encoding interleukin-10, polymorphisms in the tumor necrosis factor gene and in the CTLA-4 gene [23].

In addition to these genetic variables, different treatment-related characteristics have been implicated. Some studies suggest an increased risk in patients treated with factor VIII at a very early age compared to those who started treatment later [24, 25]. On the other hand, a protective effect of FVIII treatment in prophylaxis schemes has been observed [26, 27], although further studies are needed to corroborate this hypothesis [28]. In this respect, the most interesting data come from published data from the Canal study. This study, in which several European centers participated, firstly confirms the initial data regarding the protective effect of prophylaxis against inhibitor development and secondly clarifies the relationship between early initiation of therapy and inhibitor development. The study concludes that inhibitor development is more related to the intensity of initial treatment than to early treatment [29].

In relation to the type of factor used, the SIPPET study has undoubtedly presented the most conclusive results in this regard. The cumulative incidence of all inhibitors was 26.8% in the group of patients with plasma-derived concentrates and 44.5% in the recombinant group, with the cumulative incidence of high-titer inhibitors being 18.6% and 28.4% respectively. In the regression model, factors of recombinant origin were associated with an 87% increase in inhibitor development, with the hazard ratio for high-titer inhibitors being 1.69 [5].

3.4 Laboratory Diagnosis of Inhibitors

In most cases, the appearance of an inhibitor in a hemophilia patient is made clinically by observing a change in response to replacement therapy. However, laboratory tests are needed to confirm this suspicion.

There are several tests for the quantification of FVIII inhibitors, generally the most widely used is the Bethesda method, described in 1975 by Carol Kasper [30]. Despite its standardization, the test results depend on the cephalin reagent, the source of phospholipids used, and the contact phase activating agent used. Intra-laboratory precision is generally good, but inter-laboratory variation is important. In 1995, a modification of the Bethesda test was described that improved the specificity and efficiency of the assay for low inhibitor titers [31].

3.5 Management

The management of inhibitor patients is based on eradication of the antibody through immune tolerance (ITI) schemes and on the control and prevention of bleeding episodes. Prophylaxis in inhibitor patients has changed dramatically with the recent approval of a new drug, emicizumab, which has allowed prophylaxis of bleeding episodes in both adults and children that had not been achieved by bypass agents [32–34].

3.5.1 Prophylaxis in Inhibitor Patients

The concept of prophylaxis stems from the observation that patients with moderate hemophilia have fewer bleeds and less development of arthropathy than patients with severe involvement [35].

The concept of prophylaxis has recently been reviewed in the new hemophilia treatment guidelines issued by the World Federation of Hemophilia (WFH), suggesting a new definition [36]. While the concept applies primarily to patients without inhibitors, it could also be extrapolated to patients with inhibitors. It suggests that prophylaxis is the regular administration of a hemostatic agent(s) with the aim of preventing bleeding in people with hemophilia allowing them to maintain an active life and achieve a quality of life similar to people without hemophilia [36].

The main treatment for bleeding episodes are inhibitor bypassing agents, that is to say, activated prothrombin complex concentrates [aPCCs (factor VIII inhibitor bypassing agent—FEIBA®; Takeda)]; and recombinant factor VII activated (rFVIIa) (NovoSeven®; Novo Nordisk, Bagsvaerd, Denmark). However, the hemostatic effect of both agents is not as predictable and effective as replacement therapy as with factor deficient, therefore bleeding control is much more difficult in inhibitor patients [37].

But undoubtedly the most important change in the prophylaxis of hemophilia A inhibitor patients has come after the introduction of emicizumab into the therapeutic arsenal. Emicizumab is a humanized bispecific monoclonal antibody that substitutes the cofactor function of FVIIIa (activated factor VIII) by binding to FIXa (activated factor IX) and FX in the intrinsic tenase complex. It thus exerts its hemostatic function by facilitating the conversion of FX to FXa which goes on to activate thrombin at a later step in the coagulation cascade. Importantly, despite such favorable results in prophylaxis, emicizumab is not a monotherapy drug and requires bypassing agents for the treatment of bleeding episodes and hemostatic coverage in cases of surgery. In these circumstances, rFVIIa (rather than aPCC) is the recommended bypassing agent; this aligns with the prescribing information for emicizumab, which advises against the use of aPCC as a first choice of adjunctive therapy. Monitoring emicizumab treatment is challenging and it is hoped that ongoing research in this area will inform the best alternatives. In addition, it will be especially important to monitor patient-reported outcomes in those treated with emicizumab with a focus on bleeding frequency, joint status, pain, and physical activity levels.

3.5.2 Treatment of Bleeding Episodes

The current situation in the management of bleeding episodes in patients with hemophilia and inhibitor, except for those with low titers and high doses of FVIII, is based, as mentioned above, on the use of so-called bypass agents. Two agents are available in our setting, one is the plasma-derived aPCC (FEIBA™, Takeda) [38] and the other agent is rFVIIa (NovoSeven®, Novo Nordisk A/S) [39].

3.5.2.1 Activated Prothrombin Complex Concentrate (aPCC, FEIBA™)

The use of aPCC inhibitors in the treatment of bleeding episodes in hemophilia patients dates back more than three decades [40]. Interestingly, the therapeutic background of aPCCs is based on the experiences of clinical use of prothrombin complex concentrates (PCCs) in the late 1950s.

PCCs are plasma-derived concentrates containing the four factors that are dependent on vitamin K for their hepatic synthesis, namely factor II (FII), factor VII (FVII), factor IX (FIX), and factor X (FX). Shortly after their introduction, they were shown to be effective in the treatment of patients with hemophilia A and inhibitor.

Mechanism of Action of FEIBA

FEIBA is composed of different vitamin K-dependent coagulation factors obtained after fractionation of human plasma and separation of the cryoprecipitate. The components of FEIBA are FII (prothrombin), FVII, FIX, FX, small amounts of FIXa, FXa and thrombin, and larger amounts of FVIIa [41–43] (Figs. 3.1 and 3.2).

Due to the complexity of its composition, the mechanism of action of FEIBA has been difficult to elucidate, and remains in some respects incompletely defined. However, the most widely held view today has reverted to the concept that FEIBA acts by increasing the activity of the prothrombinase complex [43]. Thus, the mechanism of action of FEIBA appears to involve the activity of multiple procoagulant factors, but is primarily related to increased prothrombinase activity at the platelet surface (Fig. 3.3).

Clinical Efficacy of FEIBA

As defined, the primary indication for FEIBA is in the acute treatment of bleeding episodes in patients with hemophilia A or B with inhibitor. The recommended dose depends on the type and severity of the bleeding episode [44]. Single doses vary in the range of 50–100 units per kg and can be administered every 6–12 h. Because of the possible thrombotic potential, it is recommended not to exceed 200 units per kilo per day.

Several studies have shown that FEIBA offers a hemostatic effectiveness of more than 80% in different acute bleeding episodes [45–47].

FEIBA is a well-tolerated drug as described in most studies. Most of the doubts reflected in the literature over the years have been due to its possible thrombogenicity. Most thrombotic complications have been described in patients with risk factors [48]. The rate of thrombotic events is low and similar to that found with other bypass agents [49, 50].

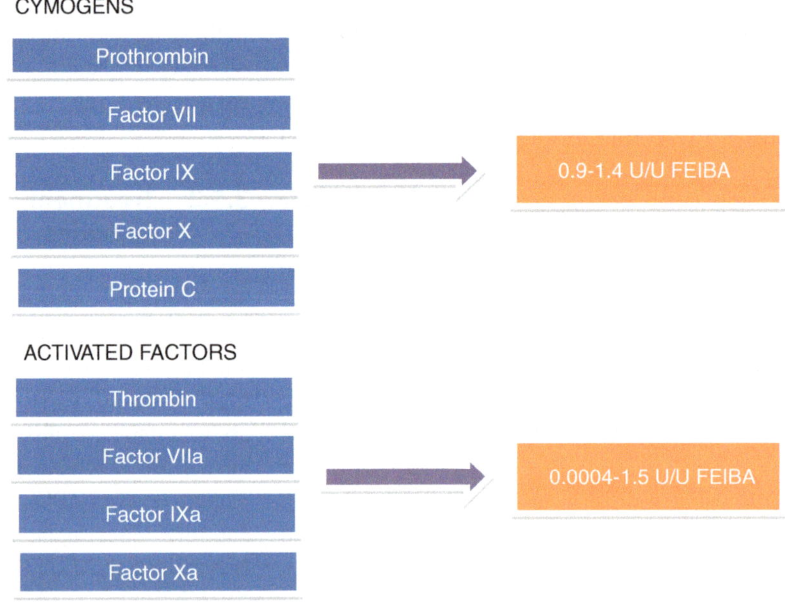

Fig. 3.1 Active components of FEIBA (factor VIII inhibitor bypassing agent)

3.5.2.2 Recombinant Factor VII Activated (rFVIIa)

Background

The first evidence that rFVIIa could be a useful agent in the treatment of hemophilia patients and inhibitor arose firstly from the identification of FVIIa as one of the clotting factors that under physiological conditions cannot be inactivated by antithrombin in the circulation [51], and from the observation of different studies that suggested that the efficacy of aPCCs could be related to the significant amount of FVII they contain [52].

It was later, however, that Hedner in collaboration with several Swedish and American groups were able to purify activated FVIIa derived from human plasma in 1981. The first doses of this FVIIa were administered to two hemophiliac patients with inhibitor in 1981 with a promising result [53, 54]. The development of a recombinant factor VII was initiated at Novo Nordisk A/S in June 1985 [54, 55]. The first patient treated with rFVIIa was in 1988, as hemorrhagic prophylaxis in a surgical synovectomy and published in Lancet the same year [56]. In 1989, the first clinical trial was initiated with the aim of finding the appropriate hemostatic dose [57].

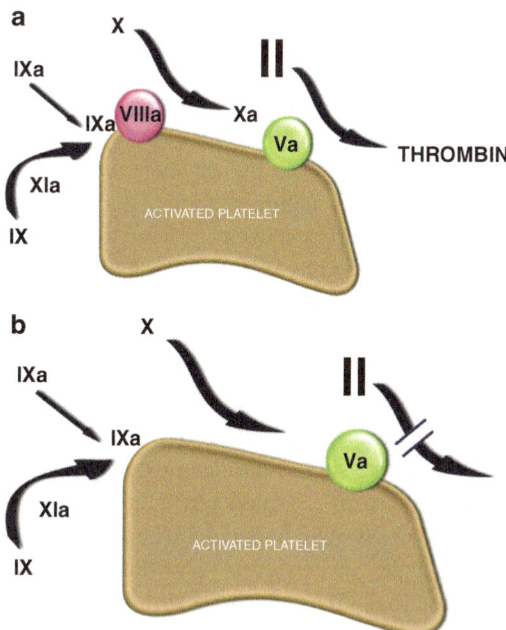

Fig. 3.2 (**a**) Thrombin generation under physiological conditions; (**b**) in patients with hemophilia A

Mechanism of Action

The initial idea underlying the use of rFVIIa as an agent capable of circumventing the effect of inhibitors was that FVIIa might be able to produce FX activation via the TF (tissue factor)/FVIIa complex in patients unable, because of the inhibitor, to initiate FX activation by the intrinsic pathway via the FIXa/FVIIIa complex and thus initiate coagulation without the need for FVIII and FIX. In the light of the cellular model of the

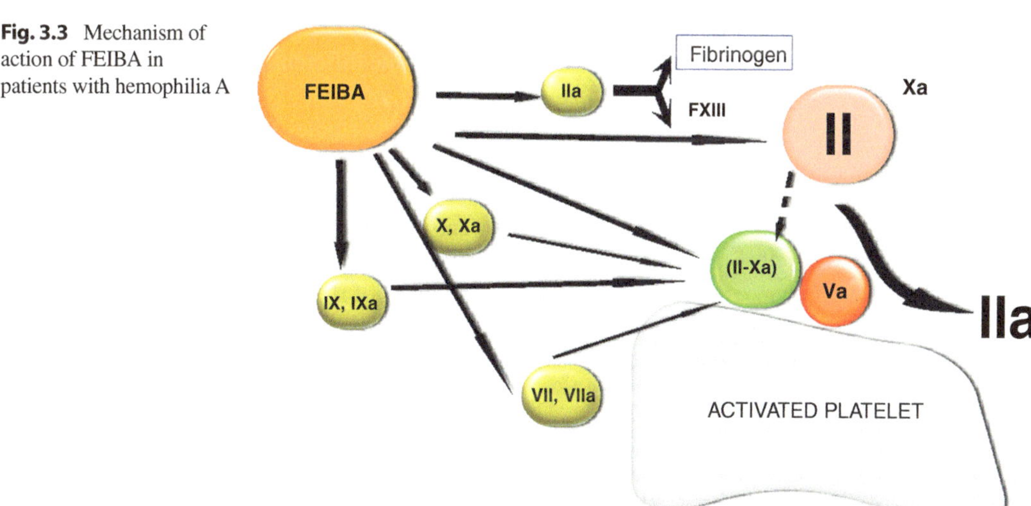

Fig. 3.3 Mechanism of action of FEIBA in patients with hemophilia A

coagulation cascade, this hypothesis seemed quite reasonable.

However, it was soon realized by different research teams that this mechanism did not seem at all as simple as initially speculated.

The cellular model of coagulation localizes the hemostatic defect in hemophilia patients to the specific generation of FXa on the platelet surface (Fig. 3.4). It thus seems explicable why high doses of rFVIIa may be effective in remedying this defect.

Therefore, without being able to definitively rule out a TF-dependent effect, the evidence we currently have suggests that a platelet surface-dependent mechanism is the major contributor to the hemostatic effect of rFVIIa in hemophilia patients.

Some aspects of the hemostatic activity of rFVIIa at the platelet surface remain to be clarified. Therefore, it can be concluded that platelets and phospholipid composition play a pivotal role in rFVIIa activity and binding. Different variations in platelet characteristics may underlie the variability found in the individual response to rFVIIa in hemophilia patients with inhibitor [43].

Clinical Efficacy of rFVIIa

As mentioned, the first description of the use of rFVIIa was in a surgical knee synovectomy in a patient with an inhibitor [56]. Subsequently, several pharmacokinetic and dose-finding studies were performed [57–59].

The overall efficacy of rFVIIa is estimated to be around 80–90%, depending on the study, the dose, the bleeding episode, the time of assessment of the process, and some individual circumstances [40].

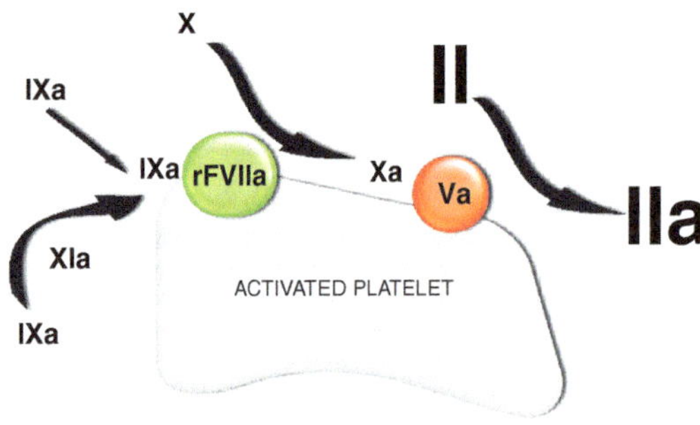

Fig. 3.4 Mechanism of hemostasis in a patient with hemophilia A and recombinant factor VII activated (rFVIIa)

The recommended doses of rFVIIa are 90–120 μg/kg every 2–3 days until resolution of the hemorrhagic process is achieved. A study conducted at home found that the mean number of doses needed to control hemostasis was 2.2 doses; however, in this study an extra dose of rFVIIa was added to consolidate hemostasis with final results of 3.2 doses per hemorrhagic episode [60].

Alternative dosing schedules have been described in the medical literature, using doses higher than 270–300 μg/kg body weight and allowing a 6-h administration interval, with increased patient acceptance. Theoretically, this would be justified by the production of a greater burst in thrombin production with a possible parallel increase in efficacy [61–63]. However, this increase in efficacy related to the use of high-dose rFVIIa has not been conclusively demonstrated in prospective studies [64].

Prospective studies have compared the use of a single dose of 270 μg/kg rFVIIa versus 2–3 standard doses of 90 μg/kg in the home treatment of moderate hemarthrosis, showing a similar response [64, 65].

3.5.2.3 Effectiveness Comparison: FEIBA Versus rFVIIa

Overall, as described, hemostatic responses to FEIBA and rFVIIa are comparable, although overall in the different papers they vary to some degree [47, 66–68].

One of the studies that directly compared the two agents was the FENOC study [69]. According to its randomized, crossover design, enrolled patients received either one dose of FEIBA 75–100 IU/kg (target dose 85 IU/kg) body weight or two doses of rFVIIa 90–120 μg/kg (target dose 105 μg/kg) administered 2 h apart. The primary endpoint for analysis was the assessment of response at 6 h, although the patient was assessed at 2, 6, 12, 24, 36, and 48 h.

At 6 h, FEIBA efficacy was 80.9% and rFVIIa efficacy 78.7%. At 12 h, FEIBA efficacy was 80.0% and rFVIIa efficacy 84.4%. Although the efficacy of both agents was similar at all hours tested, the predetermined criterion for equivalence was not achieved as the confidence interval of the efficacy percentages at 6 h (11.4–15.7) slightly exceeded the established cut-off ≤15%. Statistical criteria for equivalence may not have been obtained due to a lack of statistical power, with this being particularly evident at the 6-h point [66, 69, 70]. However, assessments made at earlier time points were more reliable than those made later, primarily because there were no other confounding factors such as underlying intra-articular inflammation in the early assessments [66, 69]. Another possible bias of the study could be due to the fact that medication administration was not masked and that a significant portion of the patient cohort (approximately 20%) was lost throughout the study.

Despite the finding that aPCC and rFVIIa are effective and safe in the treatment of bleeding episodes in inhibitor patients, it has been shown that some patients respond better to aPCC, while others respond better to rFVIIa. This is why both agents are necessary in the overall management of inhibitor patients.

The variability between different patients is underpinned by individual-specific factors in the response to bypassing agents that influence the overall efficacy of these agents. Examples of these individual characteristics that influence response include factor binding to platelet surface phospholipids, variations in platelet numbers, and the existence of platelets with increased binding capacity to these agents [68]. In addition, other factors capable of influencing bleeding tendency, such as natural anticoagulants and congenital prothrombotic factors and coagulation factors that can influence the process of hemostasis such as prothrombin levels or levels of non-inactivated FVIII, may contribute to this variability in response to aPCC and rFVIIa [66, 68].

Another important aspect is the response of the same patient in different clinical situations in which he or she responds differently to the same agent [68]. Some authors have recently described different cases of patients in these circumstances [71, 72]. In the FENOC study [69], a total of 29 patients had discordant efficacy, where one agent was effective and the other was not, especially in the first 12 h. Although the study does not analyze this discordance, 19 patients responded better to aPCC and 10 to rFVIIa [69].

Each of the agents has different mechanisms of action and different pharmacokinetics, and none is able to achieve complete normalization of thrombin generation [73]. Given these different patient responses to treatment, it is necessary to have more than one therapeutic alternative, which is why both rFVIIa and FEIBA are essential in the treatment of bleeding episodes in inhibitor patients [66].

Therefore, early identification of treatment failures is essential in order to change therapy and optimize the treatment of this group of patients.

3.6 Future

In recent years, research has revolutionized the future management of patients with hemophilia and inhibitors. The aim has been to search for mechanisms of action that differ from those currently known and that allow effective hemostasis [74]. As described above, the drug that has gained recent approval for prophylaxis by the American and European authorities is emicizumab [32, 75].

Another promising future approach in the field of hemophilia with inhibitor that could also be used in patients with hemophilia B and inhibitor is the monoclonal antibody concizumab. Concizumab (mAb 2021, Novo Nordisk), a humanized IgG4 antibody with high affinity for the K2 domain of TFPI, inhibits FXa binding and prevents tissue factor pathway inhibitor (TFPI) inhibition of the TF-FVIIa complex.

Alnylam Pharmaceuticals has developed an RNA capable of interfering with the synthesis of antithrombin (AT) by silencing its production by hepatocytes. This ALN-AT3 has been shown in animal models to decrease AT production in a dose-dependent manner by up to 90% [76]. For a period of time, trials were halted after the death of a patient from cerebral thrombosis. After detailed analysis of the data, the trial program was restarted.

3.7 Conclusions

The development of antibodies to FVIII and FIX is the most important complication of the treatment of hemophilia patients. This complication leads to an increase in morbidity and mortality and an increase in the financial resources spent on treatment. Immune tolerance is the only proven method of inhibitor eradication. However, immune tolerance may not be successful in all patients and is resource intensive. Bypassing agents are the treatment of choice in bleeding episodes. However, their efficacy is not similar to replacement therapy in the absence of inhibitor. Emicizumab is a new molecule that has brought about a radical change in the prophylaxis of patients with inhibitors. New expectations are opening up for the treatment of hemophilia patients with inhibitors with so-called non-inhibitor therapies. It remains to be elucidated who would be candidate patients for treatment with non-substitution products, most likely serious candidates being patients with failed ITI (no new planned ITI), children with newly developed high-titer inhibitor or adults with high-titer inhibitors who have not undergone ITI (due to venous access problems or reluctance to undergo ITI), older adults and/or people with co-morbidities, and finally patients with mild hemophilia and inhibitors.

While these treatments offer great promise, further research and publication of additional data (including post-authorization phase IV pharmacovigilance studies and real-world evidence in larger populations for emicizumab treatment) is required to assess expected and unexpected outcomes, such as inhibitor development, risk of thrombosis, and any other serious adverse effects.

References

1. Leissinger CA. Inhibitor development in patients with hemophilia: an overview. Semin Hematol. 2006;43(2 Suppl 4):S1–2.
2. Hoyer LW. The incidence of factor VIII inhibitors in patients with severe hemophilia A. Adv Exp Med Biol. 1995;386:35–45.
3. Wight J, Paisley S. The epidemiology of inhibitors in haemophilia A: a systematic review. Haemophilia. 2003;9:418–35.
4. Key NS. Inhibitors in congenital coagulation disorders. Br J Haematol. 2004;127:379–91.
5. Peyvandi F, Mannucci PM, Garagiola I, El-Beshlawy A, Elalfy M, Ramanan V, et al. A randomized trial of factor VIII and neutralizing antibodies in hemophilia A. N Engl J Med. 2016;374:2054–64.
6. Walsh CE, Jiménez-Yuste V, Auerswald G, Grancha S. The burden of inhibitors in haemophilia patients. Thromb Haemost. 2016;116(Suppl 1):S10–7.
7. White GC 2nd, Rosendaal F, Aledort LM, Lusher JM, Rothschild C, Ingerslev J. Definitions in hemophilia. Recommendation of the scientific subcommittee on factor VIII and factor IX of the scientific and standardization committee of the International Society on Thrombosis and Haemostasis. Thromb Haemost. 2001;85:560.
8. Blanchette VS, Key NS, Ljung LR, Manco-Johnson MJ, Berg HM, Srivastava A. Definitions in hemophilia: communication from the SSC of the ISTH. J Thromb Haemost. 2014;12:1935–9.
9. Aledort LM, Dimichele DM. Inhibitors occur more frequently in African-American and Latino haemophiliacs. Haemophilia. 1998;4:68.
10. Astermark J, Berntorp E, White GC, Kroner BL. The Malmo international brother study (MIBS): further support for genetic predisposition to inhibitor development in hemophilia patients. Haemophilia. 2001;7:267–72.
11. Shapiro SS. Genetic predisposition to inhibitor formation. Prog Clin Biol Res. 1984;150:45–55.
12. Frommel D, Allain JP. Genetic predisposition to develop factor VIII antibody in classic hemophilia. Clin Immunol Immunopathol. 1977;8:34–8.
13. Saint-Remy JM, Lacroix-Desmazes S, Oldenburg J. Inhibitors in haemophilia: pathophysiology. Haemophilia. 2004;10(Suppl 4):146–51.
14. Oldenburg J, Schroder J, Brackmann HH, Muller-Reible C, Schwaab R, Tuddenham E. Environmental and genetic factors influencing inhibitor development. Semin Hematol. 2004;41(1 Suppl 1):82–8.
15. Goodeve A. The incidence of inhibitor development according to specific mutations--and treatment? Blood Coagul Fibrinolysis. 2003;14(Suppl 1):S17–21.
16. Oldenburg J, El-Maarri O, Schwaab R. Inhibitor development in correlation to factor VIII genotypes. Haemophilia. 2002;8(Suppl 2):23–9.
17. Spena S, Garagiola I, Cannavo A, Mortarino M, Mannucci PM, Rosendaal FR, et al. Prediction of factor VIII inhibitor development in the SIPPET cohort by mutational analysis and factor VIII antigen measurement. J Thromb Haemost. 2018;16:778–90.
18. Gouw SC, van den Berg HM, Oldenburg J, Astermark J, de Groot PG, Margaglione M, et al. F8 gene mutation type and inhibitor development in patients with severe hemophilia A: systematic review and meta-analysis. Blood. 2012;119:2922–34.
19. Abdi A, Kloosterman FR, Eckhardt CL, Male C, Castaman G, Fischer K, et al. The factor VIII treatment history of non-severe hemophilia A. J Thromb Haemost. 2020;18:3203–10.

20. Oldenburg J, Picard JK, Schwaab R, Brackmann HH, Tuddenham EG, Simpson E. HLA genotype of patients with severe haemophilia a due to intron 22 inversion with and without inhibitors of factor VIII. Thromb Haemost. 1997;77:238–42.
21. Hay CR, Ollier W, Pepper L, Cumming A, Keeney S, Goodeve AC, et al. HLA class II profile: a weak determinant of factor VIII inhibitor development in severe haemophilia A. UKHCDO Inhibitor Working Party. Thromb Haemost. 1997;77:234–7.
22. White GC 2nd, Kempton CL, Grimsley A, Nielsen B, Roberts HR. Cellular immune responses in hemophilia: why do inhibitors develop in some, but not all hemophiliacs? J Thromb Haemost. 2005;3:1676–81.
23. Astermark J, Wang X, Oldenburg J, Berntorp E, Lefvert AK. Polymorphisms in the CTLA-4 gene and inhibitor development in patients with severe hemophilia A. J Thromb Haemost. 2007;5:263–5.
24. van der Bom JG, Mauser-Bunschoten EP, Fischer K, van den Berg HM. Age at first treatment and immune tolerance to factor VIII in severe hemophilia. Thromb Haemost. 2003;89:475–9.
25. Lorenzo JI, Lopez A, Altisent C, Aznar JA. Incidence of factor VIII inhibitors in severe haemophilia: the importance of patient age. Br J Haematol. 2001;113:600–3.
26. Morado M, Villar A, Jimenez Yuste V, Quintana M, Hernandez NF. Prophylactic treatment effects on inhibitor risk: experience in one Centre. Haemophilia. 2005;11:79–83.
27. Santagostino E, Mancuso ME, Rocino A, Mancuso G, Mazzucconi MG, Tagliaferri A, et al. Environmental risk factors for inhibitor development in children with haemophilia a: a case-control study. Br J Haematol. 2005;130:422–7.
28. Calvez T, Laurian Y. Protective effect of prophylaxis on inhibitor development in children with haemophilia A: more convincing studies are required. Br J Haematol. 2006;132:798–800. author reply -1
29. Gouw SC, van der Bom JG, van den Berg HM. Treatment-related risk factors of inhibitor development in previously untreated patients with hemophilia A: the CANAL cohort study. Blood. 2007;109:4648–54.
30. Kasper CK, Aledort L, Aronson D, Counts R, Edson JR, van Eys J, et al. Proceedings: a more uniform measurement of factor VIII inhibitors. Thromb Diath Haemorrh. 1975;34:612.
31. Verbruggen B, Novakova I, Wessels H, Boezeman J, van den Berg M, Mauser-Bunschoten E. The Nijmegen modification of the Bethesda assay for factor VIII:C inhibitors: improved specificity and reliability. Thromb Haemost. 1995;73:247–51.
32. Oldenburg J, Mahlangu JN, Kim B, Schmitt C, Callaghan MU, Young G, et al. Emicizumab prophylaxis in hemophilia A with inhibitors. N Engl J Med. 2017;377:809–18.
33. Pipe SW, Shima M, Lehle M, Shapiro A, Chebon S, Fukutake K, et al. Efficacy, safety, and pharmacokinetics of emicizumab prophylaxis given every 4 weeks in people with haemophilia A (HAVEN 4): a multicentre, open-label, non-randomised phase 3 study. Lancet Haematol. 2019;6:e295–305.
34. Young G, Liesner R, Chang T, Sidonio R, Oldenburg J, Jimenez-Yuste V, et al. A multicenter, open-label phase 3 study of emicizumab prophylaxis in children with hemophilia A with inhibitors. Blood. 2019;134:2127–38.
35. Gringeri A. Prospective controlled studies on prophylaxis: an Italian approach. Haemophilia. 2003;9(Suppl 1):38–42. discussion 3
36. Srivastava A, Santagostino E, Dougall A, Kitchen S, Sutherland M, Pipe SW, et al. WFH guidelines for the Management of Hemophilia, 3rd edition. Haemophilia. 2020;26(Suppl 6):1–158.
37. Leissinger CA. Prevention of bleeds in hemophilia patients with inhibitors: emerging data and clinical direction. Am J Hematol. 2004;77:187–93.
38. técnica F. [Available from: http://www.aemps.gob.es/cima/especialidad.do?metodo=verFichaWordPdf&codigo=55953&formato=pdf&formulario=PROSPECTOS.
39. Novoseven. [Available from: http://www.ema.europa.eu/ema/index.jsp?curl=pages/medicines/human/medicines/000074/human_med_000936.jsp&mid=WC0b01ac058001d124.
40. Mehta R, Parameswaran R, Shapiro AD. An overview of the history, clinical practice concerns, comparative studies and strategies to optimize therapy of bypassing agents. Haemophilia. 2006;12(Suppl 6):54–61.
41. Gallistl S, Cvirn G, Leschnik B, Muntean W. Respective roles of factors II, VII, IX, and X in the procoagulant activity of FEIBA. Blood Coagul Fibrinolysis. 2002,13:653–5.
42. Turecek PL, Varadi K, Gritsch H, Schwarz HP. FEIBA: mode of action. Haemophilia. 2004;10(Suppl 2):3–9.
43. Hoffman M, Dargaud Y. Mechanisms and monitoring of bypassing agent therapy. J Thromb Haemost. 2012;10:1478–85.
44. Negrier C, Gomperts E, Oldenburg J. The history of FEIBA: a lifetime of success in the treatment of haemophilia complicated by an inhibitor. Haemophilia. 2006;12(Suppl 5):4–13.
45. Hilgartner MW, Knatterud GL. The use of factor eight inhibitor by-passing activity (FEIBA immuno) product for treatment of bleeding episodes in hemophiliacs with inhibitors. Blood. 1983;61:36–40.
46. Hilgartner M, Aledort L, Andes A, Gill J. Efficacy and safety of vapor-heated anti-inhibitor coagulant complex in hemophilia patients. FEIBA Study Group. Transfusion. 1990;30:626–30.
47. Negrier C, Goudemand J, Sultan Y, Bertrand M, Rothschild C, Lauroua P. Multicenter retrospective study on the utilization of FEIBA in France in patients with factor VIII and factor IX inhibitors. French FEIBA study group. Factor eight bypassing activity. Thromb Haemost. 1997;77:1113–9.
48. Ehrlich HJ, Henzl MJ, Gomperts ED. Safety of factor VIII inhibitor bypass activity (FEIBA): 10-year com-

pilation of thrombotic adverse events. Haemophilia. 2002;8:83–90.
49. Aledort LM. Factor VIII inhibitor bypassing activity (FEIBA) - addressing safety issues. Haemophilia. 2008;14:39–43.
50. Aledort LM. Comparative thrombotic event incidence after infusion of recombinant factor VIIa versus factor VIII inhibitor bypass activity. J Thromb Haemost. 2004;2:1700–8.
51. Osterud B, Miller-Andersson M, Abildgaard U, Prydz H. The effect of antithrombin III on the activity of the coagulation factors VII, IX and X. Thromb Haemost. 1976;35:295–304.
52. Kurczynski EM, Penner JA. Activated prothrombin concentrate for patients with factor VIII inhibitors. N Engl J Med. 1974;291:164–7.
53. Hedner U, Kisiel W. Use of human factor VIIa in the treatment of two hemophilia A patients with high-titer inhibitors. J Clin Invest. 1983;71:1836–41.
54. Hedner U. Activated factor VII: my story. Haemophilia. 2012;18:147–51.
55. Hedner U. History of rFVIIa therapy. Thromb Res. 2010;125(Suppl 1):S4–6.
56. Hedner U, Glazer S, Pingel K, Alberts KA, Blomback M, Schulman S, et al. Successful use of recombinant factor VIIa in patient with severe haemophilia A during synovectomy. Lancet. 1988;2:1193.
57. Macik BG, Lindley CM, Lusher J, Sawyer WT, Bloom AL, Harrison JF, et al. Safety and initial clinical efficacy of three dose levels of recombinant activated factor VII (rFVIIa): results of a phase I study. Blood Coagul Fibrinolysis. 1993;4:521–7.
58. Lusher JM, Roberts HR, Davignon G, Joist JH, Smith H, Shapiro A, et al. A randomized, double-blind comparison of two dosage levels of recombinant factor VIIa in the treatment of joint, muscle and mucocutaneous haemorrhages in persons with haemophilia A and B, with and without inhibitors. rFVIIa Study Group. Haemophilia. 1998;4:790–8.
59. Lindley CM, Sawyer WT, Macik BG, Lusher J, Harrison JF, Baird-Cox K, et al. Pharmacokinetics and pharmacodynamics of recombinant factor VIIa. Clin Pharmacol Ther. 1994;55:638–48.
60. Key NS, Aledort LM, Beardsley D, Cooper HA, Davignon G, Ewenstein BM, et al. Home treatment of mild to moderate bleeding episodes using recombinant factor VIIa (Novoseven) in haemophiliacs with inhibitors. Thromb Haemost. 1998;80:912–8.
61. Hoffman M, Monroe DM 3rd, Roberts HR. Activated factor VII activates factors IX and X on the surface of activated platelets: thoughts on the mechanism of action of high-dose activated factor VII. Blood Coagul Fibrinolysis. 1998;9(Suppl 1):S61–5.
62. Parameswaran R, Shapiro AD, Gill JC, Kessler CM. Dose effect and efficacy of rFVIIa in the treatment of haemophilia patients with inhibitors: analysis from the hemophilia and thrombosis research society registry. Haemophilia. 2005;11:100–6.
63. Kenet G. High-dose recombinant factor VIIa therapy in hemophilia patients with inhibitors. Semin Hematol. 2006;43(1 Suppl 1):S108–10.
64. Kavakli K, Makris M, Zulfikar B, Erhardtsen E, Abrams ZS, Kenet G. Home treatment of haemarthroses using a single dose regimen of recombinant activated factor VII in patients with haemophilia and inhibitors. A multi-Centre, randomised, double-blind, cross-over trial. Thromb Haemost. 2006;95:600–5.
65. Santagostino E, Mancuso ME, Rocino A, Mancuso G, Scaraggi F, Mannucci PM. A prospective randomized trial of high and standard dosages of recombinant factor VIIa for treatment of hemarthroses in hemophiliacs with inhibitors. J Thromb Haemost. 2006;4:367–71.
66. Berntorp E, Collins P, D'Oiron R, Ewing N, Gringeri A, Negrier C, et al. Identifying non-responsive bleeding episodes in patients with haemophilia and inhibitors: a consensus definition. Haemophilia. 2011;17:e202–10.
67. Tjonnfjord GE, Holme PA. Factor eight inhibitor bypass activity (FEIBA) in the management of bleeds in hemophilia patients with high-titer inhibitors. Vasc Health Risk Manag. 2007;3:527–31.
68. Berntorp E. Differential response to bypassing agents complicates treatment in patients with haemophilia and inhibitors. Haemophilia. 2009;15:3–10.
69. Astermark J, Donfield SM, DiMichele DM, Gringeri A, Gilbert SA, Waters J, et al. A randomized comparison of bypassing agents in hemophilia complicated by an inhibitor: the FEIBA NovoSeven comparative (FENOC) study. Blood. 2007;109:546–51.
70. Donfield SM, Astermark J, Lail AE, Gilbert SA, Berntorp E. Value added: increasing the power to assess treatment outcome in joint haemorrhages. Haemophilia. 2008;14:276–80.
71. Watts RG. Successful use of recombinant factor VIIa for emergency fasciotomy in a patient with hemophilia A and high-titer inhibitor unresponsive to factor VIII inhibitor bypassing activity. Am J Hematol. 2005;79:58–60.
72. Young G, Blain R, Nakagawa P, Nugent DJ. Individualization of bypassing agent treatment for haemophilic patients with inhibitors utilizing thromboelastography. Haemophilia. 2006;12:598–604.
73. Negrier C, Dargaud Y, Bordet JC. Basic aspects of bypassing agents. Haemophilia. 2006;12(Suppl 6):48–53.
74. Franchini M, Mannucci PM. Non-factor replacement therapy for haemophilia: a current update. Blood Transfus. 2018;16:457–61.
75. Shima M, Hanabusa H, Taki M, Matsushita T, Sato T, Fukutake K, et al. Factor VIII-mimetic function of humanized bispecific antibody in hemophilia A. N Engl J Med. 2016;374:2044–53.
76. Pasi KJ, Rangarajan S, Georgiev P, Mant T, Creagh MD, Lissitchkov T, et al. Targeting of Antithrombin in hemophilia A or B with RNAi therapy. N Engl J Med. 2017;377:819–28.

Immune Tolerance Induction in Patients with Hemophilia A

4

M. Teresa Álvarez-Román

4.1 Introduction

The treatment in patients with hemophilia and inhibitor can be divided into two parts: prevention and treatment of episodes hemorrhagic, and eradication of the inhibitor through immune tolerance induction (ITI). Both treatments should be carried out by a comprehensive hemophilia treatment center [1]. Patients with FVIII inhibitors typically have higher rates of hospitalization, greater treatment costs, and higher mortality rates than those without inhibitors [1, 2].

The origin of the current ITI takes place in a clinical case reported by Brackmann et al. It was about a patient in which it was possible to eliminate the inhibitor with the administration of high doses of FVIII, 100 IU/Kg every 12 h [3]. This gave rise to the well-known ITI later as the Bonn protocol [4]. Subsequently, to this protocol others arose in which there were fundamentally differences in the doses, that have varied widely from less than 25 IU/kg three times a week to more than 300 IU/kg daily [5–7].

Thus, ITI treatments aim to eliminate the inhibitor permanently. Current treatments are based on exposure to the factor trigger, the FVIII or FIX, in a more or less intensive and continuous way. This treatment is maintained until the patient becomes tolerant to the administered product or, what is the same, until the incremental recovery and half-life factor infused is normal.

The objective of this chapter is to review the different immune tolerance schemes and their results as well as to summarize the new recommendations in this group of patients.

4.2 Immune Tolerance Induction (ITI) in Patients with Severe Hemophilia A

4.2.1 Definition and Objective of ITI

Immune tolerance treatment consists of the continuous administration of factor with the aim of reaching immune tolerance. Successful ITI is defined as a persistently negative Bethesda titer, accompanied by normal pharmacokinetics, including factor recovery >66% and half-life >6 h for standard FVIII concentrates (Table 4.1) [8]. Once successful ITI is achieved, FVIII prophylaxis may be initiated or resumed. There is consensus that failure of ITI is the inability to achieve successful tolerance within 2–3 years of initiation of an ITI regimen [9].

Since the number of patients with hemophilia and inhibitor is not very high, different registries have been established to collect and analyze the data. In Table 4.2, you can see the existing registries and their response rate, the overall response rate was 50–80% [10–13].

M. T. Álvarez-Román (✉)
Hemophilia Unit, Department of Hematology, La Paz University Hospital, Madrid, Spain

E. C. Rodríguez-Merchán (ed.), *Advances in Hemophilia Treatment*,
https://doi.org/10.1007/978-3-030-93990-8_4

Table 4.1 Success criteria in patients treated with immune tolerance induction (ITI)

Success	• Negative inhibitor titer (<0.6 BU) • Normal FVIII in vivo recovery (>66% of predicted FVIII concentration after infusion) • Normal FVIII half-life >6 h after a 72 h washout period • Absence of anamnesis upon further FVIII exposure
Partial response	• Inhibitor titer <5 BU/mL • FVIII recovery <66% of predicted • FVIII half-life <6 h after a 72 h washout period • Clinical response to FVIII • No increase in the inhibitor titer >5BU over 6 months of on-demand therapy or 12 months of prophylaxis
Failure	• Failure to fulfill criteria for full/partial success within 33 months • <20% reduction in inhibitor titer for any 6-month period during ITI after first 3 months of treatment, which implies that: 9 months is minimum period for ITI and 33 months is maximum duration of unsuccessful ITI (although decision may be made to continue)

Adapted from reference [8]. *BU* Bethesda units

Table 4.2 Immune tolerance induction (ITI) registries

International immune tolerance registry (IITR)	N: 314 patients. Success: 52% Mariani et al. [10]
North American immune tolerance registry (NAITR)	N: 148 patients. Success: 72% DiMichele et al. [11]
German registry	N: 126. Success: 78.6%. Partial success: 8.7% failure: 12.7% Lenk [12]
Spanish registry	N: 38. Success: 68%. Failure: 32% Haya et al. [13]

Despite this high percentage of success obtained with immune tolerance treatments, there are still several issues under debate, such as its high cost, the time necessary to achieve it, adequate venous access and what to do with those patients in whom it fails. The arrival of emicizumab has changed the way of assessing the approach to ITI as will be discussed later.

Table 4.3 Prognostic factors to achieve immune tolerance induction (ITI). BU = Bethesda units

	Good prognosis	Poor prognosis
Historical peak titer	<200 BU	>200 BU
Peak on ITI	<100 BU	>100 BU
Time inhibitor diagnosis To start	<5 years	>5 years
Interruption >2 weeks of ITI	No	Yes
Pre-ITI titer	<10 BU	>10 BU

4.2.2 Prognostic Factors to Achieve Immune Tolerance

Historical peak titer >200BU, peak on ITI >100 BU, time inhibitor diagnosis to start ITI > 5 years, and interruption >2 weeks of ITI, pre ITI titer >10 BU are outlined as poor prognostic factors [9]. In Table 4.3 we can see the predictors of successful ITI outcome.

There is controversy in some of these factors, for example, pre-ITI titer. For a long time, it was expected to start ITI until the inhibitor titer fell below 10 BU as data from registries published in 1990 and 2000 showed better results in this population. From a compilation of the data of the International Immune Tolerance Registry (IITR) and North American Immune Tolerance Registry (NAITR) it is shown that, in patients who start treatment with a titer <10 BU/mL, success is achieved in 85% of the cases and in a mean time of 11 months, compared with 33% and 15 months when the titer is >10 BU/mL. However, today ITI is started immediately after the detection of the inhibitor regardless of its titer because the sooner the inhibitor is removed, lower risk of severe bleeding or development of target joints; and because in some studies they have shown better results with early treatments [14–16].

Other factors have been implicated in the ITI results; they have not been confirmed:

- Type of mutation that causes hemophilia. Worse results have been obtained in patients with large deletions [17].
- Ethnicity, recent publications have shown worse results in reaching immune tolerance in

patients of African American origin, 57.9% versus 92% in other ethnicities [18].

4.2.3 Immune Tolerance Regimen

Table 4.4 shows principal therapeutic immune tolerance regimens. There are two principal therapeutic regimens "Bonn high-dose regimen" and the "Van Creveld Dutch low-dose" regimen [4, 5]. Other option could be the Malmö ITI-protocol which includes extracorporeal adsorption of the antibody, a procedure that is not feasible in the youngest children because the extracorporeal blood volume will be too large [6].

Perhaps two of the most interesting classic aspects of ITI are the dose to be administered and the role of VWF-containing FVIII (pdFVIII/VWF concentrates). The optimal regimen, product, or dose for ITI remains to be defined.

To analyze the benefit in the success of ITI of using high doses to the detriment of low doses, a meta-analysis of the results obtained by the International Immunotolerance Registry (IITR) and the North American Registry (NAITR) was carried out [14]. In this meta-analysis, data from 278 patients were combined and success was analyzed according to historical inhibitor titer, pre-ITI titer, and dose of FVIII used during ITI. In patients with low historical peak and low pre-ITI (patients with good prognosis) the success rate was not different in patients who received low or high doses of FVIII [14]. The IITR and NAITR meta-analysis laid the foundations for the international ITI study (ITI-study), which was the first prospective, randomized study conducted in the field of ITI in patients with hemophilia and inhibitor [19]. The main objective of the study was to compare a low-dose ITI regimen (50 IU FVIII/Kg three times a week) versus a high-dose ITI regimen (200 IU FVIII/day) in patients with hemophilia A and inhibitor. The study was based on the non-inferiority hypothesis, in which success in low-risk patients was independent of the doses of FVIII used. Even though the study was terminated early for reasons of safety and efficacy, the fundamental conclusions are that there were no differences in the success of ITI between both arms (24 out of 58 patients in the low-dose arm achieved immune tolerance vs 22 out of 57 patients in the high-dose arm dose, $P = 0.909$); time to achieve negative inhibitor detection ($P = 0.027$), normal recovery ($P = 0.002$), and tolerance ($P = 0.116$, no significance) were shorter with high doses; the historical peak ($P = 0.026$) and the ITI titer ($P = 0.002$) were inversely correlated with success; only the ITI peak predicted success in multivariate analysis and the subjects in schemes low-dose bled more frequently than high-dose (odds ratio, 2.2; $P = 0.0019$) [19]. Therefore, it seems clear that in patients with favorable prognostic factors, the dose does not influence success, although it clearly influences the time to achieve ITI and the number of bleeds.

The meta-analysis of the IITR and NAITR also provides us with useful information about patients with a poor prognosis. Large differences were observed in favor of high doses in patients with unfavorable prognostic factors (historical high inhibitor titers and/or high titers prior to initiation of ITI). These observations led to the conclusion that patients with unfavorable prognostic factors should be treated with an immunotolerance protocol based on the use of high doses of FVIII [14].

This way, several groups were in favor of using high doses of FVIII in hemophilic children and adults with unfavorable prognostic factors. The Bonn cohort (22 patients), most of them adults, with a mean pre-ITI inhibitor of 89 BU and maximum titers of 11 to 5500

Table 4.4 Immune tolerance induction (ITI) protocols

Protocol	Dosage	Reference
Bonn protocol	FVIII 100–150 IU/kg, twice daily and aPCC 50 U/kg/12 h if high risk bleeds	[4]
Van Creveld Protocol	FVIII 25 IU/kg every other day	[5]
Malmö	FVIII high doses+ high doses of FVIII and cyclophosphamide and immunoadsorption if necessary	[6]

aPCC activated prothrombin complex concentrate

obtained success rates of 95% and with a mean ITI achievement of 14.5 months (4.1.–25.4). On the other hand, the Frankfurt cohort with 21 pediatric patients (0.1–6 years) with median pre-ITI inhibitor of 42 BU and median maximum titer of 105 BU obtained response rates of 82% and a median success rate of 4 months (0.5–42) [20–22].

Different studies suggest that the presence of von Willebrand factor (VWF) in FVIII concentrates can produce an increase in the ITI efficacy rate both in primary immunotolerance and in rescue regimens. These results also suggest that it may not be necessary to perform ITI with the same product with which the patient developed the inhibitor, as is generally recommended. It is difficult to explain what the beneficial effect is played by the VWF and different hypotheses have been raised for this purpose. Under physiological conditions, FVIII forms a complex with VWF, the latter acting as a transporter in the circulatory stream. VWF could mask certain FVIII epitopes, especially the C2 domain and thus block the binding of inhibitory antibodies and/or lengthen the time that FVIII interacts with the immune system, preventing its degradation. An alternative theory is that components other than VWF found in low/intermediate purity concentrates, such as cytokines or other immunomodulatory proteins, were responsible for the observed beneficial effect.

In recent years, different publications derived from the results of the G-ITI have been published [23–26]. In the study published by Oldenburg et al., 60 patients who received a single FVIII/VWF concentrate (Fanhdi®, Grifols) from different centers in Spain, Italy, and Germany were retrospectively analyzed [23]. The use of FVIII/VWF was both in primary and salvage ITI with success rates (complete and partial) of 83%.

Until the advent of emicizumab, it was accepted that patients with hemophilia and a high inhibitor titer should undergo immunotolerance treatments. However, with the approval of emicizumab, which has a high efficacy, easier and more convenient administration for the subcutaneous patient and less frequent (weekly, every 2 weeks or once a month) it is debatable whether the eradication of the inhibitor remains necessary in all cases or even in any case [27].

4.2.4 Immune Tolerance in Patients on Prophylaxis Regimen with Emicizumab

Advocates of immune tolerance support that patients receiving emicizumab require hemostatic treatment with bypass agents for bleeding control and surgery, and this can be dangerous and difficult to monitor [28].

In one of the clinical trials with emicizumab, serious adverse events (thrombosis and thrombotic microangiopathy, TAM) were reported in inhibitor patients who required treatment with bypass agents. This occurred with the simultaneous use of emicizumab and activated prothrombin complex concentrates (aPCC) at a daily dose greater than 100 U/Kg for more than 1 day. Thrombotic/TMA events have not been reported when rFVIIa or FVIII were co-administered with emicizumab; however, there are patients with inhibitors who have a poor response to rFVIIa and need to be rescued with other hemostatic agents in case of bleeding. Clearly, the safest and most effective approach in emicizumab-treated patients requiring hemostasis is to use replacement therapy with FVIII concentrates, but this is only possible in the absence of inhibitor. Inhibitor patients who are not offered ITIs are likely to have to rely on the use of bypass agents throughout life for the scenarios mentioned above, which would not be the ideal treatment given their lower efficacy, convenience, and safety. In addition, it is very likely that despite emicizumab they have higher morbidity and mortality and cannot benefit from gene therapy [29].

Although most authors prefer to eradicate inhibitors, several questions remain regarding an optimal eradication strategy: Should patients with inhibitors undergo multiple ITI eradication attempts as has often been done in the past? Should emicizumab be given at the same time as ITI to prevent bleeding? Will ITI regimens change with the use of emicizumab? ITI regimens using high/frequent doses of FVIII (so-called high-dose ITIs) were associated with lower bleeding rates, but with a higher cost and burden of treatment. With emicizumab able to provide bleeding prophylaxis, will there be greater adoption of lower dose/lower frequency ITI regimens that are no longer hampered by higher bleeding rates? Will the health system support the cost of ITI with concomitant emicizumab? Will there remain any role for prophylaxis with traditional bypass agents using rFVIIa or aPCC? Can successful ITI patients continue to receive emicizumab? Do patients continuing emicizumab after inhibitor eradication require regular exposure to FVIII to maintain tolerance to FVIII? [30]. These uncertainties highlight the need to generate new evidence through well-conducted studies to develop new consensus recommendations based on data on ITI and the management of inhibitors.

In the absence of current data-based recommendations but recognizing that the scientific community needs guidance to drive management decisions, the Future Immunotolerance Treatment Group (FIT) was established to address these uncertainties. The group has proposed new algorithms to perform ITI with and without concomitant emicizumab [30]. Below are the main conclusions and recommendations of the FIT group regarding ITI:

- Eradication of inhibitors remains a desirable goal.
- Since ITI is the only approach that currently offers inhibitor eradication potential, all inhibitor patients should be offered at least one ITI attempt.
- Emicizumab is only an option for inhibitor patients who, for various reasons, must delay or cannot/do not want to undergo ITI.
- Where emicizumab is available, the addition of immunosuppressive therapy to ITI is no longer recommended.
- As patients with inhibitors are likely to undergo fewer cycles of ITI in the future, the choice of the initial course (source of FVIII and ITI regimen) is likely to become increasingly important.
- The ability to use emicizumab concomitantly with FVIII during ITI to prevent bleeding may influence the choice of ITI regimen.

Several studies have been initiated or will be conducted soon to further explore the use of emicizumab during ITI. An open-label trial in North America is planned to examine the safety and efficacy of concomitant use of prophylactic emicizumab in conjunction with low-dose recombinant FVIII (rFVIII). Part 1 will be to examine the incidence of inhibitor development in previously untreated patients (PUP) and minimally treated patients (MTP) (the doses used of rFVIII, simoctocog alfa (Nuwiq®) will be 25 IU / kg ±5 IU and the frequency will be every 1–2 weeks) while part 2 will focus on children and young adults <21 years with moderate/severe hemophilia A (≤2% FVIII) with inhibitor treated with the combination of emicizumab and ITI with low doses of rFVIII (ClinicalTrials.gov: NCT04030052).

A 5-year multicenter retrospective-prospective observational study called MOTIVATE (ClinicalTrials.gov: NCT04023019) is being carried out in centers in North America and Europe. MOTIVATE aims to collect the efficacy and safety of three different approaches in the management of patients with hemophilia A and inhibitor: (1) ITI without emicizumab; (2) ITI in combination with emicizumab, and (3) emicizumab alone without any attempt at ITI. The primary endpoints are the success of the ITI and bleeding rates. Recruitment started in March 2020 and the estimated inclusion is 120 participants.

Finally, a prospective European multicenter clinical trial will aim to examine the safety of the association between ITI and emicizumab prophylaxis in patients (>3 kg and < 65 years) with hemophilia A and inhibitor. The plan is for ITI to begin at enrollment in patients already receiving emicizumab or after a loading dose (3 mg/kg/week for 4 weeks) in patients new to emicizumab. Patients should receive primary or rescue ITI with pdFVIII or rFVIII at a starting dose of

50 IU/kg/IU/3 times weekly plus emicizumab prophylaxis at any approved maintenance dose. To evaluate the results after a successful ITI, these patients will continue to be evaluated for an additional 12 months, during which time they will receive an emicizumab group, another emicizumab with FVIII and finally another group with FVIII alone, depending on the decision of the investigator and the patient, the trial registration is still pending.

Regarding the concomitant use of emicizumab with FVIII after ITI, there are three possible scenarios after ITI: non-tolerization, partial tolerization, and successful tolerization [31]. For patients in whom ITI fails, treatment with emicizumab to prevent bleeding should be considered the current standard of treatment. If emicizumab is not available, treatment with bypass agents on demand or prophylactically may be considered. For patients who are partially tolerated, FVIII concentrates in doses higher than those used standard can be used to prevent bleeding or, when possible, emicizumab can be used to prevent bleeding. The clinical scenario that, paradoxically, generates the most uncertainty is how to proceed when the ITI is successful. Before the availability of emicizumab, patients would continue with FVIII, but with a different purpose: prevention of bleeding (prophylaxis) rather than maintaining immune tolerance. However, with the arrival of emicizumab, once tolerance is reached, patients have the option of using FVIII concentrates prophylactically or emicizumab. Both strategies have limitations. Continuation of FVIII indefinitely requires intravenous administrations generally 2–3 times per week with current FVIII concentrates (perhaps once a week with future FVIII concentrates), resulting in a high treatment burden that often results in poor adherence. And on the other hand, continuing only with emicizumab after a successful ITI although it can reduce the burden of treatment and improve adherence, however, it can be much more expensive than continuing with FVIII concentrates, and probably recurrence of the inhibitor if not additional exposure to the factor is provided. Inhibitor recurrence is known to be approximately 29.7%.

To try to clarify whether continued FVIII therapy is necessary to prevent inhibitor recurrence, the PRIORITY (Prevention of Inhibitor Recurrence Indefinite Recurrence), NCT04621916, study was designed. This prospective, multicenter clinical trial plans to randomize inhibitor patients who achieve successful ITI to receive emicizumab or emicizumab plus FVIII weekly. The main inclusion criteria are male patients aged ≤12 years with severe/moderate hemophilia A (FVIII ≤2%) and a history of a high-titer inhibitor (>5 BU/ml), who were successfully tolerated during the previous year using any FVIII concentrate, according to international consensus recommendations for ITI. Eligible patients must be currently receiving emicizumab or be willing to receive it. The primary outcome is the inhibitor recurrence rate at 96 weeks. Laboratory tests include the genetic study of FVIII, the measurement of the FVIII inhibitor titers by a bovine chromogenic assay (since the presence of emicizumab precludes the use of the traditional inhibitor assay) and pharmacokinetic studies (the activity of FVIII is measured before infusion and 15–30 min, 6 and 24 h after infusion) to assess FVIII half-life and FVIII recovery. Tests are scheduled for results at 24 (intermediate), 48, and 96 weeks.

4.3 Immune Tolerance in Patients with Mild or Moderate Hemophilia

In non-severe hemophilia patients, the presence of an inhibitor may exacerbate the bleeding phenotype dramatically. There are very limited data on the optimal therapeutic approach to eradicate inhibitors in these patients.

The largest study in mild patients has been published by the INSIGHT group. It includes 2709 patients, of them 101 with hemophilia and inhibitor. In 71% the inhibitor was eradicated, the majority spontaneously, 51/73 and others after treatment, 21/28. The treatments used for eradication were highly variable, including both immune tolerance induction and immunosuppression. Sustained success (no inhibitor after rechallenging with factor VIII concentrate after inhibitor disappearance) was achieved in 64% (30/47) of those patients rechallenged with FVIII concentrate. In conclusion, in non-severe HA patients most inhibitors disappear spontaneously. However, in 35% (25/72) of these patients an anamnestic response still can occur when rechallenged, thus disappearance in these patients does not always equal sustained response. Treatment for those requiring eradication must be decided case by case, as one single approach is unlikely to be appropriate for all [32]. Best results are achieved in regimens that use immunosuppression, for example rituximab [33, 34]. This may be because the inhibitor in the patient with mild hemophilia A has a behavior more like that of the autoantibodies of acquired hemophilia.

4.4 Conclusions

Since the advent of emicizumab, there have been different opinions about whether immune tolerance remains the treatment of choice for patients with severe hemophilia A who develop an inhibitor. Probably in the coming years the best strategy to follow with these patients will be defined, the dose to be used, how to continue the treatment after achieving tolerance, etc.

The therapeutic approach should be different in patients with mild-moderate and inhibitory hemophilia, who may benefit from immune suppressive treatment.

References

1. Srivastava A, Santagostino E, Dougall A, et al. WFH Guidelines for the Management of Hemophilia, 3rd edition. Haemophilia. 2020;26(S6):1–158. Special Issue: WFH Guidelines for the Management of Hemophilia, 3rd edition
2. Eckhardt CL, Loomans JI, van Velzen AS, et al. Inhibitor development and mortality in non- severe hemophilia A. J Thromb Haemost. 2015;13:1217–25.
3. Brackmann HH, Gormsen J. Massive factor-VIII infusion in haemophiliac with factor-VIII inhibitor, high responder. Lancet. 1977;2(8044):933.
4. Brackmann HH, Oldenburg J, Schwaab R. Immune tolerance for the treatment of factor VIII inhibitors--twenty years' 'bonn protocol'. Vox Sang. 1996;70(Suppl 1):30–5.
5. Mauser-Bunschoten EP, Nieuwenhuis HK, Roosendaal G, van den Berg HM. Low-dose immune tolerance induction in hemophilia A patients with inhibitors. Blood. 1995;86:983–8.
6. Nilsson IM, Berntorp E, Zettervall O. Induction of immune tolerance in patients with hemophilia and antibodies to factor VIII by combined treatment with intravenous IgG, cyclophosphamide, and factor VIII. N Engl J Med. 1988;318:947–50.
7. Mariani G, Kroner B. International immune tolerance registry, 1997 update. Vox Sang. 1999;77(Suppl 1):25–7.
8. DiMichele DM, Hoots WK, Pipe SW, Rivard GE, Santagostino E. International workshop on immune tolerance induction: consensus recommendations. Haemophilia. 2007;13(Suppl 1):1–22.
9. Ljung RCR. How I manage patients with inherited haemophilia A and B and factor inhibitors. Br J Haematol. 2018;180:501–10.
10. Mariani G, Ghirardini A, Bellocco R. Thromb Haemost. 1994;72:155–8.
11. DiMichele DM, Kroner BL, North American Immune Tolerance Study Group, et al. Thromb Haemost. 2002;87:52–7.
12. Lenk H, ITI Study Group. Haematologica. 2000;85:45–7.
13. Haya S, López MF, Aznar JA, Batlle J, Spanish Immune Tolerance Group. Haemophilia. 2001;7:154–9.
14. Kroner BL. Comparison of the international immune tolerance registry and the North American immune tolerance registry. Vox Sang. 1999;77(Suppl 1):33–7.
15. Meeks SL, Batsuli G. Hemophilia and inhibitors: current treatment options and potential new therapeutic approaches. Hematology Am Soc Hematol Educ Program. 2016;2016:657–62.
16. Collins P, Chalmers E, Alamelu J, et al. First- line immune tolerance induction for children with severe haemophilia A: a protocol from the UK Haemophilia Centre Doctors' Organisation Inhibitor and Paediatric Working Parties. Haemophilia. 2017;23:654–9.
17. Coppola A, Margaglione M, Santagostino E, et al. Factor VIII gene (F8) mutations as predictors of outcome in immune tolerance induction (ITI) of hemophilia A patients with high-responding inhibitors. J Thromb Haemost. 2009;7:1809–15.
18. Callaghan MU, Rajpurkar M, Chitlur M, et al. Immune tolerance induction in 31 children with haemophilia A: is ITI less successful in African Americans? Haemophilia. 2011;17:483–9.
19. Hay CR, DiMichele DM. The principal results of the international immune tolerance study: a randomized dose comparison. Blood. 2012;119:1335–44.
20. Brackmann HH, White GC 2nd, Berntorp E, Andersen T, Escuriola-Ettingshausen C. Immune tolerance induction: what have we learned over time? Haemophilia. 2018;24(Suppl 3):3–14.
21. Brackmann HH, Schwaab R, Effenberger W, Hess L, Hanfland P, Oldenburg J. Antibodies to factor VIII

in hemophilia A patients. Vox Sang. 2000;78(Suppl 2):187–90.

22. Ettingshausen CE, Kreuz W. The immune tolerance induction (ITI) dose debate: does the international ITI study provide a clearer picture? Haemophilia. 2013;19(Suppl 1):12–7.
23. Oldenburg J, Jimenez-Yuste V, Peiro-Jordan R, Aledort LM, Santagostino E. Primary and rescue immune tolerance induction in children and adults: a multicentre international study with a VWF-containing plasma-derived FVIII concentrate. Haemophilia. 2014;20:83–91.
24. Santagostino E, Rangarajan S, Oldenburg J, Peiro-Jordan R, Jimenez-Yuste V. Rapid and sustained immune tolerance to inhibitors induced by a plasma-derived, VWF-containing FVIII concentrate. Haemophilia. 2019;25:E110–3.
25. Jiménez-Yuste V, Oldenburg J, Rangarajan S, Peiró-Jordán R, Santagostino E. Long-term outcome of haemophilia A patients after successful immune tolerance induction therapy using a single plasma-derived FVIII/VWF product: the long-term ITI study. Haemophilia. 2016;22:859–65.
26. Jiménez-Yuste V, Oldenburg J, Rangarajan S, Kurth MH, Bozzo J, Santagostino E. Clinical overview of Fanhdi/Alphanate (plasma-derived, VWF-containing FVIII concentrate) in immune tolerance induction in haemophilia a patients with inhibitors. Haemophilia. 2016;22:e71–4.
27. Santagostino E, Young G, Escuriola Ettingshausen C, Jimenez-Yuste V, Carcao M. Inhibitors: a need for eradication? Acta Haematol. 2019;141:151–5.
28. Oldenburg J, Mahlangu JN, Kim B, Schmitt C, Callaghan MU, Young G, et al. Emicizumab prophylaxis in hemophilia A with inhibitors. N Engl J Med. 2017;377:809–18.
29. Young G. Management of children with hemophilia A: how emicizumab has changed the landscape. J Thromb Haemost. 2021 Apr 19; https://doi.org/10.1111/jth.15342. Online ahead of print
30. Carcao M, Escuriola-Ettingshausen C, Santagostino E, Oldenburg J, Liesner R, Nolan B, et al. The changing face of immune tolerance induction in haemophilia a with the advent of emicizumab. Haemophilia. 2019;25:676–84.
31. Young G. How I treat children with haemophilia and inhibitors. Br J Haematol. 2019;186:400–8.
32. Van Vellzen AS, Eckhardt CL, Hart DP, et al. Inhibitors in nonsevere haemophilia a: outcome and erradication strategies. Thromb Haemost. 2015;114:45–6.
33. Vlot AJ, Wittebol S, Strengers PF, et al. Factor VIII inhibitor in a patient with haemophilia a and an Asn618-Ser mutation responsive to immune tolerance induction and ciclophosphamide. Br J Haematol. 2002;117:136–40.
34. Dunkley S, Kershaw G, Young G, et al. Rituximab treatment of mild haemophilia a with inhibitors: a proposed treatment protocol. Haemophilia. 2006;12:663–7.

5 Hemophilia A: New Drugs

Mónica Martín-Salces

5.1 Introduction

Hemophilia A is a rare, chronic, X linked diseases characterized by a deficiency in factor VIII (FVIII) resulting in an increased bleeding tendency. The new drugs ranging from extended half-life to non-factor products, product a significant improvement in the quality of life of persons with hemophilia.

These innovative treatments have the potential to improve the level of care by decreasing the frequency of infusion, increasing adherence, promoting prophylaxis, offering alternatives to patients with inhibitors and an easy route of administration [1].

5.2 Extended Half-Life Factor VIII Products

5.2.1 Efmoroctocog Alfa, rFVIIIFc

Efmoroctocog alfa is a recombinant fusion protein comprising a single molecule of B-domain-deleted recombinant FVIII covalently fused to the Fc domain of human immunoglobulin (Ig) G1 without a linker sequencer [2]. This molecule is produced by human embryonic kidney 293 (HEK 293) and was designed to increase FVIII half-life through the IgG recycling mechanism mediated by the neonatal Fc receptor in the endosomes of endothelial cells [3].

The half-life of efmoroctocog alfa is about 1.5 times longer than that of conventional plasma-derived FVIII (pd-rFVIII) and of recombinant FVIII (rFVIII) products [4]. It is approved for the treatment and prophylaxis of bleeding in patients with hemophilia A. Clinical trials and clinical experience demonstrate that rFVIIIFc provides effective prophylaxis for previously treated patients with severe hemophilia A and is generally well tolerated. The safety and efficacy of long-term treatment (up to 5.9 years) with rFVIIIFc has been demonstrated in the phase III ASPIRE extension study. The studies also showed that rFVIIIFc can be used to manage bleeding events and to maintain perioperative hemostasis in patients with hemophilia A. Some data suggest that rFVIIIFc prophylaxis might also confer better joint protection than previous rFVIII treatment, although further data are needed to confirm these observations [5].

5.2.2 Rurioctocog Alfa Pegol, BAX 855

BAX 855 or rurioctocog alfa pegol is a pegylated molecule of full-length rFVIII produced in Chinese hamster ovary (CHO) cells. It is manu-

M. Martín-Salces (✉)
Department of Hematology, La Paz University Hospital, Madrid, Spain

E. C. Rodríguez-Merchán (ed.), *Advances in Hemophilia Treatment*,
https://doi.org/10.1007/978-3-030-93990-8_5

factured by attaching a polyethylene glycol (PEG) molecule (with a molecular weight of 20 kDa) to the B-domain of FVIII [6].

BAX 855 retains all the physiological properties of FVIII except binding to low-density lipoprotein receptor-related protein (LRP), which helps clear them from circulation; clearing FVIII from the kidneys occurs through interactions with low-density LRP, primarily in the liver [6]. This gives the pegylated molecule a prolonged half-life. In humans, the mean half-life is reported to be 14.3 h, about 1.3–1.5 times that of standard rFVIII molecules [7].

5.2.3 Damoctocog Alfa Pegol, BAY94–9027

Damoctocog alfa pegol or BAY 94–9027 is a B-domain-deleted (BDD) rFVIII that is site-specifically conjugated with a 60-kDa branched PEG at a cysteine that has been introduced into the A3 domain (K1804C) to improve its pharmacokinetics [8].

In a phase 1 study in previously treated patients with severe hemophilia A, BAY 94–9027 demonstrated decreased clearance, greater area under the curve (AUC), and a longer half-life as compared with standard half-life sucrose-formulated rFVIII [9]. The efficacy and safety of BAY 94–9027 as prophylactic and on-demand treatment for patients with hemophilia A were demonstrated in the multinational phase 2/3 PROTECT VIII study and its long-term extension [10, 11].

BAY 94–9027 has been approved for use in previously treated adults and adolescents (aged ≥12 years) with hemophilia A at dosing intervals of up to every 5–7 days.

5.2.4 Turoctocog Alfa Pegol, N8GP

Turoctocog alfa pegol or N8-GP is a recombinant human factor VIII product, synthesized in CHO cells in a serum-free production environment, with a glycopegylation on the O-linked glycan in the truncated B-domain [12]. The turoctocog alfa pegol molecule is a polypeptide containing a heavy chain and a light chain held together by non-covalent interactions [12]. In native FVIII these chains are connected by a native B-domain, while turoctocog alfa pegol has a truncated rFVIII containing 21 amino acids of the native B-domain [12]. When turoctocog alfa pegol is activated by thrombin, the B-domain containing the 40-kDa PEG and the a3-region are cleaved off, thus generating activated FVIII which is similar in structure to native FVIIIa [13].

N8-GP is developed for prophylaxis and the treatment of bleeds in hemophilia. The first in-human clinical trial demonstrated that a single dose of up to 75 IU/kg N8-GP was well tolerated in patients with hemophilia A, with no safety concerns [14].

The phase III trial demonstrates that N8-GP has a good safety profile and is well tolerated in previously treated adults and adolescents with severe hemophilia A [15]. A prophylactic effect with 50 IU/kg body weight every fourth day dosing was demonstrated (40% of patients experienced zero bleeds) and a satisfactory hemostatic effect of N8-GP in the treatment of breakthrough bleeds was confirmed [15]. Additionally, previous findings of an extended half-life of N8-GP compared with standard rFVIII products (mean terminal half-life of N8-GP was 1.6-fold longer) were confirmed in this trial [15].

5.2.5 FVIII-VWF-XTEN, BIVV001

While the other extended half-life FVIII concentrates have been authorized in the last years, FVIII-VWF-XTEN is at stage of clinical development.

The majority of FVIII in the circulation is complexed with the glycoprotein von Willebrand factor (VWF) which stabilizes and protects FVIII from proteases and clearance receptors [16]. This complex makes it difficult to extend the half-life of infused FVIII beyond that of the half-life of VWF which results in a ceiling effect on the increase in FVIII half-life [17].

An alternative approach to prolonging the half-life of FVIII involves the addition of hydrophilic protein polymers to the molecule through XTEN technology [18]. A new, investigational product, rFVIIIFc-VWF-XTEN, created by the linkage of rFVIIIFc, XTEN polypeptides and the D'D3 domain of VWF, is designed to circulate in plasma independently of VWF, thereby breaking the VWF half-life ceiling [19].

Nonclinical studies have shown that the use of BIVV001 results in a half-life of FVIII that is three to four times as long as that of rFVIII. In a phase 1–2a open-label trial a single intravenous injection of BIVV001 resulted in high sustained factor VIII activity levels, with a half-life that was up to four times the half-life associated with rFVIII, an increase that could signal a new class of FVIII replacement therapy with a weekly treatment interval [19].

5.3 Non-replacement Therapy

Despite the progress made with the development of extended plasma half-life coagulation factors, unmet needs persist. In hemophilia A patients without inhibitors, the reduction in the frequency of intravenous injections was not considered satisfactory and therapy still based on the need for a venous access continued to be unattractive. Hemophilia A patients with FVIII inhibitors remained poor candidates for prophylaxis that could only be provided by bypassing products such as activated prothrombin complex concentrate (aPCC) and recombinant activated factor VII (rFVIIa) that are very expensive and difficult to administer on a regular preventive basis. With these drawbacks in mind, therapeutic approaches that were not based on the replacement of the deficient factor were developed. This took place in two main ways: for hemophilia A, by mimicking the coagulant activity of FVIII; and for both hemophilia A and hemophilia B, by increasing defective thrombin formation through the inhibition of the naturally occurring anticoagulants (antithrombin and tissue factor pathway inhibitor). For the moment, only the monoclonal antibody emicizumab that mimics FVIII activity has been approved.

5.3.1 Emicizumab

Emicizumab is a recombinant, monoclonal antibody that functions to bring activated factor IX (FIXa) and factor X (FX) into an appropriate steric conformation to medicate the activation of FX to FXa, thereby mimicking the cofactor function of FVIIIa.

The HAVEN program of clinical trials provided evidence of the efficacy of emicizumab in preventing bleeding in persons with hemophilia with and without inhibitors. Administered subcutaneously, this drug reaches a steady state with a long plasma half-life that allows well-spaced dosing intervals of at least every week or even every 2 or 4 weeks, at a dose of 1.5 mg/kg body weight (BW) once weekly, 3 mg/kg once every 2 weeks, or 6 mg/kg BW once every 4 weeks (with a loading dose of 3 mg/kg BW per week for 4 weeks in all cases). FVIII or bypass drug treatment is also required for hemorrhages that occur during this therapy.

Emicizumab has been initially approved for routine prophylaxis of bleeding episodes in patients with hemophilia A with FVIII inhibitors [20]. The approval of emicizumab in this indication was based on the results of the HAVEN 1 study in adolescents/adults and the ongoing HAVEN 2 study in pediatrics patients under 12 years of age [21]. Emicizumab prophylaxis, when administered subcutaneously once weekly, significantly reduced the number of bleeding episodes in patients with inhibitors. However, when emicizumab was coadministered with high doses of aPCC three patients in HAVEN 1 developed thrombotic microangiopathy (TMA) and two patients showed venous thromboembolism [20]. Subsequent to these events, risk mitigation has included recommendations to use rFVIIa instead of aPCC during emicizumab prophylaxis if possible; and, if this concentrate is still required for effective hemostasis, to reduce daily dosing to less than 100 IU/kg per day when repeated doses are needed.

Following the results obtained in patients with hemophilia A and inhibitors, emicizumab has also been evaluated in hemophilia A patients without inhibitors (HAVEN 3 study).

In the HAVEN trials overall, 63–87% of patients had no treated hemorrhages [1]. This figure rose to 82.4% with longer treatment periods (121 to 144 weeks) [22]. Emicizumab was well tolerated in the HAVEN trials, with a favorable overall safety profile. The most common related adverse events were injection site reactions (15–31%). The development of antidrug antibodies with neutralizing potential was rare (<1%) [22].

5.3.2 Concizumab

Concizumab is a humanized IgG4 antibody with high affinity for the K2 domain of tissue factor pathway inhibitor (TFPI), inhibits FXa binding and prevents TFPI inhibition of the TF-FVIIa complex [23]. Anti-TFPI monoclonal antibodies restore thrombin generation by abolishing the inhibitory effect of TFPI on the initiation of coagulation [23]. On the basis of this mechanism of action, concizumab is expected to be equally effective in hemophilia A and B, regardless of inhibitor status.

The ExplorerTM studies are a series of clinical trials evaluating concizumab. In ExplorerTM1, a phase 1 randomized study in 24 patients with severe hemophilia A or B and 28 healthy volunteers, increasing concentrations of concizumab (0.5–9000 μg/kg intravenously or 50–3000 μg/kg subcutaneously) produced detectable plasma levels of the monoclonal antibody for up to 43 days, with reductions in the plasma concentrations and functional activity of TFPI for 14 or more days after the dose of concizumab had been administered. Hemophilia patients showed similar D-dimer responses compared with healthy volunteers when they received an approximately 36-fold higher dose of concizumab. No serious adverse events occurred and no anti-concizumab antibodies developed [24]. In ExplorerTM2, a multicenter, open-label, multiple dosing phase 1 clinical trial, eight doses of concizumab were given to four healthy males at a dose of 250 μg/kg every other day. This regimen improved thrombin generation and it was documented that the plasma levels of the antibody correlated directly with thrombin generation and inversely with TFPI levels. In the same study, concizumab was added ex vivo to plasma samples from 18 individuals with severe hemophilia A or B (with or without inhibitors) and restored thrombin generation in these samples to near normal level. In the ExplorerTM3 trial, which was a placebo-controlled, multiple-dose, dose-escalation study where concizumab was administered subcutaneously, the authors observed a dose-dependent decrease in concizumab free total TFPI and procoagulant effect. An analysis of the data from this phase 1, multicenter, randomized, placebo-controlled, double-blind trial investigating the safety, pharmacokinetic (PK), and pharmacodynamics (PD) of multiple doses (0.25, 0.5, 0.8 mg/kg every 4 days) of concizumab administered subcutaneously to hemophilia A patients did not reveal serious adverse events or document the development of antidrug antibodies, while confirming PK and PD relationships between the concizumab dose and TFPI levels and thrombin generation. In addition, a post-hoc analysis indicated that exposure to concizumab concentrations of at least 100 ng/mL once daily was most effective in reducing the frequency of bleeding episodes and thus better indicated for prophylaxis [25, 26]. ExplorerTM4 and ExplorerTM5 are both phase 2 trials evaluating the safety and efficacy of prophylactic administration of concizumab in hemophilia A and B patients with and without inhibitors [27]. The trials aimed to evaluate the efficacy of daily subcutaneous concizumab prophylaxis (evaluated as annualized bleeding rate [ABR] at last dose level) with secondary objectives being safety and immunogenicity (assessed as number of adverse events). The starting dose in the trials is 0.15 mg/kg with potential dose escalation to 0.20 and 0.25 mg/kg (if ≥3 spontaneous bleeding episodes within 12 weeks of concizumab treatment). In the inhibitor trial, the median ABR was 4.5 and 19.7 for concizumab and rFVIIa, respectively. In the no inhibitors trials, when assessing each patient's last dose level, a total of 70 treated bleeding episodes in 23 patients (63.9%) were reported in the main part of the trial, with a median ABR of 4.5. Concizumab was safe and well tolerated. Three patients had very low to medium titer antibodies drugs tests in each trial, with no observed clinical effect.

The trials were paused in March 2020 due to the occurrence of non-fatal thrombotic events in three patients. In August 2020 clinical trials in the concizumab phase 3 were resumed. New safety measures and guidelines, based on analysis of all available data, have been agreed.

5.3.3 Fitusiran

Fitusiran is an RNA interference therapeutic that targets antithrombin (AT) in the liver and interferes with AT translation by binding and degrading messenger RNA-AT, thereby silencing AT gene expression and preventing AT synthesis. The rationale for this strategy is that reduced antithrombin levels improve thrombin generation and promote hemostasis in hemophilia patients with and without inhibitors. In both preclinical and clinical studies, AT knockdown results in dose-dependent AT lowering when fitusiran is given weekly or monthly subcutaneously [28].

Preclinical trials showed a dose-dependent lowering of antithrombin in different animal models; in murine hemophilia models, antithrombin reduction was associated with increased thrombin generation and enhanced hemostasis. Similar results were observed in the nonhuman primates model [29].

The first study was a multicenter, international, open-label, dose-escalation study involving healthy volunteers and participants with hemophilia A or B [30]. The trial was conducted in three subsequentially enrolled phases. In the first phase (Part A), healthy volunteers received a single dose of fitusiran or placebo in a randomized, single-blind study. In the next two open-label phases, participants with hemophilia A or B were assigned to receive one of several ascending doses of fitusiran on a once-weekly basis (in Part B) or once-monthly basis (Part C). In part A, healthy male volunteers between the ages of 18 and 40 years with no history of venous thromboembolism were randomly assigned in a 3:1 ratio to receive a single subcutaneous injection of fitusiran (at a dose of 0.03 mg per kilogram of body weight) or placebo. In Parts B and C, men between the ages of 18 and 65 years who had moderate or severe hemophilia A or B and who had received previous prophylaxis were eligible to participate in the study if the prophylactic factor had been discontinued at least 5 days before the initiation of the study drug. In part B, three cohorts of participants received three once-weekly subcutaneous injections of fitusiran at doses of 0.015, 0.045, or 0.075 mg per kilogram. In part C, four cohorts of participants received three once-monthly subcutaneous injections of fitusiran at doses of 0.225, 0.45, 0.9, or 1.8 mg per kilogram, and a fifth cohort received three once-monthly subcutaneous injections of a fixed dose of 80 mg. A total of four healthy volunteers were enrolled in the first part, 12 in the second phase, and 18 in the third group. The pharmacokinetic and pharmacodynamic show that the peak of fitusiran level was observed after 2 to 6 hours, the mean elimination half-life ranged from 2.6 to 5.3 hours. The plasma level increased in a dose-proportional manner. In a post-hoc analysis evaluating the effect of fitusiran in bleeding rates, the authors observed a reduction of bleeding episodes concerning the preview period. All the bleeding episodes were managed with factor VIII or IX replacement. No thrombotic, severe adverse events and antidrug antibodies were registered. Nine of 25 enrolled patients in parts B or C had adverse events that were considered to be related to fitusiran. Monthly administration produces a lowering of the level of antithrombin level by 70–90%.

Based on these results a phase 2 study was conducted using subcutaneous administration of fitusiran at a 50 and 80 mg once monthly in 14 inhibitor patients and 19 non-inhibitors patients [28]. The overall median ABR in fitusiran treated patients without inhibitor was 1 compared with 12 and 2 in on-demand and prophylaxis, respectively. In the inhibitors patients, the median ABR was 0 compared with 38 before the trials. All breakthrough bleedings were successfully controlled with replacement therapy or bypassing agents without thromboembolic episodes but a sinus vein thrombosis in a non-inhibitor hemophilia A patient with concomitant administration of fitusiran and clotting factor VIII was observed. Following this SAE the fitusiran trial was suspended and reopened after the introduction of educational strategies for participants and protocol-specific guidelines to treat breakthrough bleeding.

Later the company paused dosing in all ongoing fitusiran clinical studies on October 30 2020, to assess reports of non-fatal thrombotic events in patients participating in the phase 3 program.

5.4 Conclusions

The new drugs for the treatment of hemophilia A include extended half-life (EHL) products and non-factor products. Among the EHL products, the following stand out: Efmoroctocog alfa, rFVIIIFc; Rurioctocog alfa pegol, BAX 855; Damoctocog alfa pegol, BAY94–9027; Turoctocog alfa pegol, N8GP; and FVIII-VWF-XTEN, BIVV001. Among the non-factor products, the following stand out: emicizumab, concizumab, and fitusiran. These new drugs have the potential to improve the level of care by decreasing the frequency of infusion, increasing adherence, promoting prophylaxis, offering alternatives to patients with inhibitors and an easy route of administration.

References

1. Morfini M, Marchesini E. The availability of new drugs for hemophilia treatment. Expert Rev Clin Pharmacol. 2020;13:721–38.
2. Peters RT, Toby G, Lu Q, Liu T, Kulman JD, Low SC, et al. Biochemical and functional characterization of a recombinant monomeric factor VIII-Fc fusion protein. J Thromb Haemost. 2013;11:132–41.
3. van der Flier A, Liu Z, Tan S, Chen K, Drager D, Liu T, et al. FcRn rescues recombinant factor VIII Fc fusion protein from a VWF independent FVIII clearance pathway in mouse hepatocytes. PLoS One. 2015;10(4):e0124930.
4. Powell JS, Josephson NC, Quon D, Ragni MV, Cheng G, Li E, et al. Safety and prolonged activity of recombinant factor VIII Fc fusion protein in hemophilia A patients. Blood. 2012;119:3031–7.
5. Hermans C, Mancuso ME, Nolan B, Pasi KJ. Recombinant factor viii fc for the treatment of haemophilia A. Eur J Haematol. 2021; https://doi.org/10.1111/ejh.13610. Online ahead of print
6. Turecek PL, Bossard MJ, Graninger M, Gritsch H, Höllriegl W, Kaliwoda M, et al. BAX 855, a PEGylated rFVIII product with prolonged half-life. Development, functional and structural characterisation. Hamostaseologie. 2012;32(Suppl 1):S29–38.
7. Konkle BA, Stasyshyn O, Chowdary P, Bevan DH, Mant T, Shima, et al. Pegylated, full-length, recombinant factor VIII for prophylactic and on-demand treatment of severe hemophilia A. Blood. 2015;126:1078–85.
8. Mei B, Pan C, Jiang H, Tjandra H, Strauss J, Chen Y, Liu T, et al. Rational design of a fully active, long-acting PEGylated factor VIII for hemophilia A treatment. Blood. 2010;116:270–9.
9. Coyle TE, Reding MT, Lin JC, Michaels LA, Shah A, Powell J. Phase I study of BAY 94-9027, a PEGylated B-domain-deleted recombinant factor VIII with an extended half-life, in subjects with hemophilia A. J Thromb Haemost. 2014;12:488–96.
10. Reding MT, Ng HJ, Poulsen LH, Eyster ME, Pabinger J, Shin H-J, et al. Safety and efficacy of BAY 94-9027, a prolonged-half-life factor VIII. J Thromb Haemost. 2017;15:411–9.
11. Mancuso ME, Reding MT, Negrier C, Kerlin BA, Rangarajan S, Simpson ML. Decreased bleeding rates in patients with hemophilia A switching from standard-half-life FVIII to BAY 94–9027 prophylaxis. Thromb Haemost. 2020; https://doi.org/10.1055/a--1333-5536. Online ahead of print
12. Thim L, Vandahl B, Karlsson J, Klausen NK, Pedersen J, Krogh TN, et al. Purification and characterization of a new recombinant factor VIII (N8). Haemophilia. 2010;16:349–59.
13. Agerso H, Stennicke HR, Pelzer H, Olsen EN, Merricks EP, Defriess NA, et al. Pharmacokinetics and pharmacodynamics of turoctocog alfa and N8-GP in haemophilia A dogs. Haemophilia. 2012;18:941–7.
14. Tiede A, Brand B, Fischer R, Kavakli K, Lentz SR, Matsushita T, et al. Enhancing the pharmacokinetic properties of recombinant factor VIII: first-in-human trial of glycoPEGylated recombinant factor VIII in patients with hemophilia a. J Thromb Haemost. 2013;11:670–8.
15. Giangrande P, Andreeva T, Chowdary P, Ehrenforth S, Hanabusa H, Leebeek FWG, et al. Clinical evaluation of glycoPEGylated recombinant FVIII: efficacy and safety in severe haemophilia A. Thromb Haemost. 2017;117:252–61.
16. Pipe SW, Montgomery RR, Pratt KP, Lenting PJ, Lillicrap D. Life in the shadow of a dominant partner: the FVIII-VWF association and its clinical implications for hemophilia A. Blood. 2016;128:2007–16.
17. Terraube V, O'Donnell JS, Jenkins PV. Factor VIII and von Willebrand factor interaction: biological, clinical and therapeutic importance. Haemophilia. 2010;16:3–13.
18. Podust VN, Balan S, Sim B-C, Coyle MP, Ernst U, Peters RT, et al. Extension of in vivo half-life of bio-

logically active molecules by XTEN protein polymers. J Control Release. 2016;240:52–66.
19. Konkle BA, Shapiro AD, Quon DV, Staber JM, Kulkarni R, Ragnie MV, et al. BIVV001 fusion protein as factor VIII replacement therapy for hemophilia A. N Engl J Med. 2020;383:1018–27.
20. Oldenburg J, Mahlangu JN, Kim B, Schmitt C, Callaghan MU, Young G, et al. Emicizumab prophylaxis in hemophilia A with inhibitors. N Engl J Med. 2017;377:809–18.
21. Le Quellec S. Clinical evidence and safety profile of emicizumab for the management of children with hemophilia a. Drug Des Devel Ther. 2020;14:469–81.
22. Callaghan MU, Negrier C, Paz-Priel I, Chang T, Chebon S, Lehle M, et al. Long-term outcomes with emicizumab prophylaxis for hemophilia a with/without FVIII inhibitors from the HAVEN 1-4 studies. Blood. 2021;137:2231–42.
23. Lauritzen B, Hilden I. Concizumab promotes haemostasis via a tissue factor-factor VIIa-dependent mechanism supporting prophylactic treatment of haemophilia: results from a rabbit haemophilia bleeding model. Haemophilia. 2019;25:e379–82.
24. Chowdary P, Lethagen S, Friedrich U, Brand B, Hay C, Karim F, et al. Safety and pharmacokinetics of anti-TFPI antibody (concizumab) in healthy volunteers and patients with hemophilia: a randomized first human dose trial. J Thromb Haemost. 2015;13:743–54.
25. Eichler H, Angchaisuksiri P, Kavakli K, Knoebl P, Windyga J, Jiménez-Yuste V, et al. A randomized trial of safety, pharmacokinetics and pharmacodynamics of concizumab in people with hemophilia a. J Thromb Haemost. 2018;16:2184–95.
26. Eichler H, Angchaisuksiri P, Kavakli K, Knoebl P, Windyga J, Jiménez-Yuste V, et al. Concizumab restores thrombin generation potential in patients with haemophilia: pharmacokinetic/pharmacodynamic modelling results of concizumab phase 1/1b data. Haemophilia. 2019;25:60–6.
27. Shapiro AD, Angchaisuksiri P, Astermark J, Benson G, Castaman G, Chowdary P, et al. Subcutaneous concizumab prophylaxis in hemophilia A and hemophilia A/B with inhibitors: phase 2 trial results. Blood. 2019;134:1973–82.
28. Machin N, Ragni MV. An investigational RNAi therapeutic targeting antithrombin for the treatment of hemophilia A and B. J Blood Med. 2018;9:135–40.
29. Sehgal A, Barros S, Ivanciu L, Cooley B, Qin J, Racie T, et al. An RNAi therapeutic targeting antithrombin to rebalance the coagulation system and promote hemostasis in hemophilia. Nat Med. 2015;21:492–7.
30. Pasi KJ, Rangarajan S, Georgiev P, Mant T, Creagh MD, Lissitchkov T, et al. Targeting of antithrombin in hemophilia A or B with RNAi therapy. N Engl J Med. 2017;377:819–28.

6 Inhibitors in Hemophilia B

Víctor Jiménez-Yuste

6.1 Introduction

Hemophilia B (HB), like hemophilia A is an X-linked recessive genetic coagulation disorder characterized by a deficit or absence of clotting factor IX (FIX) [1]. The pathophysiology of this disease is based on the insufficient generation of thrombin by the IXa/VIIIa complex in the intrinsic coagulation pathway, thus preventing proper hemostasis.

HB is much less common than hemophilia A, estimated at 15–20% of all hemophilia patients with a prevalence of 5 cases per 100,000 males [1, 2].

The two forms of hemophilia have historically been indistinguishable as the same disease, and it was not until 1952 that hemophilia B was recognized as a separate entity [3]. HB is treated using replacement intravenous FIX concentrates to elevate plasma FIX levels. Exogenous FIX replacement therapy, including recombinant FIX and plasma-derived (pd)FIX, can be administered as prophylaxis or on-demand, in addition to perioperative settings.

As in hemophilia A, the development of antibodies to FIX is the most significant complication of treatment in patients diagnosed with HB [4]. The development of this antibody results in the lack of efficacy of conventional FIX replacement therapy, precludes access to safe and effective standard treatment, especially prophylaxis in children, and leads to more uncontrolled bleeds, which has a decisive influence on increased morbidity and mortality and causes an increase in the cost of treatment [5]. In addition to these general considerations, patients with HB and inhibitor present special conditions due to the characteristics of the antibody, such as the occurrence of allergic reactions, leading to anaphylactic shock and the development of the nephrotic syndrome [6].

6.2 Epidemiology

Inhibitor rates in patients with HB differ significantly, with classic studies showing an incidence of 1–5% in HB [7] than the much higher rates occurring in hemophilia A [8].

In one review about inhibitors in hemophilia B, a set of published series is analyzed in which mostly retrospective data is referred [4]. Most inhibitors develop in severe HB, which is another difference compared to hemophilia A, where they occur in all forms from mild to severe. Most studies reflect prevalence data ranging from 1% to 5% of patients with HB, which increases to over 10% in patients with severe HB [5].

A recently published prospective study analyzed 154 patients with previously untreated patients (PUPs) with HB [9]. Fourteen patients

V. Jiménez-Yuste (✉)
Department of Hematology, La Paz University Hospital, Madrid, Spain
e-mail: vjimenezy@salud.madrid.org

E. C. Rodríguez-Merchán (ed.), *Advances in Hemophilia Treatment*,
https://doi.org/10.1007/978-3-030-93990-8_6

were diagnosed with inhibitor; seven were classified as high titer and seven as low titers. The median number of exposure days (ED) at the time of inhibitor onset was 11 (IQR 6.5–36.5), with a median age of 23.2 months (IQR 12.1–37.1). The cumulative inhibitor incidence at 75 ED was 9.3% (95% CI 4.4–14.1) for all inhibitors and 5% for high-titer inhibitors. Importantly, in which there is no selection in the inclusion of patients, this cohort were all treated with primary prophylaxis, which allowed follow-up beyond 500 ED. Between 76 and 500 EDs, only one low-titer inhibitor was diagnosed in 121 EDs. The cumulative incidence of inhibitors in the 500 EDs was 10.2% (95% CI 5.1–15.3) [9].

6.3 Pathophysiology

The development of inhibitors with hemophilia patients is a complex and multifactorial process in which there is an interplay between genetics, exogenous treatment-related factors, and the immune system's role. While these factors are not yet fully understood, they have been extensively analyzed in hemophilia A. However, in patients with HB, given the infrequency of the pathology and the lower rate of inhibitors, they have been much less extensively analyzed [7].

There have been some speculations as to why the frequency is much lower than patients with hemophilia A. On the one hand, it was speculated that the homology of the FIX protein with other vitamin K-dependent clotting factors might confer some degree of immune tolerance following administration of exogenous FIX [4]. Another essential factor influencing inhibitor development and its pharmacokinetics and clinical efficacy is the presence or absence of Cross Reacting Material (CRM) [10]. In the case of hemophilia B, it has been observed that concerning the genetic mutation, the proportion of patients with non-functioning protein but able to create tolerance (CRM+) is higher than in hemophilia A. It is estimated that 60% of patients with severe HB and 75% of all patients with HB are CRM+ [11].

Genetic alterations are another essential factor in inhibitor development and could explain this difference with hemophilia A. HB causing mutations are low-risk mutations for inhibitor development, and most inhibitors have null mutations that produce a CRM—phenotype [4]. Thus, in the Pednet series, among patients with inhibitor, the most frequent mutations were nonsense mutations in 7/14 (50.0%), four patients with low-titer inhibitors and 3 with high-titer inhibitors, and deletions with large structural changes in 5/14 (35.7%), 3 with low-risk inhibitors and 2 with high-risk inhibitors [9]. The inhibitor risk for deletions with large structural changes was 33.3% (11.8–61.6) and for nonsense mutations 26.9% (95% CI 11.6–47.8). For all other mutations, the risk of inhibition was zero [9].

Despite improvements in inhibitor development, immune responses to deficient factor and the inhibitor risk associated with replacement therapy in individual patients with hemophilia cannot be fully predicted [12]. In addition, due to the low incidence of FIX inhibitors versus FVIII inhibitors, little comparative data is available on the risk factors and immunological processes underlying their development [7]. A predictive score has been developed to estimate the risk of inhibitors in previously untreated patients with PUPs [13] to meet the need for an accurate clinical prediction tool. However, the data supporting the contribution of each risk factor is still inconclusive, and the generalized utility of the score has not been validated. Efforts are underway to develop more accurate inhibitor prediction methods [14].

6.4 Allergic and Anaphylactic Reactions

The occurrence of allergic and anaphylactic reactions after FIX infusion, which appear before or concomitant with inhibitor development, is a known phenomenon and appears exclusively in patients with HB appearing in up to 60% of the cases [7]. The exact mechanism by which these allergic reactions occur is not clearly elucidated, although several possible explanations have been described [4, 7, 15]. The immune response to FIX can be both immune globulin E (IgE)-mediated and non-IgE-mediated. Immune globulin G (IgG) pre-existence in patients with HB and previous anaphylaxis reactions results after FIX infusion in the appearance of specific IgG inhibitors, leading to complete activation of anaphylatoxins with mast cell mediators and complement activation of the formation of transient IgG1 antibodies.

Another explanation for this potential mast cell activation and IgE-mediated hypersensitivity response is due to the intravascular and extravascular localization of FIX, as most FIX resides extravascular, in the subendothelial basement membrane, it exerts vital functions for hemostasis [16]. Another possible reason is that the plasma concentration of FIX is much higher than that of FVIII, and the dose required to achieve effective plasma concentrations is much higher, with this massive dose of FIX being sufficient to trigger this allergic reaction. Although a higher dose of FIX may be associated with the development of inhibitors and an increased risk of adverse events [17], this has also been observed in some HB patients receiving low doses of FIX. In addition, the high concentration of exogenous FIX infused with treatment is probably involved in another immunological mechanism of FIX inhibitors, which is the excessive formation of circulating immune complexes [4]. The type of FIX product does not seem to play a role in the induction of allergic reactions [18]. Data from the International Society of Thrombosis and Hemostasis Scientific and Standardization Committee (ISTH-SSC) registry did not detect any difference in anaphylactic and severe allergic events after exposure to intermediate-purity or high-purity FIX products (either recombinant or plasma-derived) [4, 19].

Concerning renal involvement, nephrotic syndrome typically occurs during immunotolerance therapy and can be a severe complication. It is more frequent in patients with previous reactions to FIX infusion (allergic phenotype) [20]. Nephrotic syndrome is often unresponsive to steroids and requires discontinuation of immune tolerance induction (ITI). Renal biopsies demonstrated membranous glomerulonephritis in two patients, but immunohistochemical staining of tissue obtained from a single renal biopsy showed no association with FIX immune complexes [21].

6.5 Clinical and Laboratory Follow-Up

Detection of the development of inhibitors requires validated laboratory tests, such as the Nijmegen-Bethesda tests. Any comprehensive therapeutic management program needs to detect emerging inhibitor activity early as possible to direct appropriate medical treatment and consider inhibitor eradication [22]. Screening should be performed at least every three exposure days (EDs) during the first 20 EDs, and more frequently if there is any uncertainty due to allergic reaction or poor response. After this initial period of exposure to treatment, screening should be performed every 3–6 months up to 150 EDs and annually after that [2, 23]. Since the risk of inhibitor development is thought to be highest during the first 50–75 EDs, the number of inhibitors should be monitored [9]. EDs of patients starting treatment who have not been treated previously should be followed up to ensure that inhibitor screening is properly performed. Logistically, this may be more difficult to monitor in those receiving on-demand treatment versus patients on prophylaxis and in the case of exposures administered in care settings far from the comprehensive hemophilia treatment center. In summary, proactive monitoring of all early treatment exposures in a patient with previously untreated HB should be prioritized to detect and appropriately manage emerging inhibitors and their complications.

6.6 Treatment

The primary goal in managing hemophilia B patients with inhibitors is to treat or prevent bleeding episodes and eradicate the inhibitor. Most therapeutic recommendations are derived from studies of patients with hemophilia A and inhibitor.

The therapeutic approach to treat and/or prevent bleeding in patients with FIX inhibitor should be based on the severity of bleeding, inhibitor titer, anamnestic response, and history of allergic reactions.

There are two therapeutic options for people with inhibitors who experience spontaneous bleeding, trauma or require surgery: activated prothrombin complex concentrate (aPCC) or recombinant factor VII activated (rFVIIa). aPCC and rFVIIa [24, 25] both bypass the functional activity of FIX and have significantly improved the management of acute bleeding and quality of life in patients with chronic inhibitors, and have demonstrated acceptable efficacy and safety in those undergoing surgery and in the management of severe bleeding episodes [4, 7, 26]. Note that the most recent World Federation of Hemophilia (WFH) guideline recommends that in patients with high-responder inhibitors or those with low-responder inhibitors who develop allergic reactions or anaphylaxis, rFVIIa should be the first choice to control bleeding, as aPCC contains FIX and may stimulate an anamnestic response including further anaphylaxis [2]. As with inhibitor therapy in people with hemophilia A (PwHA), ITI is used in people with hemophilia B (PwHB) who develop high-titer FIX inhibitors, although there are some differences focused on reducing the risks of adverse reactions, which are more common in PwHB than in PwHA and are associated with its low success rate [27].

International prospective studies compiling data on the management of patients with hemophilia B and inhibitor are needed; however, different recommendations have been published on the management of bleeding in patients with HB [4, 7, 23, 26, 28].

For patients without allergic reactions, low inhibitor titer and good clinical response to FIX, it is recommended to continue FIX at higher than standard doses. For patients with high inhibitor titer and no allergic reactions or who show inadequate response to FIX concentrates, initiation of ITI is suggested. If there is a failure of ITI, initiation of treatment with rFVIIa is recommended. In those patients with allergic reactions and reasonable response to bypassing agents, the use of bypassing agents is recommended. However, if there is a severe haemorrhagic profile or failure to bypass agents, ITI is recommended after desensitisation with or without immunosuppressive agents. Since the response to ITI is highly variable in hemophilia B and is not without risk, adequate monitoring is essential (Figs. 6.1 and 6.2) [28].

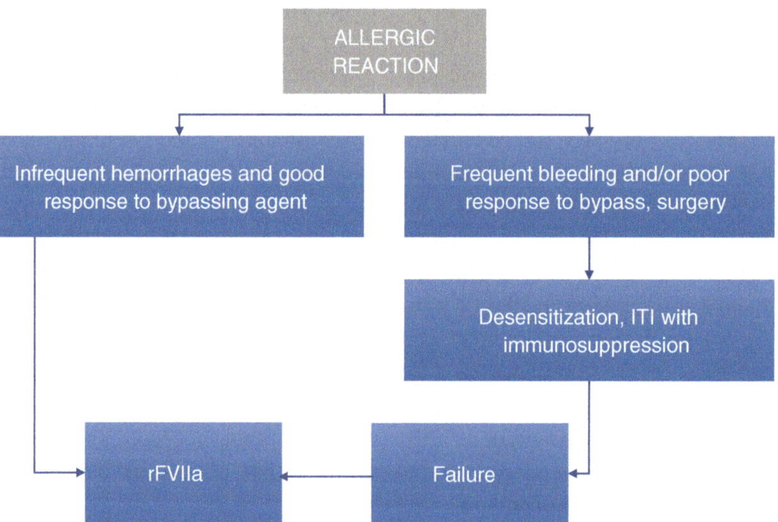

Fig. 6.1 For hemophilia B patients without allergic reactions, low inhibitor titer and good clinical response to factor IX (FIX), it is recommended to continue FIX at higher than standard doses. For patients with high inhibitor titer and no allergic reactions or who show inadequate response to FIX concentrates, initiation of immune tolerance induction (ITI) is suggested. If there is a failure of ITI, initiation of treatment with recombinant factor VII activated (rFVIIa) is recommended [28]

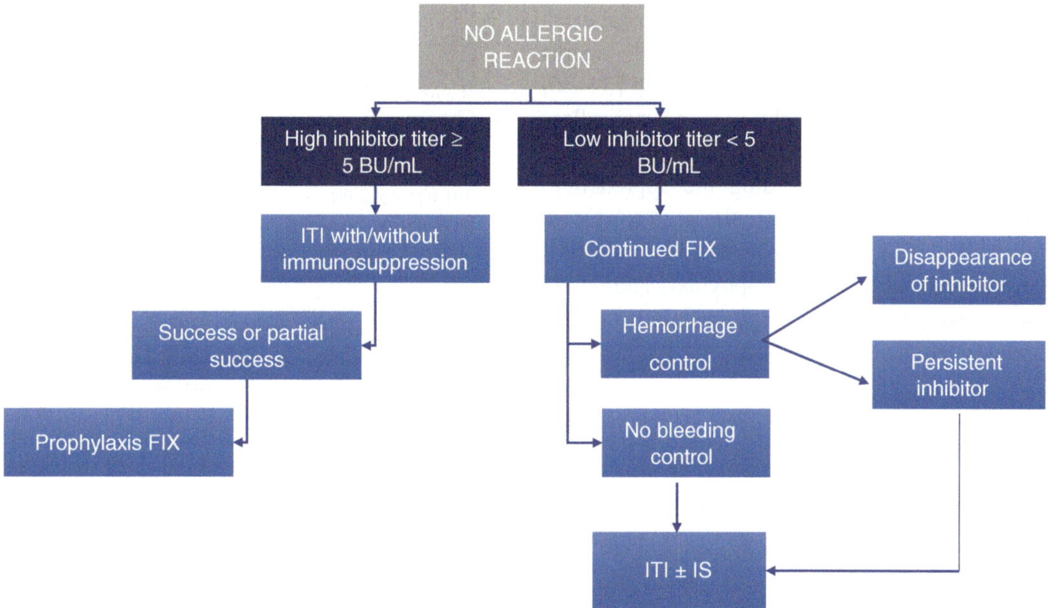

Fig. 6.2 In those hemophilia B patients with allergic reactions and reasonable response to bypassing agents, the use of bypassing agents is recommended. However, if there is a severe hemorrhagic profile or failure to bypass agents, immune tolerance induction (ITI) after desensitization or using immunosuppressive agents is recommended. Since the response to ITI is highly variable in hemophilia B and is not without risk, adequate monitoring is essential [28]. *BU* Bethesda units, IS immunosuppression

6.7 New Therapeutic Approaches

6.7.1 Gene Therapy (GT)

By reducing or eradicating the need for exogenous FIX for prolonged periods, TG by gene addition offers the potential to reduce disease burden for HB patients on single-dose GT [29]. Research efforts to date have focused on using a recombinant adeno-associated virus (AAV) vector with a functional *F9* gene cassette targeted to the liver to allow endogenous expression of FIX, replacing the otherwise missing or mutated FIX [29].

Data from mouse models for genetic or acquired diseases indicate that liver gene therapy using AAV vectors for hepatocyte-restricted transgene expression could prevent the formation of pathological antibodies against the transgene and eradicate pre-existing antibodies [30]. This apparent induction of immune tolerance was specific to the transgene without causing a systemic decrease in host immune competence. The underlying mechanisms of immune tolerance in this model involve complex and diverse pathways, and some of these strategies could be "mimicked" by pharmacological or molecular modifications [30, 31]. Although many questions remain to be answered before gene therapy can be said to be an effective treatment for patients with an inhibitor in the future, several studies point to the theoretical possibility of GT as a treatment for ITI [30].

6.7.2 Other Molecules

Since prophylaxis in patients with HB and inhibitor has been little explored and the efficacy has not been very satisfactory, other molecules are being investigated. Recently there has been increasing interest in non-factor treatments that enhance coagulation irrespective of inhibitor development, such as the FVIII-mimetic treatment emicizumab, approved for the treatment of

PwHA [32, 33]. New agents that "rebalance" hemostasis, such as investigational agents fitusiran, marstacimab, and concizumab [34–36] may be utilized in hemophilia A or B regardless of inhibitor status, and consequently may change treatment decisions regarding the approach to inhibitor management and/or the need to restore tolerance to FIX in these patients, particularly if complicated with severe anaphylaxis and/or ITI failure. However, these agents remain investigational in late-stage clinical trials.

6.8 Conclusions

Inhibitors in HB are the most critical complication of HB treatment, as in hemophilia A. Their incidence may be higher than classically estimated in the light of data from prospective studies estimating a cumulative incidence of around 10%. FIX inhibitors have two distinguishing features: anaphylactic reactions and renal damage. Current treatment is based on the use of aPCC and rFVIIa for hemorrhagic episodes and surgical prophylaxis. However, patients with HB and inhibitor are undoubtedly the group of patients with the greatest unmet need at present and who require adequate prophylactic treatment. The data emerging from the results of the clinical trials of the new molecules are exciting, opening the door to a promising future in the prevention of bleeding in patients with HB and inhibitor, improving their quality of life and morbidity.

References

1. Mannucci PM, Tuddenham EGD. The hemophilias - from royal genes to gene therapy. New Engl J Med. 2001;344:1773–9.
2. Srivastava A, Santagostino E, Dougall A, Kitchen S, Sutherland M, Pipe SW, et al. WFH guidelines for the management of haemophilia, 3rd edition. Haemophilia. 2020;26:1–158.
3. Biggs R, Douglas AS, Macfarlane RG, Dacie JV, Pitney WR, Merskey C, et al. Christmas disease: a condition previously mistaken for haemophilia. Br Med J. 1952;2:1378–82.
4. Santoro C, Quintavalle G, Castaman G, Baldacci E, Ferretti A, Riccardi F, et al. Inhibitors in hemophilia B. Semin Thromb Hemost. 2018;44:578–89.
5. Franchini M, Santoro C, Coppola A. Inhibitor incidence in previously untreated patients with severe haemophilia B: a systematic literature review. Thromb Haemost. 2016;116:201–3.
6. Castaman G, Bonetti E, Messina M, Morfini M, Rocino A, Scaraggi FA, et al. Inhibitors in haemophilia B: the Italian experience. Haemophilia. 2013;19:686–90.
7. DiMichele D. Inhibitor development in haemophilia B: an orphan disease in need of attention. Br J Haematol. 2007;138:305–15.
8. Santagostino E, Young G, Carcao M, Mannucci PM, Halimeh S, Austin S. A contemporary look at FVIII inhibitor development: still a great influence on the evolution of haemophilia therapies. Expert Rev Hematol. 2018;11:87–97.
9. Male C, Andersson NG, Rafowicz A, Liesner R, Kurnik K, Fischer K, et al. Inhibitor incidence in an unselected cohort of previously untreated patients with severe haemophilia B: a PedNet study. Haematologica. 2021;106:123–9.
10. Lollar P. Pathogenic antibodies to coagulation factors. Part one: factor VIII and factor IX. J Thromb Haemost. 2004;2:1082–95.
11. Rallapalli PM, Kemball-Cook G, Tuddenham EG, Gomez K, Perkins SJ. An interactive mutation database for human coagulation factor IX provides novel insights into the phenotypes and genetics of haemophilia B. J Thromb Haemost. 2013;11:1329–40.
12. Astermark J. FVIII inhibitors: pathogenesis and avoidance. Blood. 2015;125:2045–51.
13. ter Avest PC, Fischer F, Mancuso ME, Santagostino E, Yuste VJ, van den Berg HM, et al. Risk stratification for inhibitor development at first treatment for severe haemophilia a: a tool for clinical practice. J Thromb Haemost. 2008;6:2048–54.
14. Dolan G, Benson G, Duffy A, Hermans C, Yuste VJ, Lambert T, et al. Haemophilia B: where are we now and what does the future hold? Blood Rev. 2018;32:52–60.
15. Dioun AF, Ewenstein BM, Geha RS, Schneider LC. IgE-mediated allergy and desensitization to factor IX in haemophilia B. J Allergy Clin Immun. 1998;102:113–7.
16. Mann DM, Stafford KA, Poon M, Matino D, Stafford DW. The function of extravascular coagulation factor IX in haemostasis. Haemophilia. 2021;27:332–9.
17. Ragni MV, Ojeifo O, Feng J, Yan J, Hill KA, Sommer SS, et al. Risk factors for inhibitor formation in haemophilia: a prevalent case-control study. Haemophilia. 2009;15:1074–82.
18. Fischer K, Lassila R, Peyvandi F, Calizzani G, Gatt A, Lambert T, et al. Inhibitor development in haemophilia according to concentrate. Four-year results from the European Haemophilia safety surveillance (EUHASS) project. Thromb Haemost. 2015;113:968–75.
19. Chitlur M, Warrier I, Rajpurkar M, Lusher JM. Inhibitors in factor IX deficiency. A report of the

ISTH-SSC international FIX inhibitor registry (1997-2006). Haemophilia. 2009;15:1027–31.
20. Ewenstein BM, Takemoto C, Warrier I, Lusher J, Saidi P, Eisele J, et al. Nephrotic syndrome as a complication of immune tolerance in haemophilia B. Blood. 1997;89:1115–6.
21. Dharnidharka VR, Takemoto C, Ewenstein BM, Rosen S, Harris HW. Membranous glomerulonephritis and nephrosis post factor IX infusions in haemophilia B. Pediatr Nephrol. 1998;12:654–7.
22. Verbruggen B, Novakova I, Wessels H, Boezeman J, van den Berg M , Mauser-Bunschoten E. The Nijmegen modification of the Bethesda assay for factor VIII:C inhibitors: improved specificity and reliability. Thromb Haemost 1995;73:247–251.
23. Collins P, Chalmers E, Hart DP, Liesner R, Rangarajan S, Talks K, et al. Diagnosis and treatment of factor VIII and IX inhibitors in congenital haemophilia: (4th edition). UK Haemophilia Centre Doctors Organisation. Br J Haematol. 2013;160:153–70.
24. Negrier C, Voisin S, Baghaei F, Numerof R, Novack A, Doralt JE, et al. Global post-authorization safety surveillance study. Blood Coagul Fibrinolysis. 2016;27:551–6.
25. Batorova A, Morongova A, Tagariello G, Jankovicova D, Prigancova T, Horakova J. Challenges in the management of haemophilia B with inhibitor. Semin Thromb Hemost. 2013;39:767–71.
26. Meeks SL, Batsuli G. Hemophilia and inhibitors: current treatment options and potential new therapeutic approaches. Hematology Am Soc Hematol Educ Program. 2016;2016:657–62.
27. Di Michele DM, Kroner BL, Group NAITS. The north American immune tolerance registry: practices, outcomes, outcome predictors. Thromb Haemost. 2002;87:52–7.
28. Kempton CL, Meeks SL. Toward optimal therapy for inhibitors in hemophilia. Blood. 2014;124:3365–72.
29. Batty P, Lillicrap D. Advances and challenges for haemophilia gene therapy. Hum Mol Genet. 2019;28:R95–R101.
30. Pratt KP, Arruda VR, Lacroix-Desmazes S. Inhibitors - recent insights. Haemophilia. 2021;27:28–36.
31. Arruda VR, Samelson-Jones BJ. Gene therapy for immune tolerance induction in haemophilia with inhibitors. J Thromb Haemost. 2016;14:1121–34.
32. Oldenburg J, Mahlangu JN, Kim B, Schmitt C, Callaghan MU, Young G, et al. Emicizumab prophylaxis in hemophilia a with inhibitors. New Engl J Med. 2017;377:809–18.
33. Young G, Liesner R, Chang T, Sidonio R, Oldenburg J, Jimenez-Yuste V, et al. A multicenter, open-label phase 3 study of emicizumab prophylaxis in children with hemophilia a with inhibitors. Blood. 2019;134:2127–38.
34. Pasi KJ, Lissitchkov T, Mamonov V, Mant T, Timofeeva M, Bagot C, et al. Targeting of antithrombin in hemophilia a or B with investigational siRNA therapeutic fitusiran-results of the phase 1 inhibitor cohort. J Thromb Haemost. 2021;19:1436–46.
35. Shapiro AD, Castaman G, Cepo K, Tønder SM, Matsushita T, Poulsen LH, et al. Safety and longer-term efficacy of concizumab prophylaxis in patients with haemophilia a or B with inhibitors: results from the extension part of the phase 2 explorer4 trial. Blood. 2020;136:40–1.
36. Patel-Hett S, Martin EJ, Mohammed BM, Rahke S, Sun P, Barrett JC, et al. Marstacimab, a tissue factor pathway inhibitor neutralizing antibody, improves coagulation parameters of ex vivo dosed haemophilic blood and plasmas. Haemophilia. 2019;25:797–806.

7 Immune Tolerance Induction in Hemophilia B

María-Isabel Rivas-Pollmar, Ana Mendoza-Martínez, and M. Teresa Álvarez-Román

7.1 Introduction

Hemophilia B is a rare congenital disease defined by a deficiency of coagulation factor IX (FIX), which is much less common than hemophilia A [1]. In relation with its low incidence, there has been a lack of research in terms of diagnosis and treatment, and few evidence-based data exist.

The inhibitor frequency in hemophilia B is also uncommon and involves significant enhancement in both morbidity and mortality, with an increased risk of major bleeding and frequent development of anaphylactic reactions and nephrotic syndrome [2, 3]. The previous are unique complications of hemophilia B with inhibitors, which can occur in up to 50% of cases [4, 5], and further complicates the efforts to eradicate FIX inhibitors. These complications are often temporally related: while severe allergies against FIX concentrates are frequently found before or after inhibitor development, those patients with an allergic phenotype may also develop a nephrotic syndrome with immune tolerance induction (ITI) [6].

As a result of poor outcome and high incidence of adverse events with the treatment of hemophilia B with inhibitor [7], the primary aim should be to prevent severe hemorrhage and the development of inhibitors [2] instead of eradicating it once it is already established. ITI is still the preferred strategy for antibody eradication, but some patients do not tolerate it or are unresponsive to ITI [8]. There is limited experience with ITI in hemophilia B and the few published data has registered poor successful rate [4, 5]. Indeed, most recommendations derive from hemophilia A evidence. The currently available guidelines [6, 7, 9] suggest that initiating ITI may be justified in selected patients (high-titer inhibitors, frequent bleeding, or poor response to bypass agents), always with careful monitoring and evaluation.

7.2 Epidemiology

The published rate of inhibitors against FIX is between 1.5–3% of all patients with hemophilia B and between 9–23% of severe cases, compared with approximately 30–50% of patients in hemophilia A [2, 6]. Around 80% of the inhibitors are of the high responding type, defined as a high-titer antibody (≥5 Bethesda Units (BU)) and a strong response to antigen exposure [2].

Risk factors for inhibitor development are multifactorial, including both genetic and non-genetic influences. In contrast with hemophilia A, few comparable data exist on host, treatment and immunological variables related to FIX inhibitors [2]. Hemophilia B genotype is the

M.-I. Rivas-Pollmar (✉) · A. Mendoza-Martínez
M. T. Álvarez-Román
Department of Hematology, La Paz University Hospital, Madrid, Spain

E. C. Rodríguez-Merchán (ed.), *Advances in Hemophilia Treatment*,
https://doi.org/10.1007/978-3-030-93990-8_7

main recognized factor, wherein the highest risk of inhibitor development is the presence of null mutations, which are more prevalent in hemophilia A [1]. Most genetic disorders in hemophilia B are missense mutations, associated with a less severe phenotype and a lower incidence of inhibitors [6, 10, 11]. As a result, severe disease is less common in hemophilia B (35%), in contrast to hemophilia A (45%) [6, 12]. The available evidence for non-genetic risk factors is inconclusive for hemophilia B and should be the object of further investigation.

Overall, ITI in hemophilia B is less effective, within a success rate of 31% according to The North American Immune Tolerance Registry (NAITR) [4]. This registry was initiated to study ITI in Canada and the United States including patients with hemophilia A and B. In addition, adverse reactions to therapy had been approximately 10 times higher than in hemophilia A, including allergic reactions in 30–60% and nephrotic syndrome in 20–30% [5, 7, 8, 13].

7.3 Immunology of FIX Inhibitors

FIX is codified in gene F9, and is a vitamin K-dependent clotting factor which has conserved the amino acid sequence. This could be a reason of FIX decreased immunogenicity, while there are not contrasted trials to prove this theory [2]. FIX has a low molecular mass that may explain its extracellular distribution and the potential for mast cell activation and the IgE-mediated hypersensitivity response [14]. Alternative immune triggers proposed includes complement activation by the IgG1 antibody formation or immune complex formation. The large gene deletions have also been associated with a higher rate of allergic reactions [14].

An inhibitor is a neutralizing polyclonal IgG antibody with high affinity to FIX, which is developed as consequence of exogenous FIX infusion. It has been proven that the human anti-FIX antibody is predominantly IgG4, and transient IgG1 subclass antibodies are also detected in patients with allergic phenotype [15]. In addition, the FIX epitopes recognized by the IgG1 and IgG4 antibodies are known to include the γ-carboxyglutanic acid (GLA) and serine protease (SP) domains, which might inhibit the interaction between activated FIX with phospholipids or with FVIII light chain [16]. This mechanism may lead to decreased FX activation and could account for the FIX inhibitory antibody response [3, 17]. Accordingly, the identification of subclass antibodies has been suggested to predict those patients at high risk of immunological reaction.

7.4 Allergic Reactions, Anaphylactic Reactions, and Nephrotic Syndrome

One of the main complications of developing inhibitors in hemophilia B is the appearance of allergic reactions, which is more frequent in patients with large gene deletions, even if they can also appear in patients with nonsense mutations. This suggests that the greater impairment of FIX synthesis would be associated with a higher risk of allergic/anaphylactic reactions.

The mechanism of appearance of this severe complication remains unclear, various hypotheses have been suggested to explain this adverse event. The extracellular distribution of factor IX protein could have a potential mast cell activation. Other hypotheses suggest that it could appear due to an IgE-mediated hypersensitivity, or due to complement activation by transient IgG1 antibody formation. High amounts of exogenous FIX could also lead to the formation of immune complexes [2, 18].

This reactions don't strictly depend on the number of exposure days, they can appear concurrently with inhibitor detection or at any time of treatment, or in some cases precede the inhibitor detection [19]. It is also not related to the source of FIX replacement used (plasma-derived/recombinant) [3]. Due the risk of potentially life-threatening reactions, it has been suggested a close monitoring in the first exposures to FIX-containing products.

Nephrotic syndrome often complicates ITI in hemophilia B patients. It is more frequent in patients who have presented allergic reactions to FIX previously (allergic phenotype) [20]. It usually appears after 8–9 months from the beginning of ITI with high doses of FIX (100–325 UI/kg/day). Patients present with sepsis-like symptoms, with periorbital edema, hypoalbuminemia, and proteinuria [2]. The response to standard therapy with steroids is usually poor, forcing to stop ITI treatment. The etiology of this process is not clear; in two patients, renal biopsy showed membranous glomerulonephritis, but immunohistochemical staining of renal tissue didn't demonstrate association with FIX immune complexes [20, 21].

7.5 Management of Patients with Hemophilia B with Inhibitors

The main goal in hemophilia B patients with inhibitors is to treat/prevent bleedings and eradicate the inhibitor [3].

7.5.1 Treatment and Prevention of Bleedings

The therapeutic approach in these patients will depend on the bleeding severity, inhibitor titer, anamnestic response, and history of allergic phenotype [6].

In patients with low-titer inhibitors and no history of allergic reactions bleeding episodes can usually be managed with treatment with high doses of FIX concentrate. Patients with high-titer inhibitor will require the administration of bypassing agents to manage bleeding episodes. This bypassing agents, recombinant activated factor VII (rFVIIa) and activated prothrombin complex concentrate (APCC), have demonstrated high efficacy rates of 80–90% in the treatment of bleeding episodes in different studies. In the FEIBA Novoseven® comparative study (FENOC) which compared the efficacy of both products to treat joint bleedings in patients with hemophilia A and inhibitors, both showed similar efficacy [22]. Despite this, there are a 30% of patients who respond better to one of them than to the other.

APCC contains FVIII and FIX, which can lead to anamnestic responses or allergic reactions in patients with inhibitor.

In cases of severe bleeding episodes which cannot be managed with these agents, plasmapheresis or immunoadsorption could be an option.

Prophylaxis with bypassing agents has been shown to reduce bleeding episodes in these patients and contributes to prevent the damage of target joints, this is particularly important in children who are undergoing ITI [8]. Prophylaxis with bypassing agents has proven to be a good option before or during ITI. The International workshop on ITI, Spanish consensus guidelines, and the UKHDO guidelines recommend the use of rFVIIa prior to the initiation of ITI [2, 23, 24]. During ITI or for those patients who are not undergoing ITI, the guidelines recommend prophylactic use of either rFVIIa or APCC [2, 23, 24].

In patients undergoing ITI when inhibitor titer decreases below 5 BU, it is recommended to stop prophylaxis with bypassing agents, due to the risk of thrombosis [25].

7.5.2 Immune Tolerance Induction Treatment

The experience with ITI in hemophilia B is limited due to the low incidence of inhibitors; most of the recommendations come from series of cases or case reports and from extrapolation from studies in hemophilia A patients.

ITI is less successful in hemophilia B with inhibitors than in hemophilia A with inhibitors, with a success rate of 31% after ITI using FIX concentrates according to The North American Immune Tolerance Registry (NAITR) [4].

Before considering initiating ITI in these patients it must be considered the low success rate, and the high risk of adverse reactions.

For patients with low-titer inhibitors, no allergic symptoms and a good clinical response to

FIX concentrates, the guidelines recommend continuing treatment with FIX at a higher dose than standard dose [7]. In case of non-allergic patients with high-titer inhibitors or inadequate response to FIX concentrates, ITI should be considered [6].

Cases of patients with inhibitors and anaphylactic reactions to FIX concentrates who didn't response well to treatment with rFVIIa have been published, these patients had received treatment with FIX and hydrocortisone to control the anaphylactic reactions, FIX was increased gradually in a stepwise manner, until therapeutic levels were reached reducing the hydrocortisone doses gradually with good results [26].

The classic protocol of ITI is the Malmö protocol which nowadays has been replaced by different immunosuppressive protocols. The Malmö consists in administration of cyclophosphamide intravenously the first 2 days (12–15 mg/kg), and then orally (2–3 mg/kg body weight) for an additional 8–10 days. FIX is given daily to maintain factor concentration at 40–100 UI/dL for about 2–3 weeks. From the fourth day after the start of the treatment, IgG should be administered at dosages of 0.4 g/kg bw for 5 days. In most cases, a single dose of corticosteroids (50–150 mg) was given at the start of treatment [27]. In cases with high inhibitor titer, it could be necessary to include immunoadsorption. With this protocol, the Malmö centre reported success in 6 of 7 (86%) cases of severe hemophilia B. The limitations of this protocol include the cyclophosphamide-associated complications and the technical difficulty of performing extracorporeal immunoadsorption in young children [28].

In patients with history of allergic reactions, usually the first step of treatment consists in a desensitization protocol to abolish these reactions, increasing the dose of FIX concentrate administered gradually, using slow intravenous infusion of FIX, or eliminating the antibody from bloodstream with plasmapheresis [29, 30].

Other reported cases showed some success in the use of different immunosuppressive agents. AntiCD20 has been employed in combination with FIX with good response [31, 32], antiCD20 has also been used in combination with corticosteroids and immunoglobulins with success [28, 33].

Experience in ITI with mycophenolate has been published in combination with dexamethasone and intravenous immunoglobulin and high dose FIX replacement therapy, the complete eradication of the inhibitor was reached in 1 of the 2 patients included, but both patients benefited from the ITI treatment and FIX replacement therapy was tolerated without allergic reactions [34]. Mycophenolate mofetil can induce apoptosis of activated T lymphocytes and suppressed T-lymphocyte response to allogenetic cells and other antigens and suppresses antibody responses. Initially to avoid anaphylactic reactions and inhibitor boost patients were treated with rFVIIa, avoiding the use of FIX concentrates and the appearing of bleeding episodes. After disappearance of FIX inhibitor mycophenolate mofetil was initiated, given twice daily adjusted by serum trough levels (1.5–4.5 lg mL), dexamethasone was given twice daily (2 × 12 mg/m^2/day), and intravenous immunoglobulins (IV IG) (0.4 g/kg/day × 4 days) repeated every 4 weeks. High doses of FIX concentrate (50–100 UI/kg) were administered daily. When FIX recovery reached normal levels, dexamethasone and mycophenolate mofetil were tapered until suspension. IV IG prophylaxis was continued to counteract immunosuppression and minimize FIX replacement therapy [34].

Beutel and colleagues reported their experience in an 11-year-old patient with history of allergic reactions to FIX and to APCC, successful inhibitor eradication was reached with a combined immune modulating therapy and high dose of FIX. He received on-demand treatment with rFVIIa but he suffered multiple joint and muscle bleeds, although the inhibitor was undetectable at this time. ITI was performed with a combination of rituximab, mycophenolate mofetil, dexamethasone, intravenous immunoglobulins and high dose FIX with success, inhibitor was eradicated, and FIX half-life normalized. No allergic reactions, nephrotic syndrome, or serious infections were observed [35].

Cyclosporin A is an immunosuppressant inhibiting calcineurin which activates interleukin-2 and inhibits T-cell function. Cross and colleagues reported a case of a severe hemophilia B patient who developed an inhibitor at early age and failed several ITI regimens. He received ITI treatment with cyclosporine, increasing the level of success. A relapse occurred when cyclosporin was withdrawn after the onset of nephrotic syndrome. ITI was continued when cyclosporin was reinitiated reaching normal recoveries and negative Bethesda assays. The patient experienced relapses in recovery and rises in the inhibitor titer after needing high amounts of FIX to manage bleeds or in surgical interventions. These relapses have been managed adjusting the dose of cyclosporin A with success [36].

A case of inhibitor-associated nephrotic syndrome in a hemophilia B patient which failed to a previous ITI has been reported, who received treatment with FIX concentrate as ITI and received concomitantly 4 weekly doses of anti-CD20 and ongoing immunosuppression with mycophenolate mofetil resulting in the complete resolution of the inhibitor and of the nephrotic syndrome [37]. The inhibitor reappeared 7 years later, the same ITI protocol reached the eradication of the inhibitor again [38].

In the NAITR 17 patients with hemophilia B undergoing ITI were included (81% had high-titer inhibitors). Sixteen (16/17) patients had concluded the ITI at time of analysis. 47% of inhibitor development occurred on high purity/monoclonal FIX concentrates, and 14/17 (82%) of the ITI reported involved the use of this source of concentrates. The mean ITI dose of FIX was 100 UI/kg/day (25–200). Factor was daily administered in most of the cases (15/17(88%)). Immunosuppression was associated in 8 cases (8/17(47%)) and plasmapheresis was used in 2 occasions. The mean period of treatment in subjects who completed treatment was 11.6 months, which was significantly less time in comparison with patients included with hemophilia A. The mean time to initiate ITI in this cohort was 44 months (1–227) after inhibitor diagnosis. ITI was successful only in 31% (5/16) of the patients who completed the course, with a mean dose of 100 UI/kg/day of FIX (43–200), one of them with an inhibitor-associated allergic phenotype. Four of these 5 patients have maintained tolerance on FIX regimens (25–100 UI/kg/day). Highlights the fact that 5 of the 11 patients who failed ITI had a positive family history of inhibitors compared with none of the successes [13].

Important adverse reactions occurred in 8 of 11 patients, including allergic reactions (4/11) and venous access complications (9/11) much more frequent in patients who failed ITI [13].

Regarding adverse events, 14 of them complicated 65% (11/17) ITI regimens, which was 10 times higher than the reported in the hemophilia A group, but there was no statistically relationship between ITI factor dose and the adverse event rate. Allergic reactions were more frequent in this group (11/14(79%)) than in hemophilia A and happened in the 10 patients that had presented them before, after development of inhibitor. Three of them were severe and forced the premature cessation of ITI [13].

Three patients ongoing ITI with a known allergic diathesis developed nephrotic syndrome, in one of them it forced to immediate suspension of ITI. The symptoms that these three patients presented were periorbital edema, proteinuria, and hypoalbuminemia after 7–9 months of beginning ITI being in that moment receiving 100 UI/kg/day of FIX. All of them showed a decline in inhibitor titer at the time of diagnosis of nephrosis, and had minimal response to steroids [13].

7.5.2.1 Outcome of Immune Tolerance Induction

It is important to establish definitions of what is considered a successful or failed ITI. The International workshop on ITI published many of these definitions. Recommended duration of an ITI regimen should be of 9 months at least to a maximum of 33 months, before considering it successful or not. The UK Haemophilia Centre Doctors' Organization (UKHCDO) in their guidelines on the management of inhibitors consider defining tolerance and restoration of normal FVIII pharmacokinetics is a FVIII elimination half-life of >7 h after a 72-h wash-out period or FVIII through levels ≥1% 48 h after a dose ≤50 UI/kg (in a standard prophylaxis on alternate days). There are no similar criteria proposed for defining tolerance in hemophilia B due to the uncertainty of normal FIX half-life [8].

In the process of ITI it is important to take in count psychosocial care for patients and caregivers, to maintain an attitude of hope for the future, deal with feelings of guilt and ensure adequate educational assistance. The term of "failed ITI" could have negative connotations and it may better to use the term of "unsuccessful ITI" [8].

7.5.2.2 Predictors of Outcome of Immune Tolerance Induction

There are a lot of treatment-related and patient-related factors that are predictive for ITI outcome. Treatment-related factors that can influence ITI outcome are the inhibitor titer at ITI onset, the time between diagnosis and initiation ITI, the historical peak inhibitor titer and peak titer during ITI. Patients with <10 BU/mL of inhibitor titer at ITI onset have more probability of successful ITI and diminish the time taken to achieve success [8]. Patient-related factors include age at ITI start, ethnicity, and genotype.

7.6 Future Directions

Nowadays there are on development new therapeutics whose mechanism does not consist in replacement therapies or bypassing agents, these new therapies include the TFPI-targeting monoclonal antibodies and fitusiran (an RNAi therapy targeting AT) [39]. Both agents are administered subcutaneously and should significantly reduce treatment burden and bleeding episodes. Both are currently on phase III in investigation trials, with promising results. Fitusiran trials have recently been stopped because of thrombotic complications but will be restarted soon.

Gene therapy is a promising landscape in hemophilia B; it offers the potential for a cure for patients with hemophilia by establishing continuous expression of factor IX following the transfer of a functional gene to replace the defective gene in these patients with successful results published, but it may not be suitable for all patients. There is a need of more studies that confirm the safety and efficacy of this therapy [40].

7.7 Conclusions

Inhibitor development in patients with hemophilia B is a severe complication that represents a challenge in hemophilia and involves significant enhancement in both morbidity and mortality. Due to its low incidence, there has been a lack of research in terms of diagnosis and treatment, and few evidence-based data exist. Development of allergic/anaphylactic reactions and nephrotic syndrome supposes a serious complication in these patients which difficults management. ITI is still the preferred strategy for antibody eradication, but some patients do not tolerate it or are unresponsive to ITI. Overall, ITI in hemophilia B is less effective, within a success rate of 31%. There have been used different protocols for ITI in hemophilia B employing different types of immunosuppressive therapies. Nowadays new treatments as rebalancing therapies or the gene therapy are going to displace ITI treatment in patients with hemophilia B and inhibitors.

References

1. Bolton-Maggs PH, Pasi KJ. Haemophilias A and B. Lancet. 2003;361:1801–9.
2. DiMichele D. Inhibitor development in haemophilia B: an orphan disease in need of attention. Br J Haematol. 2007;138:305–15.
3. Santoro C, Quintavalle G, Castaman G, Baldacci E, Ferretti A, Riccardi F, et al. Inhibitors in hemophilia B. Semin Thromb Hemost. 2018;44(6):578–89.
4. DiMichele DM, Kroner BL, North American Immune Tolerance Study. The North American Immune Tolerance Registry: practices, outcomes, outcome predictors. Thromb Haemost. 2002;87(1):52–7.
5. Chitlur M, Warrier I, Rajpurkar M, Lusher JM. Inhibitors in factor IX deficiency a report of the ISTH-SSC international FIX inhibitor registry (1997-2006). Haemophilia. 2009;15:1027–31.
6. Dolan G, Benson G, Duffy A, Hermans C, Jiménez-Yuste V, Lambert T, et al. Haemophilia B: where are we now and what does the future hold? Blood Rev. 2018;32:52–60.
7. Kempton CL, Meeks SL. Toward optimal therapy for inhibitors in hemophilia. Hematology. 2014;2014:364–71.
8. Ljung R, Auerswald G, Benson G, Dolan G, Duffy A, Hermans C, et al. Inhibitors in haemophilia A and B: management of bleeds, inhibitor eradication and strat-

egies for difficult-to-treat patients. Eur J Haematol. 2019;102:111–22.
9. Hay CR, Brown S, Collins PW, Keeling DM, Liesner R. The diagnosis and management of factor VIII and IX inhibitors: a guideline from the United Kingdom Haemophilia Centre Doctors Organisation. Br J Haematol. 2006;133:591–605.
10. Nagel K, Walker I, Decker K, Chan AKC, Pai MK. Comparing bleed frequency and factor concentrate use between haemophilia A and B patients. Haemophilia. 2011;17:872–4.
11. Saini S, Hamasaki-Katagiri N, Pandey GS, Yanover C, Guelcher C, Simhadri VL, et al. Genetic determinants of immunogenicity to factor IX during the treatment of haemophilia B. Haemophilia. 2015;21:210–8.
12. High KA. Factor IX: molecular structure, epitopes, and mutations associated with inhibitor formation. Adv Exp Med Biol. 1995;386:79–86.
13. Dimichele D. The North American Immune Tolerance Registry: contributions to the thirty-year experience with immune tolerance therapy. Haemophilia. 2009;15:320–8.
14. Ketterling RP, Vielhaber EL, Lind TJ, Thorland EC, Sommer SS. The rates and patterns of deletions in the human factor IX gene. Am J Hum Genet. 1994;54:201–13.
15. Sawamoto Y, Shima M, Yamamoto M, Kamisue S, Nakai H, Tanaka I, et al. Measurement of anti-factor IX IgG subclasses in haemophilia B patients who developed inhibitors with episodes of allergic reactions to factor IX concentrates. Thromb Res. 1996;83:279–86.
16. Christophe OD, Lenting PJ, Cherel G, Boon-Spijker M, Lavergne JM, Boertjes R, et al. Functional map ping of anti-factor IX inhibitors developed in patients with severe hemophilia B. Blood. 2001;98:1416–23.
17. Smith SB, Gailani D. Update on the physiology and pathology of factor IX activation by factor XIa. Expert Rev Hematol. 2008;1:87–98.
18. Mauro M, Bonetti E, Balter R, Poli G, Cesaro S. Recurrent episodes of anaphylaxis in a patient with haemophilia B: a case report. Blood Transfus. 2016;14:582–4.
19. Yamamoto M, Kamisue S, Sawamoto Y, Nakai H, Tanaka I, Shima M, et al. Factor IX inhibition and epitope localization of factor IX inhibitor antibodies in haemophilia B patients with anaphylactoid reactions. Haemophilia. 1997;3:189–93.
20. Ewenstein BM, Takemoto C, Warrier I, Lusher J, Saidi P, Eisele J, et al. Nephrotic syndrome as a complication of immune tolerance in hemophilia B. Blood. 1997;89:1115–6.
21. Dharnidharka VR, Takemoto C, Ewenstein BM, Rosen S, Harris HW. Membranous glomerulonephritis and nephrosis post factor IX infusions in hemophilia B. Pediatr Nephrol. 1998;12:654–7.
22. Astermark J, Donfield SM, DiMichele DM, Gringeri A, Gilbert SA, Waters J, et al. A randomized comparison of bypassing agents in hemophilia complicated by an inhibitor: the FEIBA NovoSeven Comparative (FENOC) Study. Blood. 2007;109:546–51.
23. Lopez-Fernandez MF, Altisent-Roca C, Álvarez-Román MT, Canaro-Hirnyk MA, Mingot-Castellano ME, Jiménez-Yuste V, et al. Spanish consensus guidelines on prophylaxis with bypassing agents in patients with haemophilia and inhibitors. Thromb Haemost. 2016;115:872–95.
24. Collins PW, Chalmers E, Hart DP, Liesner R, Rangarajan S, Talks K, et al. Diagnosis and treatment of factor VIII and IX inhibitors in congenital haemophilia: (4th edition). UK Haemophilia Centre Doctors Organization. Br J Haematol. 2013;160:153–70.
25. Leissinger CA. Advances in the clinical management of inhibitors in hemophilia A and B. Semin Hematol. 2016;53:20–7.
26. Shibata M, Shima M, Misu H, Okimoto Y, Giddings JC, Yoshioka A. Management of haemophilia B inhibitor patients with anaphylactic reactions to FIX concentrates. Haemophilia. 2003;9:269–71.
27. Freiburghaus C, Berntorp E, Ekman M, Gunnarsson M, Kjellberg K, Nilsson IM. Tolerance induction using the Malmo treatment model 1982-1995. Haemophilia. 1999;5:32–9.
28. Di Michele DM. Immune tolerance induction in haemophilia: evidence and the way forward. J Thromb Haemost. 2011;9(1):216–25.
29. Barnes C, Rudzki Z, Ekert H. Induction of immune tolerance and suppression of anaphylaxis in a child with haemophilia B by simple plasmapheresis and antigen exposure. Haemophilia. 2000;6:693–5.
30. Barnes C, Brewin T, Ekert H. Induction of immune tolerance and suppression of anaphylaxis in a child with haemophilia B by simple plasmapheresis and antigen exposure: progress report. Haemophilia. 2001;7:439–40.
31. Kobayashi R, Sano H, Suzuki D, Kishimoto K, Yasuda K, Honjo R, et al. Successful treatment of immune tolerance induction with rituximab in a patient with severe hemophilia B and inhibitor. Blood Coagul Fibrinolysis. 2015;26:580–2.
32. Barnes C, Davis A, Furmedge J, Egan B, Donnan L, Monagle P. Induction of immune tolerance using rituximab in a child with severe haemophilia B with inhibitors and anaphylaxis to factor IX. Haemophilia. 2010;16(5):840–1.
33. Batorova A, Morongova A, Tagariello G, Jankovicova D, Prigancova T, Horakova J. Challenges in the management of hemophilia B with inhibitor. Semin Thromb Hemost. 2013;39:767–71.
34. Klarmann D, Martinez-Saguer I, Funk MB, Knoefler R, von Hentig N, Heller C, et al. Immune tolerance induction with mycophenolate-mofetil in two children with haemophilia B and inhibitor. Haemophilia. 2008;14:44–9.
35. Beutel K, Hauch H, Rischewski J, Kordes U, Schneppenheim J, Schneppenheim R. ITI with high-dose FIX and combined immunosuppressive therapy in a patient with severe haemophilia B and inhibitor. Hamostaseologie. 2009;29:155–7.

36. Cross DC, Van Der Berg HM. Cyclosporin A can achieve immune tolerance in a patient with severe haemophilia B and refractory inhibitors. Haemophilia. 2007;13:111–4.
37. Verghese P, Darrow S, Kurth MH, Reed RC, Kim Y, Kearney S. Successful management of factor IX inhibitor-associated nephrotic syndrome in a hemophilia B patient. Pediatr Nephrol. 2013;28:823–6.
38. Holstein K, Schneppenheim R, Schrum J, Bokemeyer C, Langer F. Successful second ITI with factor IX and combined immunosuppressive therapy. A patient with severe haemophilia B and recurrence of a factor IX inhibitor. Haemostaseologie. 2014;34(Suppl 1):S5–8.
39. Jiménez-Yuste V, Auerswald G, Benson G, Dolan G, Hermans C, Lambert T, et al. Practical considerations for nonfactor-replacement therapies in the treatment of haemophilia with inhibitors. Haemophilia. 2021. https://doi.org/10.1111/hae.14167.
40. Nathwani AC. Gene therapy for hemophilia. Hematology. 2019;2019:1–8.

8 Hemophilia B: New Drugs

Mónica Martín-Salces

8.1 Introduction

Hemophilia B is a rare inherited bleeding disorder caused by reduced or absent levels of factor IX (FIX). Hemophilia B can be treated with intravenous FIX replacement therapy, administered on demand to reduce bleeding episodes and as prophylaxis to prevent bleeding and joint destruction, with the aim of preserving normal musculoskeletal function.

Currently, prophylaxis is considered to be the standard of care for hemophilia. Prophylaxis is associated with a few challenges, such as need for venous access, frequent FIX administrations, variable pharmacokinetics, and increased initial cost; however, prophylaxis is considered superior to on-demand therapy as it prevents bleeding-related complications, particularly hemophilic arthropathy, in patients with severe disease [1]. Highly purified FIX concentrates [plasma-derived FIX (pdFIX) and recombinant FIX (rFIX)] are routinely used for the treatment of hemophilia B. However, as pdFIX and rFIX have a relatively short plasma half-life (*t*1/2; typically 16–19 h), they require frequent administration (2–3 times weekly) to maintain protective prophylaxis FIX levels [2].

Therefore, current development efforts have focused on extending the *t*1/2 of rFIX by modifying its physiological and pharmacokinetic properties with the aim of reducing treatment burden and thereby potentially improving treatment compliance and clinical outcomes. Approaches to prolong the *t*1/2 have included covalent attachment of a polyethylene glycol (PEG) molecule to the rFIX activation peptide or protein fusion (fusing human albumin or Ig to rFIX) [3].

Other therapeutic approaches that are not based on substitution of the deficient factor are currently being developed. In hemophilia B, those treatments are based on increasing thrombin formation by inhibiting natural anticoagulants such as antithrombin in the case of fitusiran or the tissue factor pathway inhibitor in the case of concizumab (see Chap. 5).

8.2 Extended Half-life (EHL) Factor IX Products

8.2.1 Albutrepenonacog Alfa, rFIX-FP

Albutrepenonacog alfa is a recombinant single-chain protein obtained by the fusion of recombinant human FIX with recombinant human albumin connected by a short cleavable linker peptide derived from the endogenous activation peptide of native FIX [4]. rFIX-FP is produced

M. Martín-Salces (✉)
Department of Hematology, La Paz University Hospital, Madrid, Spain

E. C. Rodríguez-Merchán (ed.), *Advances in Hemophilia Treatment*,
https://doi.org/10.1007/978-3-030-93990-8_8

by Chinese hamster ovary (CHO) cells, transfected with both the genes of recombinant human FIX and human albumin.

Pharmacokinetic (PK), efficacy, and safety of rIX-FP were evaluated in the frame of a large clinical trial program referred to as PROLONG-9FP. In a phase I, multicenter, dose-escalation trial, the safety and pharmacokinetics of rIX-FP were assessed in patients with hemophilia B. At a dose of 25–75 IU/kg, rIX-FP was well tolerated: no serious adverse events were reported and there was no evidence of hypersensitivity or immunogenic reactions. PK analysis indicated enhanced properties, including a fivefold increase in half-life, 44% higher recovery, sevenfold greater area under the curve, and sevenfold slower clearance, compared with recombinant FIX. Trough levels were maintained above 5% after 7 days when rIX-FP was administered at 25 IU/kg and after 14 days when given at 50 IU/kg [5].

In a prospective phase II, open-label study evaluated the safety and efficacy of rIX-FP for the prevention of bleeding episodes during weekly prophylaxis and assessed the hemostatic efficacy for on-demand treatment of bleeding episodes in previously treated patients with hemophilia B. The study consisted of a 10–14-day evaluation of rIX-FP PK, and an 11-month safety and efficacy evaluation period with subjects receiving weekly prophylaxis treatment. Seventeen subjects participated in the study, 13 received weekly prophylaxis, and 4 received episodic treatment only. The mean and median annualized spontaneous bleeding rate (AsBR) was 1.25 and 1.13 respectively in the weekly prophylaxis arm. All bleeding episodes were treated with 1 or 2 injections of rIX-FP. Three prophylaxis subjects who were treated on demand prior to study entry had >85% reduction in AsBR compared to the bleeding rate prior to study entry [6]. The phase 3 study evaluated the PK, efficacy, and safety of rIX-FP in 63 previously treated male patients (12–61 years) with severe hemophilia B (FIX activity ≤2%). The study included 2 groups: group 1 patients received routine prophylaxis once every 7 days for 26 weeks, followed by either 7-, 10-, or 14-day prophylaxis regimen for a mean of 50, 38, or 51 weeks, respectively; group 2 patients received on-demand treatment of bleeding episodes for 26 weeks and then switched to a 7-day prophylaxis regimen for a mean of 45 weeks. The mean terminal half-life of rIX-FP was 102 h, 4.3-fold longer than previous FIX treatment. There was 100% reduction in median AsBR and 100% resolution of target joints when subjects switched from on-demand to prophylaxis treatment with rIX-FP. The median AsBR was 0.00 for all prophylaxis regimens. Overall, 98.6% of bleeding episodes were treated successfully, including 93.6% that were treated with a single injection. Patients maintained a mean trough of 20 and 12 IU/dL FIX activity on prophylaxis with rIX-FP 40 IU/kg weekly and 75 IU/kg every 2 weeks, respectively [7].

The pediatric trial by Kenet et al. [8] was a prospective, nonrandomized, international, open-label phase 3 study, with all patients assigned to weekly prophylactic treatment. All patients participated in the PK evaluation of 50 IU/kg rIX-FP at study entry. Patients also participated in PK evaluation of 50 IU/kg of previous FIX products unless PK data were available in the medical records. The patients were assigned a dose of 35–50 IU/kg rIX-FP for weekly prophylaxis, at the investigator's discretion. All 27 patients (FIX activity ≤2%) were on weekly prophylactic treatment for a mean of 62 weeks. The total median ABR was 3.12 (range 0.91–5.91), the joint ABR was 0.99 (range 0.00–2.33), and the spontaneous ABR was 0.00 (range 0.00–0.91).

An international, multicenter extension study evaluated rIX-FP in hemophilia B (FIX ≤2%) patients previously enrolled in a phase III study or who initiated rIX-FP prophylaxis following surgery. The objective was to investigate the long-term safety and efficacy of rIX-FP prophylaxis in adult previously treated patients (PTPs) with hemophilia B. Male PTPs were treated with a 7- (35–50 IU/kg), 10- or 14-day regimen (50–75 IU/kg). Patients ≥18 years who were well-controlled on a 14-day regimen for ≥6 months could switch to a 21-day regimen (100 IU/kg). A total of 59 patients (aged 13–63 years) participated in the study. Following a single dose of 100 IU/kg rIX-FP, in patients eligible for the 21-day regimen, the mean terminal half-life was 143.2 h.

Mean steady-state FIX trough activity levels ranged from 22% with the 7-day regimen to 7.6% with the 21-day regimen. Median (Q1, Q3) annualized spontaneous bleeding rates were 0.00 (0.00, 1.67), 0.28 (0.00, 1.10), 0.37 (0.00, 1.68), and 0.00 (0.00, 0.45) for the 7-, 10-, 14-, and 21-day regimens, respectively. Comparable efficacy was demonstrated for both the 14- and 21-day regimens compared to the 7-day regimen. Overall, 96.5% of bleeding episodes were treated successfully with 1 to 2 rIX-FP infusions [9].

8.2.2 Nonacog Beta Pegol, N9-GP

N9-GP is a recombinant coagulation factor IX derivative. It is produced without animal-derived materials and with an attached 40 kDa polyethylene glycol (PEG) molecule for peptide activation by a site-directed glycoPEGylation. Once activated, the activation molecule with PEG are cleaved to leave the activated factor IX (FIXa) [10].

The first human dose trial in patients with severe or moderate hemophilia B investigated the safety and pharmacokinetic properties of a single IV dose of N9-GP. Sixteen previously treated patients received one dose of their previous FIX product followed by one dose of N9-GP at the same dose level (25, 50, or 100 U/kg). None of the patients developed inhibitors. One patient developed transient hypersensitivity symptoms during administration of N9-GP and was excluded from PK analyses. In the remaining 15 patients, N9-GP was well tolerated. The half-life was 93 h, which was 5 times higher than the patient's previous product. The incremental recovery of N9-GP was 94% and 20% higher compared with recombinant and plasma-derived products, respectively [11].

The source data of the first phase I was used to developing a population PK model, based on a linear two-compartment model, to describe the PK behavior of N9-GP, pd- and rFIX concentrates on different prophylaxis regimens, 10 IU/kg or 40 IU/kg once weekly. The first scheme achieved a C_{max} of 18 IU/dL and a trough of 4.2 IU/dL. In contrast, the second one achieved a C_{max} of 72 IU/dL and a trough of 17 IU/dL [12].

The Paradigm TM3 trial was a multinational, randomized, single-blind trial investigated the safety and efficacy of N9-GP, in 74 previously treated patients with hemophilia B (FIX activity ≤2 IU/dL). Patients received prophylaxis for 52 weeks, randomized to either 10 IU/kg or 40 IU/kg once weekly or to on-demand treatment of 28 weeks. Three hundred forty-five bleeding episodes were treated, with an estimated success rate of 92.2%. The median annualized bleeding rates (ABRs) were 1.04 in the 40 IU/kg prophylaxis group, 2.93 in the 10 IU/kg prophylaxis group, and 15.58 in the on-demand treatment group. In the 40 IU/kg group, 10 (66.7%) of 15 patients experienced no bleeding episodes into target joints compared with 1 (7.7%) of 13 patients in the 10 IU/kg group [13].

In the Paradigm TM5 trial, 25 children (aged ≤12 years) with hemophilia B (FIX ≤2%) were enrolled and treated. Patients were stratified by age (0–6 years and 7–12 years), and received once-weekly prophylaxis with 40 IU/kg N9-GP for 50 exposure days. Forty-two bleeds in 15 patients were reported to have been treated; the overall success rate was 92.9%, and most bleeds (85.7%) resolved after one dose. The ABRs were 1.0 in the total population, 0.0 in the 0–6-year group, and 2.0 in the 7–12-year group; the estimated mean ABRs were 1.44 in the total population, 0.87 in the 0–6-year group, and 1.88 in the 7–12-year group. For 22 patients who had previously been receiving prophylaxis, the estimated mean ABR was 1.38 versus a historical ABR of 2.51. Estimated mean steady-state FIX trough levels were 0.153 IU/ mL (0–6 years) and 0.190 IU/mL (7–12 years) [14].

8.2.3 Eftrenonacog Alfa, rFIXFc

Eftrenonacog alfa is a recombinant fusion protein comprising human FIX covalently linked to the constant region (Fc) domain of human IgG1. The presence of the Fc domain extends the terminal half-life of rFIXFc, permitting prolonged treatment intervals [15].

In a phase I/IIa trial, fourteen subjects received a single dose of rFIXFc; 1 subject each received

1, 5, 12.5, or 25 IU/kg, and 5 subjects each received 50 or 100 IU/kg. Blood samples have been collected up to 10 or even 14 days, and the data were analyzed using the two-compartment model. C_{max} (20.4, 47.5, and 98.5 IU/dL) and AUC (766, 1700, and 4020 h × IU/dL) were proportional to the injected doses, alfa distribution half-life was 3.31 ± 3.13 and 10.3 ± 5.64 h, beta elimination half-life 56.7 ± 10.4 and 57.6 ± 8.27 h, clearance 2.84 ± 0.66 and 3.44 ± 0.83 mL/h/kg, volume of distribution 183 ± 28 and 262 ± 54 mL/kg. With baseline subtraction, mean activity terminal $t1/2$ and mean residence time for rFIXFc were 56.7 and 71.8 h, respectively. This is threefold longer than that reported for standard half-life rFIX products. The incremental recovery of rFIXFc was 0.93 IU/dL per IU/kg, similar to plasma-derived FIX [16].

The phase 3 clinical trial was a nonrandomized, open-label study of the safety, efficacy, and pharmacokinetics of rFIXFc for prophylaxis, treatment of bleeding, and perioperative hemostasis in 123 previously treated male patients. All participants were 12 years of age or older and had severe hemophilia B. The study included four treatment groups: group 1 received weekly dose-adjusted prophylaxis (50 IU/kg of rFIXFc), group 2 received interval-adjusted prophylaxis (100 IU/kg every 10 days), group 3 received treatment as needed for bleeding episodes (20–100 IU/kg), and group 4 received treatment in the perioperative period. A total of 115 participants completed the study. As compared with recombinant FIX, rFIXFc exhibited a prolonged terminal half-life (82.1 h). Prophylactic treatment significantly reduced the annualized rate of bleeding in group 1 (by 83%) and group 2 (by 87%) as compared with the rate in the group receiving episodic treatment. Among the participants receiving prophylaxis, 23.0% in group 1 and 42.3% in group 2 had no bleeding episodes during the study. The median spontaneous ABR was 1.0 (range 0.0–2.2) and 0.9 (range 0.0–2.3) for group 1 and group 2, respectively. And the median joint ABR was 1.0 (0.0–2.1) and 0.0 (range 0.0–1.7) for group 1 and group 2, respectively. In group 2, 53.8% of participants had dosing intervals of 14 days or more during the last 3 months of the study. In groups 1, 2, and 3, 90.4% of bleeding episodes resolved after one injection. Hemostasis was rated as excellent or good during all major surgeries [17].

Kids B-LONG was a multicenter, open-label, phase 3 study assessing the safety, efficacy, and PK of rFIXFc in 30 previously treated pediatric patients younger than 12 years with severe hemophilia B. All patients were initially given rFIXFc prophylaxis (50–60 IU/kg) once per week with adjustments to dose (≤100 IU/kg per infusion) or dosing frequency (up to two times per week) as needed. Overall, rFIXFc exhibited a prolonged half-life of 68.6 h. Ten patients (33%) reported no bleeding, and 19 (63%) reported no joint bleeding events during the study. The overall median ABR was 2.0 (IQR 0.0–3.1). The median ABR of patients younger than 6 years was 1.1 (0.0–2.9) and 2.1 (0.0–4.2) for patients aged 6–11 years. The median average prophylactic dose of rFIXFc was 58.6 IU/kg (IQR 52.3–64.8) per week. Throughout the study, 29 (97%) of 30 patients remained on once per week infusions [18].

In the B-YOND extension study ninety-three subjects from B-LONG and 27 from Kids B-LONG were enrolled. Most subjects received weekly prophylaxis (B-LONG: n = 51; Kids B-LONG: n = 23). For subjects from B-LONG, median (range) treatment duration was 4.0 (0.3–5.4) years and for pediatric subjects were 2.6 (0.2–3.9) years. No inhibitors were observed and the overall rFIXFc safety profile was consistent with prior studies. Annualized bleed rates remained low and extended-dosing intervals were maintained for most subjects. The median dosing interval for the individualized interval prophylaxis group was approximately 14 days for adults and adolescents (n = 31) and 10 days for pediatric subjects (n = 5) [19].

8.3 Conclusions

In hemophilia B, current development efforts have focused on extending the $t1/2$ of recombinant FIX by modifying its physiological and pharmacokinetic properties with the aim of reducing treatment burden and thereby potentially ameliorating treatment compliance and clinical results. Approaches to prolong the *t*1/2 have included covalent attachment of a polyethylene glycol (PEG) molecule to the rFIX activation peptide or protein fusion (fusing human albumin or Ig to rFIX). Among the extended half-life factor IX products, the following stand out: albutrepenonacog alfa, rFIX-FP; nonacog beta pegol, N9-GP: and eftrenonacog alfa, rFIXFc. Other therapeutic approaches that are not based on substitution of the deficient factor are currently being developed. In hemophilia B, those treatments are based on augmenting thrombin formation by inhibiting natural anticoagulants such as antithrombin in the case of fitusiran or the tissue factor pathway inhibitor in the case of concizumab.

References

1. Oladapo AO, Epstein JD, Williams E, Ito D, Gringeri A, Valentino LA. Health-related quality of life assessment in haemophilia patients on prophylaxis therapy: a systematic review of results from prospective clinical trials. Haemophilia. 2015;21:344–58.
2. Peyvandi F, Garagiola I, Young G. The past and future of haemophilia: diagnosis, treatments, and its complications. Lancet. 2016;388:187–97.
3. Mannucci PM. Half-life extension technologies for haemostatic agents. Thromb Haemost. 2015;113:165–76.
4. Metzner HJ, Weimer T, Kronthaler U, Lang W, Schulteet S. Genetic fusion to albumin improves the pharmacokinetic properties of factor IX. Thromb Haemost. 2009;102:634–44.
5. Santagostino E. PROLONG-9FP clinical development program—phase I results of recombinant fusion protein linking coagulation factor IX with recombinant albumin (rIX-FP). Thromb Res. 2013;131(2):7–10.
6. Martinowitz U, Lissitchkov T, Lubetsky A, Jotov G, Barazani-Brutman T, Voigtet C, et al. Results of a phase I/II open-label, safety and efficacy trial of coagulation factor IX (recombinant), albumin fusion protein in haemophilia B patients. Haemophilia. 2015;21:784–90.
7. Santagostino E, Martinowitz U, Lissitchkov T, Pan-Petesch B, Hanabusa H, Oldenburg J, et al. Long-acting recombinant coagulation factor IX albumin fusion protein (rIX-FP) in hemophilia B: results of a phase 3 trial. Blood. 2016;127:1761–9.
8. Kenet G, Chambost H, Male C, Lambert T, Halimeh S, Chernova T, et al. Long-acting recombinant fusion protein linking coagulation factor IX with albumin (rIX-FP) in children. Results of a phase 3 trial. Thromb Haemost. 2016;116:659–68.
9. Mancuso ME, Lubetsky A, Pan-Petesch B, Lissitchkov T, Nagao A, Seifert W, et al. Long-term safety and efficacy of rIX-FP prophylaxis with extended dosing intervals up to 21 days in adults/adolescents with hemophilia B. J Thromb Haemost. 2020;18:1065–74.
10. Ostergaard H, Bjelke JR, Hansen L, Petersen LC, Pedersen AA, Elmet T, et al. Prolonged half-life and preserved enzymatic properties of factor IX selectively PEGylated on native N-glycans in the activation peptide. Blood. 2011;118:2333–41.
11. Negrier C, Knobe K, Tiede A, Giangrande P, Møss J. Enhanced pharmacokinetic properties of a glycoPEGylated recombinant factor IX: a first human dose trial in patients with hemophilia B. Blood. 2011;118:2695–701.
12. Collins PW, Møss J, Knobe K, Groth A, Colberg T, Watson E. Population pharmacokinetic modeling for dose setting of nonacog beta pegol (N9-GP), a glycoPEGylated recombinant factor IX. J Thromb Haemost. 2012;10:2305–112.
13. Collins PW, Young G, Knobe K, Karim FA, Angchaisuksiri P, Banner C, et al. Recombinant long-acting glycoPEGylated factor IX in hemophilia B: a multinational randomized phase 3 trial. Blood. 2014;124:3880–6.
14. Carcao M, Zak M, Karim FA, Hanabusa H, Kearney S, Lu M-Y, et al. Nonacog beta pegol in previously treated children with hemophilia B: results from an international open-label phase 3 trial. J Thromb Haemost. 2016;14:1521–9.
15. Peters RT, Low SC, Kamphaus GD, Dumont JA, Amari JV, Luet Q, et al. Prolonged activity of factor IX as a monomeric Fc fusion protein. Blood. 2010;115:2057–64.
16. Shapiro AD, Ragni MV, Valentino LA, Key NS, Josephson NC, Powellet JS, et al. Recombinant factor IX-Fc fusion protein (rFIXFc) demonstrates safety and prolonged activity in a phase 1/2a study in hemophilia B patients. Blood. 2012;119:666–72.
17. Powell JS, Pasi KJ, Ragni MV, Ozelo MC, Valentino LA, Mahlangu JN, et al. Phase 3 study of recombinant factor IX Fc fusion protein in hemophilia B. N Engl J Med. 2013;369:2313–23.
18. Fischer K, Kulkarni R, Nolan B, Mahlangu J, Rangarajan S, Gambino G, et al. Recombinant factor IX Fc fusion protein in children with haemophilia B (Kids B-LONG): results from a multicentre, non-randomised phase 3 study. Lancet Haematol. 2017;4:e75–82.
19. Pasi KJ, Fischer K, Ragni M, Kulkarni R, Ozelo MC, Mahlangu J, et al. Long-term safety and sustained efficacy for up to 5 years of treatment with recombinant factor IX Fc fusion protein in subjects with haemophilia B: Results from the B-YOND extension study. Haemophilia. 2020;26:262–71.

9 Management of Hemophilia Carriers

Miguel A. Escobar, Joanna Larson, and Natalie Montanez

9.1 Introduction and Epidemiology

Hemophilia A and B are X-linked bleeding disorders that clinically affect more males than females given the homozygosity of the inheritance. The majority of female carriers are heterozygous for hemophilia alleles and historically have not been classified and treated as their male counterpart due to the presumption that they have a milder phenotype. The variability in the phenotype of women with hemophilia can partially be explained by the broad distribution of factor levels. When compared to normal women (non-hemophilia carriers) that have a mean FVIII/FIX level of 100 IU/dL, carriers have a mean level near to 50 IU/dL. This variability may be explained in part by X-chromosome inactivation; the type of genetic mutation does not seem to influence factor levels.

The true prevalence of hemophilia carriers is unknown but it is estimated that for every male with hemophilia, there are 3–5 hemophilia carriers [1]. Approximately thirty percent of hemophilia carriers have low FVIII/FIX levels (<40 IU/dL), with the same proportion of carriers presenting with bleeding symptoms. However, there is a poor correlation between bleeding symptomatology and basal factor levels [2, 3].

In most reports describing bleeding symptoms in hemophilia carriers, pregnancy-related complications, surgical procedures, and menorrhagia are prevalent and deserve special consideration [4].

Reduced health related quality of life (HR-QOL) has been well described in males with hemophilia, but data in female carriers is very limited. In the few studies that have been published, hemophilia carriers had poorer HR-QOL scores due to menorrhagia, dysmenorrhea, joint bleeding, pain, and general health [5–7].

Since 2011, The Community Counts program collects de-identified data from 135 hemophilia centers in the USA. From the total number of patients, 6.1% of hemophilia A and 8.5% of hemophilia B patients are females for a total of 1672 (6.7%) hemophilia carriers. The proportion of severe and moderate is low, accounting for 0.48% and 1.4% respectively. On the other hand, the number of mild female patients is significant (16% for hemophilia A and 23.7% for hemophilia B) (https://www.cdc.gov/ncbddd/hemophilia/communitycounts/data-reports/2020-9/table-2-factor.html).

M. A. Escobar (✉)
Department of Internal Medicine and Pediatrics, University of Texas Health Science Center and the McGovern Medical School, Gulf States Hemophilia and Thrombophilia Center, Houston, TX, USA
e-mail: miguel.escobar@uth.tmc.edu

J. Larson · N. Montanez
Department of Pediatrics, University of Texas Health Science Center and the McGovern Medical School, Gulf States Hemophilia and Thrombophilia Center, Houston, TX, USA

E. C. Rodríguez-Merchán (ed.), *Advances in Hemophilia Treatment*,
https://doi.org/10.1007/978-3-030-93990-8_9

9.1.1 Definition of a "Carrier"

A hemophilia carrier is defined as a female who carries a mutated FVIII or FIX gene that causes hemophilia A or hemophilia B. Since there is so much variability among the symptoms hemophilia women report, and there is lack of correlation with factor levels, a new nomenclature for carriers has been defined for clinical care and research studies.

The Thrombosis and Hemostasis ISTH Scientific and Standardization Committees recommends that the term "hemophilia carrier" be reserved for genetic counseling and terms such as "symptomatic/asymptomatic hemophilia carrier" and "women and girls with hemophilia" be used in the clinical setting. This nomenclature is similar to the one used for males with hemophilia. It differentiates five clinically relevant hemophilia carrier phenotypes. Females with clotting factor levels >40% without a bleeding phenotype are often referred to as asymptomatic carriers, while women and girls with a bleeding phenotype with clotting factor levels >40% are considered to be symptomatic carriers. Women and girls with levels ranging from 5% to 40% may be referred to as having mild hemophilia. Factor levels less than 5% may be noted in some women, and are thus classified as having moderate hemophilia 1–5% or having severe hemophilia <1%. This variability is thought to be attributed to the lyonization phenomenon (skewed X-chromosome inactivation pattern) [8] (Table 9.1).

Table 9.1 New definition for hemophilia carriers

Factor level of Hemophilia A/B carrier	Hemophilia carrier type
<1%	Woman/girl with severe hemophilia
1–5%	Woman/girl with moderate hemophilia
>5–40%	Woman/girl with mild hemophilia
>40% with bleeding phenotype	Symptomatic hemophilia carrier
>40% without bleeding phenotype	Asymptomatic hemophilia carrier

9.2 Symptoms

Hemophilia carriers have a broad variety of bleeding symptoms, which are more prevalent with clotting factor levels within the lower normal range. However, there is evidence that, even despite normal factor VIII and factor IX levels, hemophilia carriers can be at increased bleeding risk. This includes prolonged skin bleeding, heavy menstrual bleeding, oral bleeding, postpartum hemorrhage, and excessive bleeding following dental procedures and surgery (Table 9.2).

Olsson et al. evaluated a cohort of 126 carriers of severe and moderate hemophilia and compared it to 90 female controls. They found a high occurrence of bleeding symptoms in the carrier cohort compared to the healthy controls. This bleeding tendency was present not only in carriers with clotting factor levels comparable to those in mild hemophilia, but also in carriers with factor levels within the normal range [9]. The bleeding score (BAT) was significantly higher in the carriers when compared to the controls but was weakly correlated to FVIII levels in the carriers of hemophilia A. Thirty two percent of carriers reported bleeding complications during surgery and 12% of them required blood transfusion when compared to 7% and 4% of controls, respectively. Menorrhagia and postpartum bleeding were also more common in the female carriers (Fig. 9.1).

Paroskie and colleagues performed a prospective cross-sectional study of bleeding phenotype, comparing 44 hemophilia A carriers to 43 normal women. Hemophilia carriers had higher bleeding scores reporting increased cutaneous bruising, postpartum hemorrhage, post-surgical bleeding, atraumatic hemarthrosis, and menorrhagia when compared to normal controls [10]. Plug et al. also studied the effect of hemophilia A and B carriership in the Netherlands with comparison to normal women. Of a total of 274 carriers and 245 noncarriers, the median clotting factor level was 0.60 IU/mL (range, 0.05–2.19 IU/mL) and 1.02 IU/mL (range, 0.45–3.28 IU/mL), respectively. Interestingly, 8% of the carriers reported joint bleeds. Overall, carriers experience a higher risk of prolonged bleeding after trauma and procedures [2] (Fig. 9.2).

Table 9.2 Variability of bleeding symptoms in carriers among multiple studies

Ref	Population	Hemarthrosis (%)	Minor wound bleeding (%)	Oral cavity bleeding (%)	Tooth extraction (%)	Post-surgical bleeding (%)	Postpartum bleeding (%)	Menorrhagia (%)
Plug et al. [2]	274 HA/HB	8	21	60	27	28	NA	57
Olsson et al. [9]	126 107HA/19HB	3	32	12	30	32	24	37
Paroskie et al. [10]	44 HA	19	25	50	72	48	30	67
James et al. [11]	168 155HA/13 HB	9	16	49	39	20	30	64

HA hemophilia A, *HB* hemophilia B, *NA* not available

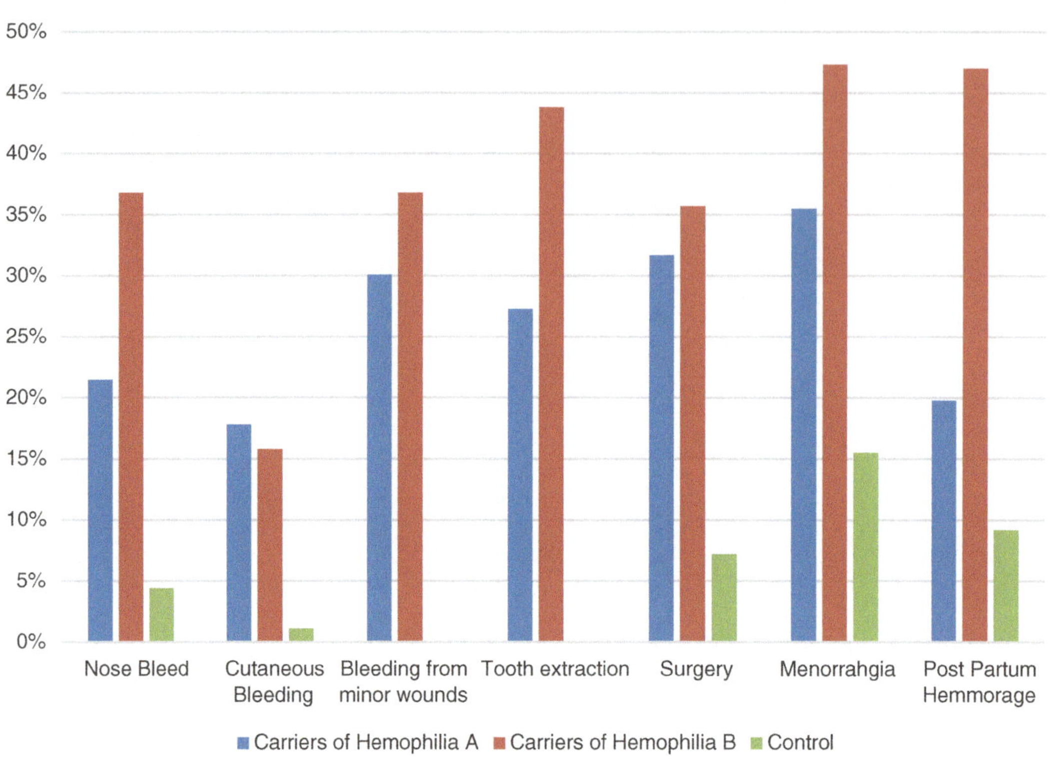

Fig. 9.1 Hemorrhagic symptoms among hemophilia carriers and controls (adapted from Olsson et al. [9])

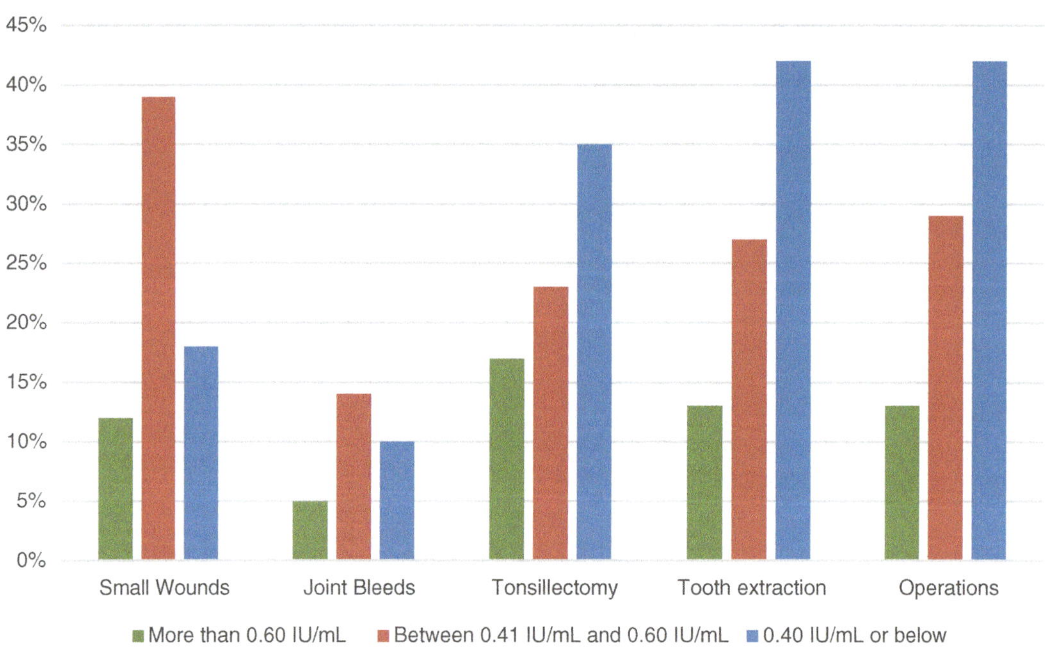

Fig. 9.2 Bleeding symptoms according to clotting factor level in hemophilia carriers and noncarriers (adapted from Plug et al. [2])

9.2.1 Surgeries

A complex and chronic condition like hemophilia requires specialized treatment throughout the individual's lifespan and can only be achieved in a comprehensive care setting with access to a multidisciplinary team of specialist. This is the standard of care for our male patients with hemophilia, and the same recommendation should apply to hemophilia carriers. For years many clinicians have underestimated the bleeding risk of carriers, especially during trauma and surgery, putting them at increased risk of bleeding complications. For this reason, preoperative planning is crucial for a successful outcome [12].

In regard to treatment, hemophilia carriers should be managed with the same medications and dosing as male carriers when it comes to surgical procedures (Table 9.3).

9.2.2 Pregnancy

Carriers of hemophilia remain at an increased risk of bleeding during pregnancy and delivery when compared to noncarriers, despite a natural shift towards a procoagulant state in the hemostatic balance that occurs during the course of a pregnancy with the physiological increase of many coagulation factors, including factor VIII, von Willebrand factor, and to a lesser extent, factor IX. The increase in FVIII level is variable and although it might be within normal range, levels may still be insufficient in some women. In the postpartum period, FVIII levels decrease by the third day and return to basal levels between 7 and 21 days [4]. Factor IX levels during pregnancy have minimal variation, which could pose an increased risk of hemorrhagic complications in hemophilia B carriers. Challenges with hemostasis most often occur at time of delivery, third stage of labor, and postpartum period, and not typically during the antepartum period. Carriers are not believed to be at an increased risk of pregnancy loss; however, establishment of care with a Hemophilia Treatment Center early in pregnancy is recommended for anticipatory guidance in the event of spontaneous early pregnancy loss with need for possible uterine evacuation, in which hemostatic therapy may be indicated. Bleeding risk associated with pregnancy in the general population (non-hemophilia) varies between 6% and 18%.

Table 9.3 Hemophilia carriers: management of pregnancy, delivery, and postpartum period

Stages of pregnancy	Management
Preconception	• Counseled prior to pregnancy regarding carrier status • Causative mutation identified through genetic testing • Baseline clotting factor level measured
Antepartum[a]	• Determine sex of fetus by ultrasound • Delivery plan dictated by sex of fetus • Assess clotting factor level in 3rd trimester (30–34 weeks), ≥80% sufficient for delivery
Delivery[b]	• Male fetus—avoid instrumental vaginal deliveries • Female fetus—no restrictions during delivery • Unassisted vaginal delivery recommended, emergency cesarean if second stage of labor prolonged or suspected fetal distress • Factor concentrate for hemostatic support indicated if FVIII/FIX levels <50%. Targeted peak clotting factor level at delivery 100% • Option of neuraxial anesthesia with factor levels >80%
Postpartum	• Factor concentrate for hemostatic support indicated if FVIII/FIX levels <50%. Targeted trough level >50% for 3 days (vaginal delivery) and 5 days (cesarean delivery) • Tranexamic acid 1300 mg po every 8 h for 7 days

[a] If minor bleeding symptoms occur, DDAVP may be safely used in first and second trimester for FVIII carriers. Aminocaproic acid and tranexamic acid are not recommended for use during pregnancy

[b] DDAVP should be avoided at time of delivery, given risk for hypotension in mother and hyponatremia in both mother and infant

Nau et al. described a multicenter study looking at complications during pregnancy and delivery in 104 hemophilia carriers. During the 5-year study, 30% of women had bleeding events from a total of 124 pregnancies and 117 deliveries.

Sixteen percent of the deliveries had bleeding complications during pregnancy or primary postpartum or both, and cesarean section was the only variable independently associated with bleeding in this period. Eleven percent of the bleeding occurred during secondary postpartum and low basal factor level, cesarean section, and age (younger women at higher risk) were independently associated with bleeding. Low basal factor level (<0.4 IU/mL) was also a risk factor for secondary postpartum bleeding [4].

In another study, Chi and collaborators review the complications, management, and outcome of pregnant hemophilia carriers over a 10-year period following the development of multidisciplinary guidelines in the United Kingdom. Fifty-three carriers (41 hemophilia A and 12 hemophilia B) were included in the study. Interestingly, 8% of the hemophilia A carriers and 50% of hemophilia B carriers had factor levels ≤50 IU/dL at term, requiring treatment with FVIII or FIX during labor and delivery. Primary postpartum hemorrhage was reported in 19% of the patients, two which occurred after vaginal delivery complicated with retained placenta and seven with cesarean section [13].

Overall, pregnant female carriers seem to have a higher risk of bleeding complications when compared to the general population. Delivery should occur in a facility with appropriate laboratory, pharmacy, and transfusion services support, as well as consulting Hematology service and Neonatology. Clotting factor replacement and other hemostatic agents must be available on-site. Given the unpredictability of labor a spontaneous vaginal delivery cannot be guaranteed. Therefore, discussion regarding alternative birth plan such as cesarean delivery should be considered when an affected or potentially affected infant is anticipated. Infants of hemophilia carriers can be safely delivered vaginally, although forceps and vacuum extraction should be avoided, as well as fetal scalp electrode monitoring, as invasive interventions increase the risk of intracranial hemorrhage in affected infants.

Third stage of labor requires active management to reduce blood loss and incidence of postpartum hemorrhage. Following delivery, clotting factors begin their return to baseline levels, possibly abruptly, therefore women who require clotting factor replacement therapy should continue to receive prophylaxis 3–5 days postpartum. Use of antifibrinolytic therapy is recommended as delayed postpartum hemorrhage is not uncommon and may occur more than two weeks following delivery (Table 9.3).

These are some guidelines for the obstetric management of carriers with hemophilia (adapted from [13]):

1. Establish care in a hemophilia treatment center with multidisciplinary care.
2. Pre-pregnancy counseling.
3. Prenatal diagnosis and fetal gender determination.
4. Measure basal non-pregnant factor levels, at I and III trimester and before any invasive procedure.
5. If pre-labor factor level <50 IU/mL, administer FVIII or FIX accordingly for delivery and postpartum.
6. After delivery, check factor levels once a day if non-pregnant baseline levels are <50 IU/mL and administer FVIII or FIX if necessary.
7. Avoid invasive fetal monitoring techniques and instrumental deliveries in affected male fetuses or when fetal sex or coagulation status, if male, is unknown.
8. Regional block or neuraxial anesthesia can be allowed if factor level is normal.
9. Obtain umbilical cord sample to assess the coagulation status of the newborn.
10. Consider a pediatric hematology consult.
11. Avoid intramuscular injection in affected male infants or if coagulation status is unknown. Can give oral vitamin K and subcutaneous vaccinations.
12. Follow-up care with the hemophilia treatment center.

9.2.3 Other Types of Bleeding

Joint bleeding in hemophilia males is the hallmark of the disease. However, in female carriers hemarthrosis has been taken with skepticism among treaters despite published reports available since 1976 [14]. In the last decade, the number of studies describing joint bleeding in carriers is more defined, although the true prevalence of joint disease in carriers is unknown. Osooli et al. conducted a retrospective study in 539 female carriers from Sweden, where the main study outcomes included joint diagnosis, joint surgery and related hospital admissions. By the age of 60, 37% of the hemophilia A and B carriers with factor levels <40 IU/dL or unknown factor levels had a diagnosis of joint disease compared to only 23% of carriers with a normal factor activity [15]. In the same cohort, similar observation was found in patients requiring joint surgery, those with lower levels were 10 times more likely of having orthopedic surgery compared to normal women. About 1.5% of the carriers underwent hip surgery and 1.0% knee surgery. Sidonio and collaborators reported a cross-sectional study looking at data from the United States public health surveillance project (Universal Data Collection System) from 1998 to 2011. A total of 148 carriers of hemophilia A or B and 303 female controls between the ages of 2–69 years were compared. The mean overall joint range of motion (ROM) was significantly lower in carriers with FVIII levels ≤5% compared to carriers with FVIII levels ≥40%. Loss of ROM was seen as early as 2–8 years of age and more limited, with increasing hemophilia severity. The authors suggest that these patients may be having subclinical bleeding as early as the pre-teen years [16].

9.3 Diagnosis

Similar to the diagnosis of males with hemophilia, assessment of baseline clotting factor is pursued in women thought to be obligatory and possible carriers. The expected mean clotting factor level in carriers of hemophilia is 50% of normal, consistent with exactly 50% suppression of each X-chromosome. However, a wide range in clotting Factor VIII or Factor IX levels can be observed in hemophilia carriers, from <1% to >150%, independent of disease severity within the family. Clotting factor within normal limits should not exclude the diagnosis of carriership. Factor VIII clotting assay variability is often noted with fluctuating estrogen levels, such as in pregnancy or hormonal contraceptive use, as well as in the setting of physical and mental stress, exercise, and infections. Factor IX clotting assay has less variability, with fluctuation typically noted in the setting of liver impairment. Increasing utilization of chromogenic clotting Factor VIII and Factor IX has also suggested a discrepancy between one-stage assay levels and chromogenic. Suggesting a carrier's baseline level may be lower than initial laboratory assessment, given that one-stage assay has demonstrated a high intra-laboratory variation as compared to chromogenic assays.

Given considerable clotting factor variability in hemophilia carriers, with approximately only one-third of hemophilia carriers manifesting deficient Factor VIII or Factor IX levels [16], genetic testing is now considered the standard for hemophilia carrier diagnosis. Diagnosis is made by gene mutation analysis, identifying the specific disease-causing variant in either the Factor VIII or Factor IX gene, thereby providing the most accurate method of carriership diagnosis.

Prior to the availability of DNA analysis in the 1980s, pedigree analysis and clotting Factor VIII and Factor IX levels were applied for diagnosing hemophilia carrier status. Pedigree analysis is important in the detection of obligatory and potential carriers, by identifying females that would benefit from clotting factor studies and bleeding symptom assessment. Family history may also guide genetic testing options, such as targeted-variant testing in instances where a specific mutation has been previously identified in affected family members (Table 9.4).

Assessment of carrier status is often recommended in early childhood prior to menarche to allow establishment of care with a hemophilia treatment center that can provide adequate treatment and management of potential bleeding symptoms. Therefore, assessing bleeding risk is standard in all obligate or potential carriers. As genotyping has become increasingly routine in the diagnosis of hemophilia carriers, there is interest in determining whether genotype influ-

Table 9.4 Carrier detection

Obligatory carriers	Possible carriers
• Daughters of a male with hemophilia • Mothers of one son with hemophilia and at least one other family member with hemophilia (brother, maternal grandfather, uncle, nephew, or cousin) • Mothers of one son with hemophilia and a family member who is a carrier of the hemophilia gene (mother, sister, maternal grandmother, aunt, niece, or cousin) • Mothers of two or more sons with hemophilia	• All daughters of a carrier • Mothers of one son with hemophilia who have no other family members who either have or are carriers of hemophilia • Sisters, mothers, maternal grandmothers, aunts, nieces, and female cousins of carriers
Genetic testing	
Factor VIII gene mutation previously identified in family? • Yes—perform targeted familial mutation testing • No—determine clinical severity of affected family member – Unknown or Severe hemophilia A—intron 1 and 22 inversion mutation analysis – Mild or moderate hemophilia A—factor VIII next-generation sequencing Factor IX gene mutation previously identified in family? • Yes—perform targeted familial mutation testing • No—factor IX next-generation sequencing – Recommend performing baseline clotting factor levels both one-stage and chromogenic prior to or at the time of genetic testing	

ences the bleeding phenotype of carriers. Although new data is constantly emerging, thus far the clinical phenotype of a carrier is not solely determined by genotype or clotting factor levels.

9.4 Bleeding Tools: The International Society on Thrombosis and Hemostasis (ISTH)-Bleeding Assessment Tool (BAT)

Hemophilia carriers were previously considered to be clinically asymptomatic in terms of bleeding symptoms; however, emerging studies have demonstrated that despite a variability in clotting factor activity and no clear correlation between genotype and phenotype, carriers do in fact express a bleeding phenotype. Therefore, a distinctive bleeding history should guide treatment and management, as severity of previous bleeding symptoms correlates with the risk of future bleeds.

The ISTH-BAT, originally designed for von Willebrand disease (VWD) patients, has been validated for use in hemophilia carriers [11], and is endorsed by the ISTH and has been widely accepted and used by the hemophilia community. The ISTH-BAT is an expert-administered questionnaire, which covers both mucocutaneous and musculoskeletal bleeding using a 0–4 scoring system for each bleeding symptom. The overall bleeding score (BS) is summative, and scores of ≥4 for men and ≥6 for women are considered positive or abnormal [17]. Alternatively, a Self-BAT may be utilized with recent studies suggesting correlating bleed scores between Self-BAT and those generated from an expert-administered BAT. Cutaneous bleeding, heavy menstrual bleeding, and prolonged bleeding after invasive procedures and childbirth are common findings noted on ISTH-BAT assessment in hemophilia carriers [11]. As with any assessment tool, there are limitations of the ISTH-BAT, with inevitable subjective bias influenced by symptom awareness, barriers to healthcare, as well as cultural and education backgrounds. Symptoms may be unrecognized, as well as undertreated, thus lowering overall bleeding score.

ISTH-BAT should be performed prior to or at the time of pursuing clotting factor assay and/or genetic testing. ISTH-SCC Bleeding Assessment Tool can be accessed: https://bleedingscore.certe.nl/

9.5 Treatment

Bleeding symptoms should be treated similarly to males diagnosed with hemophilia and although there is a wide range of clotting factor level variability noted in carriers, previous bleeding history established through the use of a standardized bleeding assessment tool such as the ISTH-BAT can assist with formulation of treatment strategies. Bleeding symptom management is best

Table 9.5 Management of bleeding symptoms

Types of bleeding	
Gynecological and obstetrical bleeding	Other types of bleeding
• Heavy, prolonged menstrual bleeding • Abnormal, irregular vaginal bleeding • Hemorrhagic ovarian cyst • Postpartum bleeding	• Easy bruising • Epistaxis • Bleeding from minor wounds • Prolonged bleeding after tooth extraction • Significant bleeding after trauma or surgery • Bleeding into joints and muscles
Treatment	
Hemostatic therapies	Route, dose, frequency
Antifibrinolytic agents	Minor bleeding symptoms Oral • Tranexamic acid 1300 mg po every 8 h • Aminocaproic acid 100 mg/kg po every 6 h Major bleeding symptoms (surgical prophylaxis) Intravenous • Tranexamic acid 10 mg/kg IV every 6–8 h for 5–7 days • Aminocaproic acid 100 mg/kg IV every 4–6 h for 5–7 days
Hormonal therapies	• Combined hormonal contraceptives • Progesterone only contraceptives • Levonorgestrel releasing IUD
Desmopressin • Only indicated for hemophilia A carriers • DDAVP trial recommended	Minor bleeding symptoms Intranasal >50 kg: 150 mcg spray in each nostril daily for no more than 3 consecutive days ≤50 kg: single 150 mcg spray daily for no more than 3 consecutive days Major bleeding symptoms (Surgical prophylaxis) Intravenous 0.3 mcg/kg IV in 30–50 ml of NS over 30 min • Hyponatremia may complicate repeated DDAVP dosing
Factor concentrates • 1 IU/kg will increase FVIII level approximately 2% • 1 IU/kg will increase FIX level approximately 0.8–1%	Minor bleeding symptoms Hemophilia A carriers 25–50 IU/kg IV Hemophilia B carriers 20–40 IU/kg IV Major bleeding symptoms Hemophilia A carriers 50 IU/kg IV Hemophilia B carriers 50–100 IU/kg IV Surgical prophylaxis Hemophilia A carriers 50 IU/kg IV Hemophilia B carriers 80–100 IU/kg IV

provided by a Hemophilia Treatment Center care team, as non-hemophilia specialists often underestimate severity of bleeding symptoms. Bleeding in carriers can be grouped into two general categories: gynecological and obstetrical bleeding, and other types of bleeding with severity of symptoms dictating treatment (Table 9.5).

9.6 Conclusion

Hemophilia carrier status is a diagnosis that requires a multidisciplinary team that can develop a treatment plan and share management of congenital bleeding disorder with both patient and family. Women and young girls face specific challenges associated with reproduction and menses that require a care team, all of whom are knowledgeable in the management of women with bleeding disorders. Appropriate treatment strategies can effectively reduce bleeding symptoms, thereby reducing overall morbidity, hospitalizations, and mortality, as well as improving quality of life. Similar to males diagnosed with hemophilia, a carrier's care team should include a Hematologist, Nurse, Social Worker, and Genetic Counselor. A physician specialized in physical and rehabilitation medicine and a physical therapist may be required for carriers who may experience a musculoskeletal bleed event. Comprehensive care with a Hemophilia Treatment Center is recommended for carriers at least once a year with supportive services accessible as needed.

References

1. Iorio A, Stonebraker JS, Chambost H, Makris M, Coffin D, Herr C, et al. Establishing the prevalence and prevalence at birth of hemophilia in males: a meta-analytic approach using national registries. Ann Intern Med. 2019;171:540–6.
2. Plug I, Mauser-Bunschoten EP, Bröcker-Vriends AH, Ploos van Amstel HK, van der Bom JG, van Diemen-Homanet JEM, et al. Bleeding in carriers of hemophilia. Blood. 2006;108:52–6.
3. Shahbazi S, Moghaddam-Banaem L, Ekhtesari F, Ala FA. Impact of inherited bleeding disorders on pregnancy and postpartum hemorrhage. Blood Coagul Fibrinolysis. 2012;23:603–7.
4. Nau A, Gillet B, Guillet B, Beurrier P, Ardillon L, Cussac V, et al. Bleeding complications during pregnancy and delivery in haemophilia carriers and their neonates in Western France: an observational study. Haemophilia. 2020;26:1046–55.
5. Di Michele DM, Gibb C, Lefkowitz JM, Ni Q, Gerber LM, Ganguly A. Severe and moderate haemophilia A and B in US females. Haemophilia. 2014;20:e136–43.
6. Gilbert L, Paroskie A, Gailani D, Debaun MR, Sidonio RF. Haemophilia A carriers experience reduced health-related quality of life. Haemophiliia. 2015;21:761–5.
7. Kadir RA, Sabin CA, Pollard D, Lee CA, Economides DL. Quality of life during menstruation in patients with inherited bleeding disorders. Haemophilia. 1998;4:836–41.
8. James P. Women and bleeding disorders: diagnostic challenges. Hematology. 2020;2020:547–52.
9. Olsson A, Hellgren M, Berntorp E, Ljung R, Baghaei F. Clotting factor level is not a good predictor of bleeding in carriers of haemophilia A and B. Blood Coagul Fibrinolysis. 2014;25:471–5.
10. Paroskie A, Gailani D, DeBaun MR, Sidonio RF Jr. A cross-sectional study of bleeding phenotype in haemophilia A carriers. Br J Haematol. 2015;170:223–8.
11. James PD, Mahlangu J, Bidlingmaier C, Mingot-Castellano ME, Chitlur M, Fogarty PF, et al. Evaluation of the utility of the ISTH-BAT in haemophilia carriers: a multinational study. Haemophilia. 2016;22:912–8.
12. Escobar M, Brewer A, Caviglia H, Forsyth A, Jimenez-Yuste V, Laudenbach L, et al. Recommendations on multidisciplinary management of elective surgery in people with haemophilia. Haemophilia. 2018;24:693–702.
13. Chi C, Lee CA, Shiltagh N, Khan A, Pollard D, Kadir RA. Pregnancy in carriers of haemophilia. Haemophilia. 2008;14:56–64.
14. Graham JB, Miller CH, Reisner HM, Elston RC, Olive JA. The phenotypic range of hemophilia A carriers. Am J Hum Genet. 1976;28:482–8.
15. Osooli M, Donfield SM, Carlsson DS, Baghaei F, Holmström M, Berntorp E, et al. Joint comorbidities among Swedish carriers of haemophilia: a register-based cohort study over 22 years. Haemophilia. 2019;25:845–50.
16. Sidonio R, Mili F, Li T, Miller C, Miller CH, Hooper WC, DeBaun MR, et al. Females with FVIII and FIX deficiency have reduced joint range of motion. Am J Hematol. 2014;89:831–6.
17. Elbatarny M, Mollah S, Grabell J, Bae S, Deforest M, Tuttle A, et al. Normal range of bleeding scores for the ISTH-BAT: adult and pediatric data from the merging project. Haemophilia. 2014;20:831–5.

Suggested Reading

d'Oirin R, O'Brien S, James A. Women and girls with haemophilia: Lessons learned. Haemophilia. 2021;27(3):75–81.

Noone D, Skouw-Rasmussen N, Lavin M, van Galen KPM, Kadir RA. Barriers and challenges faced by women with congenital bleeding disorders in Europe: Results of a patient survey conducted by the European Haemophilia Consortium. Haemophilia. 2019;25:468–74.

Rodeghiero F, Tosetto A, Abshire T, Arnold DM, Coller B, James P, et al. ISTH/SSC bleeding assessment tool: a standardized questionnaire and a proposal for a new bleeding score for inherited bleeding disorders. J Thromb Haemost. 2010;8:2063–5.

Street AM, Ljung R, Lavery AS. Management of carriers and babies with haemophilia. Haemophilia. 2008;14(3):181–7.

Young J, Grabell J, Tuttle A, Bowman M, Hopman WM, Good D, et al. Evaluation of the self-administered bleeding assessment tool (Self-BAT) in haemophilia carriers and correlations with quality of life. Haemophilia. 2017;23:536–8.

Pharmacoeconomic Aspects in Hemophilia

10

Jose A. Romero-Garrido, Marta Ayllón-Morales, Nuria Blázquez-Ramos, and Miguel Escario-Gómez

10.1 Introduction

Hemophilia is a genetic disease characterized by a deficit or absence of clotting factors due to mutations occurring on chromosome X. The main types of hemophilia are hemophilia A, caused by a deficiency of factor VIII (FVIII) and hemophilia B caused by a deficiency of Factor IX (FIX). The characteristic phenotype in both hemophilias is the bleeding tendency. The severity of bleeding manifestations in hemophilia generally correlates with the degree of the clotting factor deficiency [1]:

- Severe hemophilia: clotting factor level is less than 1%. It is usually characterized by spontaneous bleeding episodes.
- Moderate hemophilia: clotting activity factor is between 1 and 5%. It is characterized by the occurrence of spontaneous bleeding episodes occasionally, and in cases of severe trauma or surgery.
- Mild hemophilia: clotting factor level exceeds 5%. Bleeding is infrequent and typically occurs only after injury, trauma, or surgery.

J. A. Romero-Garrido (✉) · M. Ayllón-Morales
N. Blázquez-Ramos · M. Escario-Gómez
Department of Pharmacy, La Paz University Hospital, Madrid, Spain
e-mail: josea.romero@salud.madrid.org

Bleeding episodes can occur in any part of the body but most often occur in the muscles and joints such as knees, ankles, elbows, and hips. Repeated bleeding in the joints causes, in the medium and long term, highly disabling sequelae known as hemophilic arthropathy. Hemophilic arthropathy may significantly limit mobility and generate severe deformities that sometimes require minimally invasive surgical techniques such as synoviorthesis or complex surgical techniques such as the implantation of joint prostheses [2–4].

The therapeutic management of hemophilic patients is complicated, especially if they suffer from hemophilic arthropathy because the therapeutic options are limited. The optimal treatment for patients with hemophilia is the prevention of hemorrhagic episodes through prophylactic treatment to avoid the appearance of joint and muscular sequelae. When joint health degenerates, the administration of exogenous coagulation factor does not solve mobility problems. In addition, this therapeutic option involves a high economic cost, due to the constant administration of high-priced factor concentrates. Surgical techniques have the advantage of being able to recover, at least in part, the patient's mobility, relieving pain and stopping the constant bleeding from the affected joint. However, in order to perform the surgical technique, it is necessary to strictly control the patient's perioperative and postoperative hemostasis. This hemostatic control must be car-

E. C. Rodríguez-Merchán (ed.), *Advances in Hemophilia Treatment*,
https://doi.org/10.1007/978-3-030-93990-8_10

ried out by administering factor concentrates, which has a high economic impact.

In this respect, the pharmacoeconomic analysis of hemophilia treatments may be interesting, mainly due to the high costs that the different therapeutic options can entail, which are not always affordable for healthcare systems.

10.2 Economic Evaluations in Healthcare

Healthcare systems in different countries have the need to cope with an ever-increasing healthcare demand with increasingly limited resources. The economic evaluations of health interventions are the essential tools for carrying out this work.

The economic evaluation studies are very important although they can be very complex, as they involve the quantification of each of the factors that may be affected by a particular intervention.

However, there are other simpler studies that may provide a closer view of the economic reality of a health intervention, warning of possible overspending.

Canada was one of the pioneering countries in conducting health economic evaluations. The Canadian Coordinating for Health Technology Assessment (CCOHTA) draft "Guidelines for economic evaluation of pharmaceuticals" that describe the methodology of the different economic evaluation models to encourage the appropriate use of health technology by influencing decision-maker [5].

There are other national agencies that establish criteria for the selection and use of drugs financed by national health systems. In Europe, the main agencies are the British National Institute for Health and Clinical Excellence (NICE), the Scottish Medicines Consortium (SMC), the Institut für Qualität und im Wirtschaftlichkeit Gesundheitswesen (IQWIG) in Germany and Haute Authorité de Santé (HAS) in France.

In Spain, there is no official agency that includes economic evaluation to establish health interventions such as financing by the National Health System. However, the Spanish Ministry of Health elaborated two publications that address economic evaluations: "Methods for the economic evaluation of new supplies," published in 2003 and "Proposed guideline for economic evaluation of health technologies," published in 2006 [6, 7].

A high percentage of the economic resources in healthcare is the cost of medicines used in the different pathologies. This fact and the absence of Spanish agency to carry out the economic evaluation has highlighted the fundamental role of Pharmacy Services of Spanish medical centers in the search for pharmacological efficiency (greater therapeutic benefit at lower cost), using the pharmacoeconomic as a toll. In this analysis, therapeutic alternatives will be compared in terms of costs and benefits [8].

10.3 Types of Economic Evaluations

The term "economic evaluations" usually implies the economic comparison of various therapeutic alternatives. However, there are other types of studies that, without comparing therapeutic alternatives, can improve the efficiency of pharmacological therapy such as the analysis of the pharmaceutical bill and budget impact studies. These evaluations are of great interest in pharmacological groups that have a high economic impact on the pharmaceutical budget for treatment of a small number of patients. This situation occurs with the pharmacological treatment of hemophiliac patients, whose annual cost per patient can exceed 200,000 €, being even higher if orthopedic surgery is performed. Consumption of clotting factor concentrates implies more than 90% of the cost of surgery.

Budget impact analysis can be defined as a quantitative estimate of the expected deviation in healthcare expenditure for a healthcare intervention [9, 10]. To determine the budgetary impact must know the total number of patients undergoing this health intervention or the total number of health interventions. These estimates are useful for decision-making and are the most valued by the Directors and Managers of healthcare centers.

Complete economic evaluations include comparison of at least two alternatives and involve the analysis of costs and the health consequences of both. The choice of comparator is crucial to obtain an incremental cost-effectiveness value. The comparator should be the best therapeutic alternative. If the economic assessment is based on clinical trials, the outcome variable would be efficacy and if it is based on data obtained in routine clinical practice, it would be the effectiveness.

A major concept in economics is opportunity cost, in other words, the forgone benefit that would have been derived by an option not chosen. To properly evaluate opportunity costs, the costs and benefits of every option available must be considered and weighed against the others. Cost information can be obtained from official publications, analytical accounting of healthcare facilities or market prices.

Economic evaluations approach costs in a common format, they differ in the way they approach benefits. The main forms of economic evaluation include cost-minimization analysis (CMA), cost–benefit analysis (CBA), cost-effectiveness análisis (CEA), and cost–utility analysis (CUA) (Table 10.1).

CMA refers to the simple comparison of cost between two interventions. This form of analysis should only be used when the consequences between two interventions are assumed to be the same, which is unusual and therefore infrequently used.

In CBA, the costs and benefits of an intervention are valued in monetary terms. This type of analysis is not useful in healthcare because it is difficult to assign monetary values to health outcomes.

CEA assesses the consequences of alternative interventions using clinical outcomes in "natural units." In hemophilia, intermediate clinical outcomes can be measured as the number of avoided bleeding, or clinical outcomes such as years of life gained in case of orthopedic surgery. This type of economic evaluation should compare incremental costs and effects, meaning the additional cost that one alternative imposes compared to the additional benefit it delivers. It is expressed as the "Incremental Cost-Effectiveness Ratio" (ICER), which is calculated by dividing the incremental cost of the new intervention by the incremental change in effectiveness.

$$\text{ICER} = \frac{\text{Costs}_1 - \text{Costs}_2}{\text{Effects}_1 - \text{Effects}_2}$$

A variant of the CEA is the CUA that considers the patient's quality of life as an outcome in addition to efficacy. In this economic evaluation, the benefit is usually measured in quality-adjusted life year (QALY). The interpretation of the results is very similar to that of the CEA, and an incremental analysis should be performed.

Table 10.2 shows an example of a cost–utility analysis to compare the cost and effectiveness of a new treatment. The scenario involves an adult hemophiliac patient with advanced knee arthropathy with an indication for total knee replacement. The patient's four alternatives are:

1. Keep the patient without treatment at zero cost but without any QALY.
2. Maintain with prophylaxis replacement therapy at an annual cost of €200,000 to correct the bleeding from the injured joint. In this case we assume that he would have 10 QALY gained. The result would be an incremental cost of €200,000 over the first assumption (no treatment). Each QALY would cost €20,000.
3. Maintain the patient with on-demand replacement therapy at a cost of €100,000 and 9 QALY gained. The results compared to prophylaxis treatment would be a cost increase of €100,000 with 1 QALY gained. The cost of each QALY gained from prophylaxis treatment versus demand would cost €100,000.
4. Perform knee prosthesis implantation with an assumed cost of €300,000 but with 20 QALY gained. The surgery versus prophylaxis replacement therapy would mean an increase of 10 QALY gained and a cost of €10,000 for each QALY gained.

In this case, the most favorable option from the pharmacoeconomic point of view would be the implantation of a knee prosthesis.

Table 10.1 Types of economic evaluation

Type of evaluation	Cost measurement	Outcome measurement	Focus
Cost-minimization analysis	Any currency	Assumed or demonstrated equivalent effects	Efficiency
Cost–benefit analysis	Any currency	Money	Most beneficial use of limited resources
Cost-effectiveness analysis	Any currency	Usual clinical units (e.g., life-years gained)	Least costly way to achieve an objective
Cost–utility analysis	Any currency	Usual clinical units (QALY)	Least costly way to achieve an QALY gain

Table 10.2 Costs, outcomes, and cost-effectiveness of different treatment alternatives for a supposed adult hemophiliac patient with knee arthropathy who is a candidate for total knee prosthesis implantation

Bought alternatives	Costs (€)	Results (QALY)	Rising costs	Increased QALY	ICER (€/QALY)
Without pretreatment	0	0	200,000	10	20.000
Replacement therapy prophylaxis	200,000	10			
Replacement therapy demand	100,000	9	100,000	1	100.000
Replacement therapy prophylaxis	200,000	10			
Replacement therapy prophylaxis	200,000	10	100,000	10	10.000
Treatment of prosthetic implant	300,000	20			

Cost-effectiveness studies alone are not valid for decision-making, since it is not the same to assume high costs in a context of economic prosperity as in situations of economic crisis. Therefore, economic evaluations are not intended to determine whether a treatment or technique should be applied. Their sole purpose is to facilitate decision-making in the choice of an alternative in an efficient manner.

One issue to be taken into account in economic evaluations is the temporal space. Costs and benefits rarely occur at the same time. In this regard, the introduction of a prophylactic treatment or the implantation of a joint prosthesis in a hemophilic patient involves an immediate increase in cost, but a long-term benefit. This can be an obstacle, since immediate benefits are usually preferred. Therefore, benefits and costs cannot be separated from the time period in which they occur.

The application of the so-called discount rate in economic evaluation takes into account these temporary circumstances, since costs and benefits arising in the future are valued less. The discount rate applied usually varies from country to country, although it ranges between 3% and 5%. This is of great importance when transferring the results of a pharmacoeconomic study carried out in one country to another country. These results should be interpreted with caution.

The robustness of the results in economic evaluation studies is supported by sensitivity analyses. This type of analysis is necessary in CEA, because the very nature of the studies assumes values of variables that are not verified in the analysis, creating uncertainties in the results. To minimize these uncertainties, it is necessary to accompany the results of the variables involved with a range of estimates, keeping the others constant. If, after incorporation of the different estimates, the conclusions do not change substantially, the study can be considered very reliable and solid conclusions.

10.4 Costs of Prophylaxis in Hemophilia

The optimal treatment for hemophilia, and especially for severe hemophilia, is prophylaxis treatment. This consists of frequent intravenous administration of deficient clotting factor with the aim of achieving blood levels of factor always above 1%. In patients at higher risk this minimum value can be increased, for example, in patients with advanced arthropathy or with high levels of physical activity.

These frequent doses represent a high cost and require careful individualization to provide adequate care at the lowest cost.

The high cost of these treatments has limited their widespread use, especially in countries with fewer resources, and has represented a significant percentage of the total pharmaceutical expenditure of many hospital centers.

The budgetary impact of hemophilia prophylaxis treatment is influenced by several factors:

a. The number of patients susceptible to be treated with this type of treatment. Centers with many hemophilia patients on prophylaxis must make a significant economic effort to maintain these treatments adequately.
b. The age of the patients. Since treatment is dosed by weight, the budgetary impact of treatment of patients before adolescence is lower and more affordable than the treatment in adult patients.

   It would be possible, in patients over 35–40 years of age and with low physical activity, to readjust the dosing regimens by spacing them out and thus reduce the cost of treatment without increasing the risk for the patient.

   Analyses carried out in our center have shown over the years that the cost per hemophilic patient in prophylaxis is minimal from 0 to 5 years of age and increases with age until it reaches a maximum at 20 years of age. After this age, the cost decreases slightly until 45–50 years of age and then is maintained. Therefore, the distribution of patients to be treated according to age is another important parameter to consider in the distribution of economic resources to maintain the prophylaxis treatment of patients with hemophilia.
c. The type of drug used. Patients treated with recombinant drugs involve a greater economic effort than those treated with plasma derivatives.

The cost differences between recombinant and plasma treatments in children are small, but care must be taken if starting with recombinant treatments, since the differences between the two options will be much greater as the child grows.

In recent years, new extended half-life recombinant therapies have emerged. These drugs allow less frequent administrations as they remain longer in the blood. A good optimization of the dosage of these drugs, using pharmacokinetic tools, can reduce the costs of treatment with recombinant drugs, although they will always exceed the costs of plasma treatments.

A new prophylactic treatment for subcutaneous administration has recently become available. This new therapeutic option also involves a high cost, although in adults with high doses of recombinant treatments, this new therapeutic option, administered weekly or fortnightly, can lead to savings.

To optimize economic resources in the prophylaxis treatment of patients with hemophilia, an individualized analysis of each of the factors analyzed in this section is necessary. In this way the cost of hemophilia prophylaxis can be optimized according to weight and age, type of drug, pharmacokinetic adjustment, and adherence control. Considering these factors, we can improve the efficiency of prophylaxis treatment of hemophilia patients, improving their musculoskeletal health and quality of life.

10.5 Costs of Orthopedic Surgery in Patients with Hemophilia

Most patients diagnosed with hemophilia who undergo orthopedic surgery should be treated throughout the surgical procedure with concentrated clotting factor to control its hemostasis. The high cost of drugs used as concentrates of clotting factors increases the total cost of the process significantly. In this sense it can be assumed that over 90% of the total cost of the intervention is due to the drug therapy used. Thus, considering only the costs of concentrates drugs used, one can obtain a fairly accurate estimate of the economic realities involved in such interventions in this group of patients.

Our experience, as a team that attends to the processes of these patients, includes more than 100 surgical processes, which in the Spanish context, have involved a total cost of more than 5 million euros in the last 10 years.

Among the surgeries performed are mainly: minor surgery such as arthroscopy and major surgery such as orthopedic knee or hip implants. The cost of each of these surgeries can vary greatly (Fig. 10.1).

These costs may vary depending on several factors. These include: the severity of the coagulopathy, the patient's weight, the type of surgery, and the type of medication used.

Depending on these factors, the cost of arthroscopic surgery can be between 20,000 and 30,000 euros and that of major surgery between 40,000 and 50,000 euros. The implantation of a hip prosthesis, in turn, is 2–3% more expensive than that of a knee prosthesis.

These costs are estimates, include only the perioperative period and do not consider postoperative hemostatic requirements such as those necessary for the rehabilitation process.

10.6 Quality and Cost of Drug Replacement Therapy Used During Orthopedic Surgeries in Patients with Hemophilia

The problems in the efficient use of drug therapies can be classified into three categories: underuse, overuse, and inadequate use.

- Underuse can be defined as the omission of a care intervention when it would have produced a clear benefit for the patient and possibly a subsequent cost saving.
- For example, not starting a prophylactic treatment or not performing a surgical intervention for the implantation of a joint prosthesis in a hemophilic patient at a specified time can lead to the need t o overuse other pharmacological resources. In this sense, a patient without prophylaxis who develops successive bleeds in a target joint, would require high amounts of coagulation factor to control them, which would have a significant budgetary impact, and a deterioration in the patient's quality of life. However, the introduction of prophylaxis or the implantation of a hip or knee prosthesis, at the appropriate time, could mean the

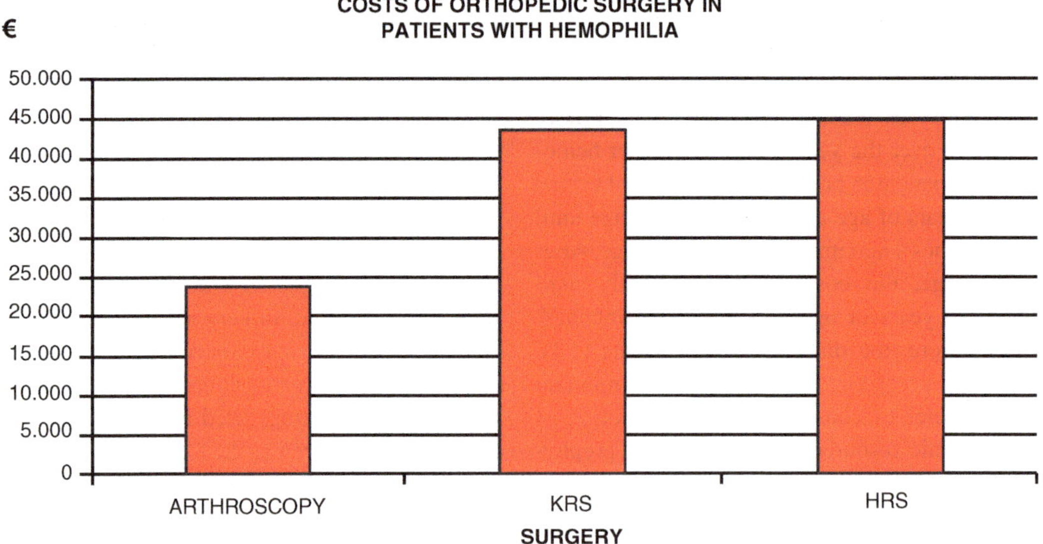

Fig. 10.1 Fee associated with each type of surgery, in the Spanish context. *HRS* hip replacements surgery, *KRS* knee replacement surgery

absence or cessation of bleeding in that target joint, and therefore a subsequent decrease in the consumption of coagulation factor in that patient. Although initially the prophylaxis or surgery would suppose an important economic expense, this could be amortized, in a reasonable period and would manage to improve the patient's quality of life.

- In our center, in recent years, the number of patients with prophylactic treatment has increased and numerous surgeries have been performed4, which initially meant a significant increase in cost. But at present practically all patients with prophylaxis or who have undergone surgery have reduced their consumption of coagulation factor very significantly. This has meant an important economic saving and a notable increase in the quality of life of these patients.
- Overuse is defined as the utilization of pharmacological resources in circumstances in which the cost exceeds the potential benefits. This increases the expenditure of economic resources unnecessarily.
- In these situations and taking again the example of orthopedic surgeries in hemophiliac patients, the administration of coagulation factors in continuous infusion during the postoperative period can save money compared to bolus administration, achieving adequate plasma factor levels without fluctuations. In this case, bolus administration is more costly because to maintain adequate plasma levels it requires administration with peaks exceeding the desired concentration.
- Inappropriate use of drugs can produce avoidable undesirable effects in patients and lead to increased costs. Poor adherence to treatment, inadequate doses or type of factor can lead to complications in patient management.

An example of this case may be the administration of insufficient doses of clotting factor during surgery. Due to the low factor coverage, the injury would be more likely to bleed and become complicated with an infection. This would require further surgery to resolve it.

The economic evaluation of the different alternatives that may occur in each process, represented by decision trees, allows us to take the most appropriate and cost-effective decision to achieve the best results for the patient at the lowest cost.

The appropriate use of pharmacological therapies requires close monitoring of patients, the development of treatment protocols, and adequate economic forecasting and evaluation.

- Analyze the short- and long-term benefits and costs of pharmacological therapies.
- In surgeries is fundamental:
  - Anticipate the pharmacological needs of the surgery to make its provisioning. Consider the increase in expenditure and what it may mean if several surgeries coincide in time.
  - Consider the possibility of simultaneously more than one surgical intervention on the patient, under the same factor coverage.
  - Careful monitoring of the patient, taking advantage of pharmacokinetic information, to maintain adequate factor concentrations in the blood, avoiding peaks or insufficient coverage (Fig. 10.2).

10.7 Economic Evaluations as a Tool in Decision-Making

Decision-making by the professionals involved in healthcare processes is usually complex and subject to doubts, risks, and uncertainties. These situations require the establishment of systematic procedures that facilitate the finding of the most convenient solution to the problem posed.

Conceptually, decision-making in healthcare refers to any process by which a health professional, a manager, or an institutional authority adopts a particular solution to a specific problem, choosing the most appropriate strategy from among all the possibilities.

It is reasonable to accept that the logical sequence to be adopted in the decision-making process, within a context of limited information, would be as follows:

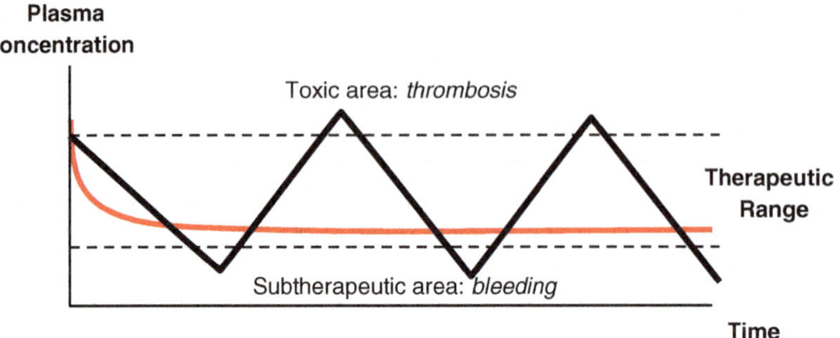

Fig. 10.2 Plasma factor concentration during continuous intravenous infusion (red); plasma factor concentration after bolus administration (black)

a. Identification and definition of the problem.
b. Strategic search for alternative solutions.
c. Evaluation of the benefits and risks of each one.
d. Selection of the most appropriate alternative.

The following case can serve as a model in the use of economic evaluations for decision support in patients with hemophilia who may develop hemophilic arthropathy and be susceptible to orthopedic surgeries.

If considering the case of patients with severe hemophilia, we can decide on two therapeutic options: the establishment of an on-demand treatment when bleeding episodes occur, or the establishment of a prophylactic drug treatment. Prophylactic treatment may involve a higher cost in the short term; however, it may result in cost savings and an increase in quality of life throughout the patient's life.

Identifying the problem: the appearance of bleeding that develops arthropathy and eventually requires orthopedic surgery. We must consider a therapeutic alternative such as prophylaxis, which even though it may initially imply a higher cost per patient, it will neutralize the appearance of arthropathy and subsequent orthopedic surgeries, reducing the consumption of drugs used for these procedures. Therefore, the most appropriate solution would be the establishment of a prophylaxis treatment to avoid the appearance of arthropathies.

On the other hand, and analyzing the context of an established arthropathy, we have two therapeutic options: maintenance with coagulation factor replacement therapy or orthopedic surgery for the implantation of a joint prosthesis. We recognize that lifelong maintenance with replacement therapy for successive hemorrhagic episodes in a target joint may involve a higher cost than surgery for the implantation of a joint prosthesis.

We identified the problem: those patients with high consumption of coagulation factor due to successive bleeding in a target joint susceptible to prosthesis implantation. We must develop a strategy that will allow us to find a solution that can minimize the cost for these patients.

Among the solutions, orthopedic surgery for the implantation of a prosthesis to replace the bleeding joint could be considered. In this way, the absence of bleeding in this joint would mean a decrease in the cost of the patient's medication. With this decision, we would obtain the benefit for the patient in relation to his mobility and well-being, in addition to a reduction in the administration of drugs due to the absence of repeated bleeding in the replaced joint. However, it would be necessary to assume a high cost in this patient in a timely manner, to approach the surgery that would have to be covered with coagulation factor in an intensive way in the perioperative process. We would certainly be adopting a decision that would allow us both to increase the patient's well-being in terms of morbidity and to reduce the overall cost of the patient's treatment in the medium and long term, as the patient would no longer require successive administrations of coagulation factor. In this case, we would be selecting the most due to the appropriate alternative to the problem posed.

Therefore, an economic evaluation would lead us to adopt an appropriate decision to solve a problem by analyzing possible alternatives, considering the benefit to the patient at a lower overall cost.

10.8 Pharmacoeconomy and Health Management in the Pharmacological Treatment of Hemophilia

Healthcare represents one of the basic pillars in the social structure of developed countries. Healthcare is one of the fundamental rights of citizens, and therefore one of the priority commitments to be addressed by governments through healthcare managers at all levels:

a. Macro-management: ministries and departments of health.
b. Meso-management: hospital managers, drug information centers and health technology assessment agencies.
c. Micro-management: heads of services and clinical units. Pharmacy and therapeutics commissions, specialized care teams.

Public financing of healthcare is one of the most representative achievements of the welfare state. Its development has contributed to improving health and preventing disease. A very important part of the cost of healthcare in these pathologies is pharmacological therapy, which is the essential basis for the healthcare of patients with hemophilia. Prophylactic therapy with coagulation drugs and orthopedic surgery have reduced morbidity and mortality and improved the quality of life of these patients.

Cost-of-illness studies aim to evaluate the economic impact of healthcare. The results of these studies, combined with epidemiological studies of morbidity and mortality, constitute a useful tool for determining the magnitude of the cost of healthcare. For this reason, the results of health technology and drug evaluations are considered very valuable information prior to the analysis of therapeutic alternatives or available health interventions, as in the case of prophylaxis treatments or orthopedic surgery in patients with hemophilia.

Economic evaluation of drugs identifies, analyzes and compares the costs, benefits, and risks of pharmacological treatments. The cost-effectiveness ratio allows different therapeutic alternatives to be considered in order to achieve a more efficient use of resources.

The drugs used in these treatments have a very important economic impact on the public health system, which is a cause for concern. A universal public health system, which produces welfare without obtaining economic benefits, is obliged to minimize costs in order to ensure its survival.

10.9 Conclusions

Healthcare systems in different countries have the need to cope with an ever-increasing healthcare demand with increasingly limited resources. The pharmacoeconomic analysis of hemophilia treatments is paramount, mainly due to the high costs that the different therapeutic options can entail, which are not always affordable for healthcare systems. There are national agencies that establish criteria for the selection and use of drugs financed by national health systems. A high percentage of the economic resources in healthcare is the cost of medicines used in the different pathologies. This fact and the absence of Spanish agency to carry out the economic evaluation has highlighted the fundamental role of Pharmacy Derpartments of Spanish medical centers in the search for pharmacological efficiency.

References

1. Srivastava A, Santagostino E, Dougall A, Kitchen S, Sutherland M, Pipe SW, et al. WFH guidelines for the management of hemophilia. In: Haemophilia. 3rd ed. Hoboken: Wiley; 2020.
2. Rodriguez-Merchan EC, Jiménez-Yuste V, Goddard NJ. Initial and advanced stages of hemophilic arthropathy and other musculo-skeletal problems: the role of orthopedic surgery. In: Rodriguez-Merchan EC, Valentino LA, editors. Current and future issues in hemophilia care. Oxford: Wiley; 2011. p. 127–32.
3. Rodriguez-Merchan EC. Aspects of current management: orthopedic surgery in haemophilia. Haemophilia. 2012;18:8–16.

4. Quintana-Molina M, Martínez-Bahamonde F, González-García E, Romero-Garrido JA, Villar-Camacho A, Jiménez-Yuste V, et al. Surgey in haemophilic patients with inhibitor: 20 years of experience. Haemophilia. 2004;10(2):30–40.
5. Canadian Coordinating Office for Health Technology Assessment. Guidelines for economic evaluations of pharmaceuticals. 2nd ed. Ottawa: Canadian Coordinating Office; 1997.
6. Pinto Prades JL, Sánchez Martinez FL. Métodos para la evaluación económica de nuevas prestaciones. Madrid: Ministerio de Sanidad y Consumo; 2003.
7. López Bastida J, Oliva J, Antoñanzas F, et al. Propuesta de guía para la evaluación económica aplicada a las tecnologías sanitarias. Madrid: Servicio de Evaluación del Servicio Canario de Salud; 2008.
8. Brosa M, Gisbert R, Rodriguez JM, Soto J. Principios, Métodos, y aplicaciones del análisis del impacto presupuestario en el sector sanitario. PharmacoEconomics. 2002;2:65–78.
9. Romero Garrido JA, Lucia Cuesta JF, Febrer L, Trabal I, Sabater FJ, Lindner L, Herrero A. Study of the costs of inhibitor development in patients with severe haemophilia in Spain. Pharmaoeconomy. https://doi.org/10.1007/s40277-013-0016.
10. Jiménez-Yuste V, Núnez R, Romero JA, Montoro B, Espinós B. Cost-effectiveness of recombinant activated factor VII vs. Plasma-derived prothrombin complex concentrate in the treatment of mild-to-moderate bleeding episodes in patients with severe haemophilia A and inhibitors in Spain. Haemophilia. 2013;19:841–6.

Assessment of Joint Health and Outcome Measures in Hemophilia

11

Hortensia De la Corte-Rodríguez,
Alexander D. Liddle,
and E. Carlos Rodríguez-Merchán

11.1 Introduction

Before commencing therapy in a patient with hemophilia, a global, systematic and complete evaluation of the musculoskeletal (MSK) system should be performed, and information gathered as to the type of hemophilia the patient has and any treatment that is being administered [1]. It is important to approach the MSK system from a holistic perspective, as these patients present with polyarticular bleeds which may involve other parts of the MSK system aside from that the clinician may be focusing upon.

As the development of hemophilic arthropathy is slow and progressive over time, it is essential to comprehensively analyze the MSK aspects of the patient from an early age and to follow them closely throughout life. Detecting and avoiding adverse consequences of each bleeding event is essential.

With the advent of modern hematologic prophylaxis, the hemorrhagic profile of patients has changed radically. Patients may suffer subclinical hemarthrosis that may be undetectable with routine physical or functional tests, but which nonetheless trigger the cascade of hemophilic arthropathy. In this regard it will be possible to detect indirect changes secondary to subclinical bleeds, such as synovitis and articular cartilage damage. These changes, in the early stages, are basically asymptomatic; therefore, it is necessary to make an evaluation aimed at their early detection, with sensitive methods such as ultrasonography (US).

Early recognition of joint damage and disability caused by hemophilia (i.e., in infancy) is essential in order to optimize treatment and make economically sound clinical decisions. Objective evidence of short- and long-term sequelae of disease, and response to different treatment regimens, is required to guide appropriate patient care [2].

The aim of this chapter is to review joint health assessment tools. In addition, the characteristics of the outcome measures used in hemophilia from the perspective of both the health care provider and the patient are reviewed [3].

H. De la Corte-Rodríguez
Department of Physical and Rehabilitation Medicine, La Paz University Hospital, Madrid, Spain

A. D. Liddle
MSK Lab, Imperial College, London, UK

E. C. Rodríguez-Merchán (✉)
Department of Orthopedic Surgery, La Paz University Hospital, Madrid, Spain

11.2 Joint Health and Outcome Assessment Tools in Hemophilia

In patients with hemophilia, a detailed history, clinical examination, instrumented tools, imaging tests, assessment of disease-specific structure

E. C. Rodríguez-Merchán (ed.), *Advances in Hemophilia Treatment*,
https://doi.org/10.1007/978-3-030-93990-8_11

and function, and activity, participation, and quality of life scores are important and should be performed on a regular basis according to the patient's age and clinical status [4].

The assessment of joint health and treatment outcomes is a complex task involving many factors. To include the full spectrum of potential consequences of hemophilia, outcome assessments should follow the International Classification of Functioning, Disability and Health (ICF) proposed by the World Health Organization (WHO) [2, 5]. According to ICF, disability and health assessment should focus on the impact of the disease on body structures and functions, activities, and participation. These domains can be affected by individual contextual factors, which represent a person's circumstances and background. Contextual factors include both environmental factors (facilitating factors and barriers to treatment) and personal factors (which might include co-morbidities, disabilities, and psychological factors) [6], as depicted in the schematic in Fig. 11.1. The ratings for each of these areas are described below. Table 11.1 summarizes the most recommended scales for assessing MSK problems in hemophilia.

11.2.1 Body Structure and Function

Body structure and function refers to changes in anatomical structures and physiological functions of systems. In hemophilia, this refers, for example, to a clotting factor deficit or deficiency or altered range of motion of the joints.

11.2.1.1 Annual Joint Bleeding Rate (AJBR)

The AJBR assesses the number of bleeding episodes over 12 months. Since bleeding rates in patients on hematologic prophylaxis or those with mild to moderate hemophilia are generally low, it is advisable to collect bleeding data prospectively, over a minimum of 12 months in order to ascertain reliable annual bleeding rates. Furthermore, it is recommended to distinguish between major and minor bleeding, and between spontaneous and posttraumatic bleeding [5].

However, AJBR is difficult to assess and has limitations. Patient reports of bleeding, particularly joint bleeding, are by nature subjective, as pain and other joint symptoms may be more reflective of pathologies other than bleeding (such as osteoarthritis, injury, or inflammation). For that reason, AJBR is an imperfect surrogate measure of future joint deterioration, as it only captures clinically recognized bleeding episodes and not subclinical bleeding, which may occur despite intensive hematologic prophylaxis [3]. However, still in many centers, it is the main parameter for making therapeutic decisions, which can lead to incorrect decisions [3, 5].

Fortunately, we currently have simple tools that allow accurate diagnosis of intra-articular bleeding, such as US. US has been shown to be sensitive to soft tissue changes (bleeding, effusions, and synovial hyperplasia), even in those hemarthroses with small volume or blood concentration [7]. Its systematic use when patients present with symptoms suggestive of bleeding

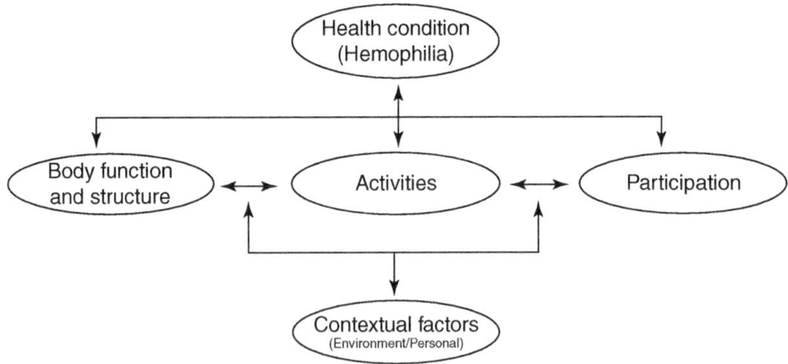

Fig. 11.1 Multidirectional model adopted in the international classification of functioning, disability and health (ICF)

Table 11.1 Recommended scales for assessing musculoskeletal problems in hemophilia

	Specific	Generic
Bleeding	Annual joint bleeding rate (AJBR)	
Pain	Multidimensional Hemophilia Pain Questionnaire (MHPQ) Can be scored through subscales within the quality of life or physical examination tools.	Visual analog scale (VAS) Wong–Baker (FACES) scale McGill Pain Questionnaire Brief Pain Inventory (BPI)
Physical examination	Hemophilia Joint Health Score (HJHS) Gilbert score Colorado Physical Examination Score (CPES) Petrini Joint Score (PJS)	
Echography	Hemophilia Early Arthropathy Detection with Ultrasound (HEAD-US)	
Radiology	Pettersson scale Arnold and Hilgartner scale	
MRI	IPSG compatible scale Denver scale (progressive) European scale (additive)	
Activities and participation	Functional Independence Score in Hemophilia (FISH) Hemophilia Activity List (HAL) Pediatric version of HAL (PedHAL) for children Reported Outcomes, Burdens and Experiences (PROBE)	Up and go test (UGT) Canadian Occupational Performance Measure (COPM) McMaster Toronto Patient Disability Questionnaire (MACTAR) Health Assessment Questionnaire-Disability Index (HAQ-DI)
Quality of life	Hemophilia Well-Being Index Hemophilia-specific QoL questionnaire for adults (HAEMO-QoL-A) Reported Outcomes, Burdens and Experiences (PROBE) Outcomes-Kids Life Assessment Tool (CHO-KLAT) for children	EuroQoL 5 Dimensions (EQ-5D) *Short Form-36* Health Survey (SF-36)
Patient-reported outcomes	Hemophilia Activity List (HAL) Outcomes-Kids Life Assessment Tool (CHO-KLAT) Hemophilia-specific QoL questionnaire for adults (HAEMO-QoL-A) Reported Outcomes, Burdens and Experiences (PROBE) Comprehensive assessment tool of challenges in hemophilia (CATCH)	5-level EuroQoL 5 Dimensions (EQ-5D-5L) Brief Pain Inventory v2 (BPI) International Physical Activity Questionnaire (IPAQ) Short Form 36 Health Survey v2 (SF-36v2) Patient-Reported Outcomes Measurement Information System (PROMIS)

QoL quality of life, *IPSG* International Prophylaxis Study Group

will help us to make a more accurate quantification of the AJBR.

11.2.1.2 Pain Assessment in Hemophilia

In hemophilia, pain is often underdiagnosed and therefore undertreated. It is important to carefully determine the cause of the pain in order to be able to treat the cause. Pain should be assessed and addressed in the context of a comprehensive care setting. Although pain can be scored through subscales within quality of life questionnaires or physical examination instruments, the use of specific pain assessment tools is helpful to be able to give more focused attention to this problem [8].

Hemophilia-related pain can be assessed using unidimensional numerical or visual rating scales, such as the visual analog scale (VAS), the Wong–Baker FACES Scale, or multidimensional pain questionnaires such as the generic McGill Pain

Questionnaire or the Brief Pain Inventory (BPI), or specific instruments such as the Multidimensional Hemophilia Pain Questionnaire (MHPQ) [2].

11.2.1.3 Physical Examination Measurements

In hemophilia patients with arthropathy, physical fitness, muscular strength, aerobic endurance, bone mineralization, and balance are decreased [9]. Hemophilia-specific physical examination scales exist to measure these items, such as the Gilbert scale for adults [10] (Table 11.2) and the Hemophilia Joint Health Score (HJHS) for children and young adults (Table 11.3) [11].

These tools include parameters such as swelling, muscle hypotrophy, crepitus, joint deficit, pain, strength, stability, and gait. But it is also advisable to analyze other aspects that are not reflected in these scales such as postural strength, proprioceptive and balance status, support anomalies, lower limb length discrepancy, rotational anomalies, spinal deformity, neurovascular status, and bimanual ability. These assessments may be especially necessary in children.

The Gilbert joint score, although widely used in clinical and research studies, was never designed for use in patients with minimal arthropathy. It is an additive scale, collecting several parameters to be assessed for each joint [10].

Subsequently, the HJHS was developed which is more sensitive to changes in early joint function. The HJHS underwent formal reliability and validation studies in children with hemophilia aged 4–18 years [11]. Its current version (HJHS 2.1) consists of 8 items for elbows, knees, and ankles, and another for gait, with a maximum global score of 124.

On the other hand, when the patient presents with joint signs and symptoms, these are not specific to hemarthrosis or arthropathy. This is due to the demonstrated overlap of symptoms common to both joint problems, such as pain, swelling, deficits in mobility, and increased temperature, among others [12]. Therefore, although pain is often used as an indicator of increased bleeding, it is not a reliable indicator as to the actual cause of the painful episode [13].

Table 11.2 World federation of hemophilia physical examination score (also called the Gilbert score)

	Score
Swelling	0
None	2
Present	(S)
Added after score if chronic synovitis is present	
Muscle atrophy	0
None or minimal (<1 cm)	1
Present	
Axial deformity (measured only at knee or	0
ankle)	1
Knee	2
Normal (0–7° valgus)	0
8–15° valgus or 0–5° varus	1
>15° valgus or >5° varus	2
Ankle	
No deformity	
Up to 10° valgus or up to 5° varus	
>10° valgus or >5° varus	
Crepitus on motion	0
None	1
Present	
Range of motion	0
Loss of 10% of total FROM	1
Loss of 10–33% of total FROM	2
Loss of >33% of total FROM	
Flexion contracture	0
Measured only at hip, knee, or ankle	2
<15° FFC	
15° or greater FFC at hip or knee or equines at ankle	
Instability	0
None	1
Noted on examination but neither interferes with function nor requires bracing	2
Instability that creates a functional deficit or requires bracing	

FROM full range of motion, *FFC* fixed flexion contracture

Available at: http://www1.wfh.org/docs/en/Publications/Assessment_Tools/Gilbert_Score.pdf

11.2.1.4 Imaging Tests

In recent decades, the ability to assess soft tissue changes has improved dramatically [5]. While bleeding, pain, or physical status have classically driven most clinical decisions in hemophilia care, imaging offers a more accurate objective assessment of joint structural findings that can be directly compared at various times for individual patients or between patients. The most commonly used imaging tests in hemophilia are discussed below.

Table 11.3 Hemophilia joint health score 2.1 (HJHS)—summary score sheet

	Score
Swelling No Mild Moderate Severe	0 1 2 3
Duration (swelling) No or >6 months >6 months	0 1
Muscle atrophy None Mild Severe	0 1 2
Crepitus on motion None Mild Severe	0 1 2
Flexion loss <5° 5–10° 11–20° >20°	0 1 2 3
Extension loss <5° 5–10° 11–20° >20°	0 1 2 3
Joint pain No pain through active ROM No pain through active ROM, only pain on gentle overpressure or palpation Pain through active ROM	0 1 2
Strength Holds test position against gravity with maximum resistance Holds test position against gravity with moderate resistance Holds test position against gravity with minimal resistance or against gravity Able to partially complete ROM against or to move through ROM gravity eliminated Trace or not muscle contraction	0 1 2 3 4
All these items should be evaluated for both elbows, knees, and ankles, with a maximum score per joint of 20 and overall of 120	
Global gait (walking, stairs, running, hopping in 1 leg) All skills are within normal limits One skill is not within normal limits Two skills are not within normal limits Three skills are not within normal limits No skills are within normal limits	0 1 2 3 4

The maximum score for the assessment of the 6 joints plus gait is 124. For all items, if it cannot be scored, there is the option of non-evaluable (NE)

ROM range of motion

Available at: http://www1.wfh.org/docs/en/Publications/Assessment_Tools/HJHS_Summary_Score.pdf

Ultrasound

Currently, ultrasound tends to be the imaging method of choice because it is fast, noninvasive and accessible, and is ideal for early detection of activity and damage in multiple joints, even in asymptomatic patients [14].

In addition, it allows differential diagnosis with other intraarticular disorders [15]. The use of imaging techniques, specifically ultrasound, is recommended along with physical assessment of synovial status after each reported bleeding event until the situation is controlled [2].

POCUS is very useful for the diagnosis of intraarticular bleeding, synovitis, or osteochondral damage. This approach can be used in the clinic and can be performed by hematologists and other professionals caring for people with hemophilia (PWH), making it an easy-to-use imaging modality that allows for direct therapeutic actions [16]. POCUS is of great value for early detection of subclinical hemorrhage and synovial proliferation as markers of activity, as well as osteochondral damage [14, 17].

It is a user-dependent technique; therefore, the development of standardized protocols improves its reproducibility. There are new protocols to systematize joint ultrasound scanning, which reduce interobserver variability and are useful for use by physicians who are not experts in radiodiagnosis. Hemophilia Early Arthropathy Detection with Ultrasound (HEAD-US) is the most widely used, with standardized interpretation of its results (Table 11.4) [18]. It allows evaluation of the elbow, knee, and ankle joints for early detection of synovitis or osteochondral damage. In addition, it includes an additive scoring method according to the damage patterns detected, with a maximum score of 8 per joint [15]. Its high sensitivity, specificity and positive predictive value for detecting the presence of hemophilic arthropathy (synovial proliferation and osteochondral damage) in both adults and children, when compared with magnetic resonance imaging (MRI), have been published [19].

Therefore, US would be an ideal imaging test to be used as a first joint screening. If necessary, other tests can help in diagnosis, such as plain radiography, MRI, computed tomography (CT) scan, and electromyography.

Table 11.4 Hemophilia early arthropathy detection with ultrasound (HEAD-US) scoring method

		Score
Hypertrophic synovium	Absent/minimal	0
	Mild/moderate	1
	Severe	2
Cartilage	Normal	0
	Echotexture abnormalities, focal partial-/full-thickness loss of the articular cartilage involving <25% of the target surface	1
	Partial- /full-thickness loss of the articular cartilage involving ≤50% of the target surface	2
	Partial-/full-thickness loss of the articular cartilage involving >50% of the target surface	3
	Complete cartilage destruction or absent visualization of the articular cartilage on the target bony surface	4
Bone	Normal	0
	Mild irregularities of the subchondral bone with/without initial osteophytes around the joint	1
	Deranged subchondral bone with/without erosions and presence of prominent osteophytes around the joint	2

Elbow anterior aspect of the distal humeral epiphysis, *knee* femoral trochlea, *ankle* anterior aspect of the talar dome

Available at: Martinoli et al. [18]

Radiology

Radiography (conventional X-ray) was one of the first imaging modalities used to evaluate hemophilic arthropathy. It allows detection of advanced structural changes in the joints. To standardize the evaluations, two scoring systems were developed; one progressive [20] and one additive [21]. The Pettersson score has been more widely used in research as it has excellent reliability when used by experienced radiologists (Table 11.5) [22].

However, in light of the evolution of other imaging modalities, comparison of X-ray with MRI and US imaging has shown that radiology is not accurate enough to assess early pathologic changes in joints, primarily affecting articular cartilage and synovial membrane [23]. Therefore, its usefulness would be reserved for adult patients with advanced arthropathy, or when other skeletal evaluations, such as alignments, bone cysts, fractures, deformities, etc., are desired.

Magnetic Resonance Imaging (MRI)

MRI is sensitive for the detection of early intraarticular soft tissue changes, including synovial hypertrophy, hemosiderin deposition, and early osteochondral changes in people with MSK dis-

Table 11.5 Radiological Pettersson score

Radiologic findings	Score
Osteoporosis	0
Absent	1
Present	0
Enlargement of epiphysis	1
Absent	0
Present	1
Irregularity of subchondral surface	2
Absent	0
Slight	1
Pronounced	2
Narrowing of joint space	0
Absent	1
<50%	2
>50%	0
Subchondral cyst formation	1
Absent	0
1 cyst	1
>1 cyst	2
Erosions at joint margin	0
Absent	1
Present	2
Incongruence between joint surfaces	
Absent	
Slight	
Pronounced	
Deformity (angulation and/or displacement of articulating bones)	
Absent	
Slight	
Pronounced	

Possible joint score: 0–13 points for each joint (total possible score, 6 × 13 = 78)
Available at: Pettersson et al. [21]

ease [23], so it is considered the gold standard in the joint study of hemophilia. In addition, MRI can assess response to treatment by capturing changes in the joint over time after treatment has been administered [24].

MRI scoring scales have also been developed for hemophilia. Initially, as with plain radiographs, a progressive scoring system [25] and an additive scoring system [26] were described. Subsequently, the International Prophylaxis Study Group (IPSG) combined these systems into a single MRI scoring system with good measurement properties, which should be applied by experienced radiologists (Table 11.6).

However, MRI has practical disadvantages, such as high cost, limited availability, and the need for sedation in young children, which limit its use for research and evaluation of specific clinical situations [5].

Table 11.6 IPSG MRI scale to assess hemophilic arthropathy

		Score
Soft tissue changes (maximum 9 points)	Effusion/hemarthrosis	1
	Small	2
	Moderate	3
	Large	
	Synovial hypertrophy	1
	Small	2
	Moderate	3
	Large	
	Hemosiderin	1
	Small	2
	Moderate	3
	Large	
Osteochondral changes (maximum 8 points)	Surface erosions involving	1
	subchondral cortex or joint	1
	margins	1
	Any surface erosion	1
	Half or more of the	1
	articular surface eroded	1
	in at least one bone	1
	Subchondral cysts	1
	At least one subchondral cyst	
	Subchondral cysts in at least two bones, or cystic changes involving a third or more of the articular surface in at least one bone	
	Cartilage degradation	
	Any loss of joint cartilage height	
	Loss of half or more of the total volume of joint cartilage in at least one bone	
	Full-thickness loss of joint cartilage in at least some area in at least one bone	
	Full-thickness loss of joint cartilage including at least one half of the joint surface in at least one bone	

IPSG International Prophylaxis Study Group, *MRI* magnetic resonance imaging
Lundin B, Babyn P, Doria AS, Kilcoyne R, Ljung R, Miller S, et al. Compatible scales for progressive and additive MRI assessments of haemophilic arthropathy. Haemophilia 2005;11:109–115

The correlation for quantification of hemophilic arthropathy between US and MRI is high. Therefore, with US being more readily available and offering the possibility of analyzing multiple joints, it should be used to make an initial assessment of the patient's joint damage [27, 28].

11.2.2 Activities and Participation

It is undoubtedly essential to assess the extent to which MSK health problems have an impact on patients' lives. Activities and participation are very closely related, although they are defined differently according to the ICF model. Activity refers to an individual's performance of an action of instrumental activities of daily living (e.g., walking, eating, using the toilet). Participation refers to an individual's performance of activities in the context of social interactions [2, 6]. Measures of activities and participation used in hemophilia include both objective and self-reported assessments [5].

Of interest is also the use of validated scales to objectively assess the ability of PWH to perform certain tasks. These include the Functional Independence Score in Hemophilia (FISH) and the Hemophilia Activities List (HAL) within the specific ones. If we cannot apply these scales, we will resort to generic scales.

The FISH is a specific instrument developed to assess the ability of persons with hemophilia to perform activities of daily living (Table 11.7) [29]. It is the most widely studied validated measure of observed activities for people with hemophilia. The FISH includes eight activities in three categories: self-care, transfers, and locomotion. Each activity is scored according to the amount of assistance needed to perform the task.

The HAL can identify problematic activities for individuals with hemophilia (Table 11.8) [30]. It is the best-studied measure of self-reported activities for adults and has been translated into many languages. The questionnaire has seven domains; it also generates three subscores (upper extremity, basic lower extremity, and complex lower extremity). The PedHAL is a version of the HAL that has been validated for pediatric patients [31]. The internal consistency and convergent validity of the HAL were tested in several countries in Europe and America, and it is available in many languages. However, being an instrument developed in Western Europe, it may not apply as well when used in other cultural settings [5].

Although FISH and HAL are the most widely used, there are other instruments as well. The reported outcomes, burdens and experiences (PROBE) questionnaire also includes measures that assess activities and participation, such as school/education, employment, family life, and impact on activities of daily living [2].

The Canadian Occupational Performance Measure (COPM), the McMaster Toronto Arthritis Patient Preference Disability Questionnaire (MACTAR), and the Health Assessment Questionnaire (HAQ) are generic instruments that have been used for daily assessment of a person's perception of changes in the

Table 11.7 Functional independence score in hemophilia (FISH)

	List of activities tested
Self-care	Eating Grooming Bathing Dressing
Transfers	Chair transferring Squatting
Locomotion	Walking Climbing stairs Running

Scores range from 1 to 4 for each activity depending on the degree of independence: 1, unable to perform; 2, requires the help of an assistant/aid; 3, able to perform the activity without an aid but not like a healthy subject; 4, able to perform the activity like other healthy subjects

Available at: http://www1.wfh.org/docs/en/Publications/AssessmentTools/FISHupdatedJan2017.pdf

Table 11.8 Hemophilia activities list (HAL)

HAL domains
Lying/sitting/kneeling/standing
Functions of the legs
Functions of the arms
Use of transportation
Self-care
Household tasks
Leisure activities and sports
HAL components
Upper extremity
Basic lower extremity
Complex lower extremity

Available in multiple languages at: https://elearning.wfh.org/resource/hemophilia-activities-list-hal/

domains of activities and participation. They can be used for target scaling [2]. Three-dimensional gait analysis (3DGA) provides information on functional performance but requires specialized equipment. There is also some experience in hemophilia with the 6-min walk (6MWT) and 50-m walk (50WT) tests [5].

Indirect "objective" assessment of activities and participation is provided by recording work participation and days missed from work or school due to hemophilia. These parameters can also be used for economic evaluations [32]. How small differences in radiological and clinical scores translate into patient function and quality of life remains to be determined [29].

11.2.3 Health-Related Quality of Life (HRQoL)

HRQoL refers to an individual's perception of his or her life situation. It is therefore a subjective parameter related to their goals, expectations, standards, and concerns, which is self-reported or reported by the family. Therefore, even more so than in functional scores, HRQoL questionnaires should be validated in the language and social and cultural contexts in which they are to be applied [2].

Multiple scales measuring quality of life in PWH are available, including specific and generic tools for adults and children. For adults with hemophilia, the Hemophilia Wellbeing Index and the hemophilia-specific quality of life questionnaire for adults with hemophilia (HAEMO-QoL-A) have been widely used. The PROBE questionnaire assesses HRQoL in addition to disease burden in persons with hemophilia. For children with hemophilia, the Canadian Hemophilia Outcomes-Kids Life Assessment Tool (CHO-KLAT) has been widely used. The most widely used generic tools for assessing HRQoL in hemophilia are the EuroQoL 5 Dimensions (EQ-5D) [2, 3] and the Short-form-36 Health Survey (SF-36) (Table 11.9) [2]. Given their global nature, it is recommended to apply them in combination with domain-specific assessments of ICF and not in isolation.

Table 11.9 36-item short form survey instrument (SF-36)

Eight domains described in SF-36
Physical functioning
Role limitations due to physical health problems
Role limitations due to personal or emotional problems
Energy/fatigue
Emotional well-being
Social functioning
Pain
General health

Available at: https://clinmedjournals.org/articles/jmdt/jmdt-2-023-figure-1.pdf

11.2.4 Patient-Reported Outcomes

Increasingly, and as in other subspecialities within orthopedics, outcome measures are looking to place more importance on patient satisfaction versus clinician satisfaction with treatment outcomes.

In light of new therapies, there is an evolution toward "patient-centered" definition of health status and outcomes. Patient-reported outcomes (PROs) encompass unidimensional and multidimensional measures of health status, treatment adherence, treatment satisfaction, quality of life, and other measures. PROs include disease-specific instruments such as the HAL, HRQoL measures such as CHO-KLAT, HAEMO-QoL-A, burden of disease questionnaires such as PROBE or the comprehensive assessment tool of challenges in hemophilia (CATCH). There are also generic instruments such as the 5-level EuroQoL 5 Dimensions (EQ-5D-5L), Brief Pain Inventory v2 (BPI), International Physical Activity Questionnaire (IPAQ), Short Form 36 Health Survey v2 (SF-36v2), or the Patient-Reported Outcomes Measurement Information System (PROMIS) [2].

These PRO instruments can provide evidence of a treatment benefit from the patient's point of view [33]. One issue to consider with PROs is that the questionnaires are dependent on literacy and cultural issues, and beyond simple translation, cultural adaptation is necessary [5].

11.2.5 Economic Factors

The health problems associated with hemophilia can also be quantified in terms of costs and benefits. Direct costs include disease care, representing hematological therapies. We know that in patients with severe hemophilia, more than 90% of the costs are related to this treatment [34]. To which must be added the cost of other treatments, health services, and surgical and medical supplies. In addition, there are indirect costs generated by the loss of work productivity of adult patients and parents of pediatric patients due to the problems resulting from hemophilia.

11.2.6 Other Measures

In recent years, other methods have been sought to assess the joint health of PWH. Among them laboratory biomarkers are the most studied, as they would offer a very simple assessment, focused on blood analysis or other samples. However, to date, although interesting from a scientific point of view, they do not seem to provide benefits from a practical point of view [35].

Moreover, current biomarkers are not accurate enough to assess actual joint health, as they do not measure exactly when joint damage and bleeding occurred [36]. Furthermore, the current literature does not clarify whether biomarkers can detect cartilage destruction in the child with suboptimal hematologic prophylaxis [35].

Some biomarkers have been implicated in different stages of hemophilic joint deterioration and disease development; however, there is still a need to quantify correlations between biomarkers and physical and radiological examination [35, 37]. In short, while potentially promising for the future, biomarkers in hemophilia add little, if anything, to our current diagnostic armamentarium.

11.3 Which Tools to Choose?

Standardized and validated assessments of hemophilia outcomes are essential for personalized clinical management of the patient, as well as for research into the optimization of new therapies.

When choosing instruments, it is very important to consider the purpose of the assessment, patient characteristics, and the environment. The environment includes aspects such as access to replacement therapy and the use of prophylaxis. The age of the population and the duration of follow-up should also be taken into account [5].

The assessments mentioned in this chapter should be done periodically. If possible, it is recommended to evaluate every 6 months during osteoarticular development in the pediatric population and annually in adulthood. Follow-up of musculoskeletal bleeding should be done more closely, at shorter times, e.g., weekly. These serial assessments should be made throughout the patient's life. This will provide us with the necessary data to better direct hematologic, rehabilitation and orthopedic therapeutic strategies. In this way we will also be able to measure the efficacy of the interventions performed.

When using a combination of different outcome tools, it is important to combine professionally collected and patient-reported outcomes (PROs), which can provide an objective basis for comparison over time and with other patients [5].

To select the scale we need, it is useful to ask the following questions: What information do I need and what for? What is the best scale available? It is necessary to understand the information it provides, its ease of administration and its metric characteristics. In hemophilia the choice will also depend on the objective of outcome assessment, the setting, the patient's age, the joint status, and the duration of follow-up [5].

With several options available, the choice will depend on the objective being pursued. For example, measurement of HRQoL may help clinicians determine the effectiveness of treatment in terms of patient perception, but may not reflect the intraarticular pathophysiologic changes following hemarthrosis.

The most appropriate scales are always those that are valid, reliable, and sensitive and measure the problem adequately. Whenever possible we should use a scale that already exists and is appropriate for our environment, which requires cross-cultural validation.

11.4 Future Perspectives

In the new era of hemophilia treatments with long-acting coagulation factor concentrates, gene therapy or bypassing agents, it is necessary to evaluate whether traditional assessment measures will be appropriate in the coming decades to define the response to treatment in patients with hemophilia. Researchers have observed that several assessment methods that have been used for many years require updating to accommodate joint damage that occurs before the patient presents symptoms. In this regard tools such as POCUS, which allows early diagnosis of joint injuries in hemophilia, is expanding [17].

We physicians continue to strive to optimize treatment, which can only be achieved by prospective evaluation of different treatment protocols. International collaboration is mandatory to enable research into optimal treatment strategies. Standardization of outcome assessment measures is critical. Details of both the treatment and the outcome should be collected [5]. Defining a standardized core set of outcome assessment measures for specific clinical settings will allow meaningful comparison across studies and reduce heterogeneity in advancing knowledge and clinical care of PWH.

11.5 Conclusions

It is important to have a basic set of tools to measure joint health in hemophilia in the clinical or research setting. The assessment of joint health and outcome measures in hemophilia should include bleeding rate, assessment of body structure and function, activity levels and participation, in accordance with the ICF of the WHO. It is recommended that MSK health assessment be evaluated and documented at least annually and preferably semi-annually in the pediatric age group. As far as possible, valid, reliable and sensitive scales should be used. The most recommended scales for body structure and function include the AJBR taken with sensitive methods, the HJHS for children and adolescents, and US or MRI as imaging tests. Hemarthroses and early osteochondral changes in the joints are adequately evaluated with the use of US and MRI. Late joint changes can be evaluated on plain radiographs. The most recommended scales for activity and involvement levels should be FISH and HAL. HRQoL can be assessed in combination with the other ICF domains. In addition, there is a growing focus on patient feedback, so the use of PRO instruments is increasing. With advances in hemophilia treatments, it is foreseeable that updates to several of the markers used so far will be required in the coming years. This will require the joint collaboration of the scientific community and hemophilia patients.

References

1. De la Corte-Rodriguez H, Rodriguez-Merchan EC. The role of physical medicine and rehabilitation in haemophiliac patients. Blood Coagul Fibrinolysis. 2013;24:1–9.
2. Srivastava A, Santagostino E, Dougall A, Kitchen S, Sutherland M, Pipe SW, et al. WFH guidelines for the management of hemophilia panelists and co-authors. Haemophilia. 2020;26(6):1–158.
3. Konkle BA, Skinner M, Iorio A. Hemophilia trials in the twenty-first century: defining patient important outcomes. Res Pract Thromb Haemost. 2019;3:184–92.
4. Seuser A, Djambas Khayat C, Negrier C, Sabbour A, Heijnen L. Evaluation of early musculoskeletal disease in patients with haemophilia: results from an expert consensus. Blood Coagul Fibrinolysis. 2018;29:509–20.
5. Fischer K, Poonnoose P, Dunn AL, Babyn P, Manco-Johnson MJ, David JA, et al. Choosing outcome assessment tools in haemophilia care and research: a multidisciplinary perspective. Haemophilia. 2017;23:11–24.
6. De la Corte-Rodriguez H, Rodriguez-Merchan EC. The ICF (International Classification of Functioning, Disability and Health) developed by the WHO for measuring function in hemophilia. Expert Rev Hematol. 2016;9:661–8.
7. Nguyen S, Lu X, Ma Y, Du J, Chang EY, von Drygalski A. Musculoskeletal ultrasound for intra-articular bleed detection: a highly sensitive imaging modality compared with conventional magnetic resonance imaging. J Thromb Haemost. 2018;16:490–9.
8. Rodriguez-Merchan EC. Treatment of musculoskeletal pain in haemophilia. Blood Rev. 2018;32:116–21.

9. Hilberg T. Programmed sports therapy (PST) in people with Haemophilia (PwH) "sports therapy model for rare diseases". Orphanet J Rare Dis. 2018;13(1):38.
10. Gilbert MS. Prophylaxis: musculoskeletal evaluation. Semin Hematol. 1993;30(3):3–6.
11. Feldman BM, Funk SM, Bergstrom BM, Zourikian N, Hilliard P, van der Net J, et al. Validation of a new pediatric joint scoring system from the International Hemophilia Prophylaxis Study Group: validity of the hemophilia joint health score. Arthritis Care Res. 2011;63:223–30.
12. Timmer MA, Pisters MF, de Kleijn P, de Bie RA, Fischer K, Schutgens RE. Differentiating between signs of intra-articular joint bleeding and chronic arthropathy in haemophilia: a narrative review of the literature. Haemophilia. 2015;21:289–96.
13. Ceponis A, Wong-Sefidan I, Glass CS, von Drygalski A. Rapid musculoskeletal ultrasound for painful episodes in adult haemophilia patients. Haemophilia. 2013;19:790–8.
14. De la Corte-Rodriguez H, Rodriguez-Merchan EC, Alvarez-Roman MT, Martin-Salces M, Martinoli C, Jimenez-Yuste V. HJHS 2.1 and HEAD-US assessment in the hemophilic joints: how do their findings compare? Blood Coagul Fibrinolysis. 2020;31:387–92.
15. Kidder W, Nguyen S, Larios J, Bergstrom J, Ceponis A, von Drygalski A. Point-of-care musculoskeletal ultrasound is critical for the diagnosis of hemarthroses, inflammation and soft tissue abnormalities in adult patients with painful haemophilic arthropathy. Haemophilia. 2015;21:530–7.
16. Lisi C, Di Natali G, Sala V, Tinelli C, Canepari M, Gamba G, et al. Interobserver reliability of ultrasound assessment of haemophilic arthropathy: radiologist vs. non-radiologist. Haemophilia. 2016;22:211–4.
17. Bakeer N, Shapiro AD. Merging into the mainstream: the evolution of the role of point-of-care musculoskeletal ultrasound in hemophilia. F1000Res. 2019;8:1029.
18. Martinoli C, Casa D, Di Minno G, Graziano E, Molinari AC, Pasta G, et al. Development and definition of a simplified scanning procedure and scoring method for Haemophilia Early Arthropathy Detection with Ultrasound. Thromb Haemost. 2013;109:1170–9.
19. Plut D, Faganel Kotnik B, Preložnik Zupan I, Ključevšek D, Vidmar G, Snoj Ž, et al. Detection and evaluation of haemophilic arthropathy: which tools may be considered more reliable. Haemophilia. 2020. https://doi.org/10.1111/hae.14153.
20. Arnold WD, Hilgartner MW. Hemophilic arthropathy. Current concepts of pathogenesis and management. J Bone Jt Surg Am. 1977;59:287–305.
21. Pettersson H, Nilsson IM, Hedner U, Norehn K, Ahlberg A. Radiologic evaluation of prophylaxis in severe haemophilia. Acta Paediatr Scand. 1981;70:565–70.
22. Erlemann R, Rosenthal H, Walthers EM, Almeida P, Calleja R. Reproducibility of the Pettersson scoring system. An interobserver study. Acta Radiol. 1989;30:147–51.
23. Poonnoose PM, Hilliard P, Doria AS, Keshava SN, Gibikote S, Kavitha ML, et al. Correlating clinical and radiological assessment of joints in haemophilia: results of a cross sectional study. Haemophilia. 2016;22:925–33.
24. Manco-Johnson MJ, Abshire TC, Shapiro AD, Riske B, Hacker MR, Kylcoine R, et al. Prophylaxis versus episodic treatment to prevent joint disease in boys with severe hemophilia. N Engl J Med. 2007;357:535–44.
25. Nuss R, Kilcoyne RF, Geraghty S, Shroyer AL, Rosky JW, Mawhinney S, et al. MRI findings in haemophilic joints treated with radiosynoviorthesis with development of an MRI scale of joint damage. Haemophilia. 2000;6:162–9.
26. Lundin B, Pettersson H, Ljung R. A new magnetic resonance imaging scoring method for assessment of haemophilic arthropathy. Haemophilia. 2004;10:383–9.
27. Lundin B, Manco-Johnson ML, Ignas DM, Moinnedin R, Blanchette VS, Dunn AL, et al. An MRI scale for assessment of haemophilic arthropathy from the International Prophylaxis Study Group. Haemophilia. 2012;18:962–70.
28. Doria AS, Keshava SN, Mohanta A, Jarrin J, Blanchette V, Srivastava A, et al. Diagnostic accuracy of ultrasound for assessment of hemophilic arthropathy: MRI correlation. AJR Am J Roentgenol. 2015;204:336–47.
29. Poonnoose PM, Manigandan C, Thomas R, Shyamkumar NK, Kavitha ML, Bhattacharji S, et al. Functional independence score in haemophilia: a new performance-based instrument to measure disability. Haemophilia. 2005;11:598–602.
30. van Genderen FR, van Meeteren NL, van der Bom JG, Heijnen L, van den Berg HM, Helders PJM. Functional consequences of haemophilia in adults: the development of the haemophilia activities list. Haemophilia. 2004;10:565–71.
31. Groen WG, van der Net J, Helders PJ, Fischer K. Development and preliminary testing of a paediatric version of the haemophilia activities list (pedhal). Haemophilia. 2010;16:281–9.
32. Nicholson A, Berger K, Bohn R, Carcao M, Fischer K, Gringeri A, et al. Recommendations for reporting economic evaluations of haemophilia prophylaxis: a nominal groups consensus statement on behalf of the Economics Expert Working Group of The International Prophylaxis Study Group. Haemophilia. 2008;14:127–32.
33. Beeton K, De Kleijn P, Hilliard P, Funk S, Zourikian N, Bergstrom BM, et al. Recent developments in clinimetric instruments. Haemophilia. 2006;12(3):102–7.
34. Globe DR, Curtis RG, Koerper MA. Utilization of care in haemophilia: a resource- based method for cost analysis from the Haemophilia Utilization Group Study (HUGS). Haemophilia. 2004;10(1):63–70.

35. Rodriguez-Merchan EC. Serological biomarkers in hemophilic arthropathy: Can they be used to monitor bleeding and ongoing progression of blood-induced joint disease in patients with hemophilia? Blood Rev. 2020;41:100642.
36. van Vulpen LF, van Meegeren ME, Roosendaal G, Jansen NWD, van Laar JM, Schutgens REG, et al. Biochemical markers of joint tissue damage increase shortly after a joint bleed; an explorative human and canine in vivo study. Osteoarthr Cartil. 2015;23:63–9.
37. Pasta G, Annunziata S, Polizzi A, Caliogna L, Jannelli E, Minen A, et al. The progression of hemophilic arthropathy: the role of biomarkers. Int J Mol Sci. 2020;21:7292.

Musculoskeletal Medicine in Hemophilia (Including Pain Control)

12

Hortensia De la Corte-Rodríguez, Alexander D. Liddle, and E. Carlos Rodríguez-Merchán

12.1 Introduction

The current approach to managing hemophilia is multidisciplinary, with both orthopedic and rehabilitation clinicians working with hematologists in preventing and treating musculoskeletal (MSK) lesions and maintaining the MSK system in optimal condition. This involves the prevention of bleeding and its consequences on the MSK system, as well as working to maintain an adequate physical condition to promote the autonomy and independence of the patient [1]. Education and promotion of physical activity, adjusted to the physical characteristics and age of each patient, is important.

When bleeding or other MSK injuries inevitably appear, they should be treated effectively and early to avoid medium- and long-term sequelae, thus shortening recovery periods and hospitalizations. The therapeutic objectives of Physical and Rehabilitation Medicine in the case of MSK injuries in patients with hemophilia are shown in Table 12.1. Special attention should be paid to the problems that patients present in their activities of daily living (ADL) and in their social participation, so that they maintain as much independence and autonomy as possible.

The design of a rehabilitation-orthopedic treatment program requires knowledge of the hematologic condition, the cause of the injury, the functional anatomy, the different methods of treatment, and almost most importantly, the specific characteristics of each patient. This will allow the treating clinician to develop a treatment program adjusted not only to the clinical situation, but also to the personal and social situation of each patient. Therefore, before indicating a therapy in a patient, it is necessary to perform a global, systematic and complete evaluation of the MSK system, as well as to know the hematologic treatment that the patient is undergoing [1].

This chapter will analyze the most frequent MSK manifestations of hemophilia, as well as the recommended non-surgical therapies, working always with a multidisciplinary approach.

12.2 Musculoskeletal (MSK) Clinical Manifestations

In the MSK system, the vast majority of clinical manifestations of hemophilia are the result of episodes of bleeding. Recurrent hemarthroses are the most frequent manifestations in hemophilia, causing chronic inflammation of the synovial membrane as well as osteochondral

H. De la Corte-Rodríguez
Department of Physical and Rehabilitation Medicine, La Paz University Hospital, Madrid, Spain

A. D. Liddle
MSK Lab, Imperial College, London, UK

E. C. Rodríguez-Merchán (✉)
Department of Orthopedic Surgery, La Paz University Hospital, Madrid, Spain

E. C. Rodríguez-Merchán (ed.), *Advances in Hemophilia Treatment*,
https://doi.org/10.1007/978-3-030-93990-8_12

Table 12.1 Objectives of rehabilitation treatment in musculoskeletal injuries in patients with hemophilia

Pain relief
Restore tissue flexibility and joint range of motion
Prevent muscle atrophy and improve muscle power and endurance
Recovery of proprioception and balance
Prevent sequelae and deformities
Improve manual skills
Maintain an adequate gait pattern
Reduce the frequency of joint bleeds
Encourage activities of daily living (ADL) and social participation
In general, improving the quality of life

Table 12.2 Frequency of bleeding by location in hemophilia

Bleeding site	Approximate frequency (%)
Hemarthrosis More frequent in hinge joints: ankles, knees, and elbows. Less frequent in multiaxial joints: shoulders, wrists, and hips	70–80
Muscles	10–20
Other locations	5–10
Central nervous system	<5

damage leading to hemophilic arthropathy, with biomechanical sequelae that affect the patient's mobility and functionality. As well as the joints, bleeding can also occur within the muscles and in other locations (Table 12.2). Each of the hemorrhagic manifestations in the musculoskeletal system, their initial approach, useful imaging tests and non-surgical treatment from the point of view of MSK Medicine are mentioned below.

12.2.1 Hemarthrosis

Hemarthrosis is defined as the presence of free intra-articular blood from the synovial membrane. The most affected joints in which hemorrhages usually occur are the ankles, knees, and elbows, although the possibility of their occurrence in other joints should not be forgotten. A "target joint" is a joint which suffers three or more hemarthroses in a 6-month period [2]. In children with severe hemophilia and without hematologic prophylactic treatment, the first spontaneous episode of hemarthrosis usually occurs before 2 years of age. If not adequately treated, repeated hemarthroses lead to a dose-dependent effect of blood on the intra-articular tissues, leading to an inflammatory process (chronic synovitis) and a degenerative process (arthropathy) that will be irreversible [3].

When hemarthrosis is expected clinically, confirmation can be made using physical examination and imaging tests. The joint presents as inflamed, with pain, palpable swelling and loss of function. Ultrasound is a useful tool to determine the presence and extent of hemarthrosis, based on its echogenic characteristics and sonopalpation. It is also a very useful tool to follow up bleeding until its resolution, as well as to rule out rebleeding.

The goal of hemarthrosis treatment is to stop the bleeding as soon as possible and to avoid its sequelae. Most important in the treatment of acute hemarthrosis is the administration of clotting factor replacement. The most effective way to administer the factor early is through home programs that allow the patient to self-infuse the factor from the first symptoms. In hemophilia patients with inhibitors, other appropriate hemostatics should be used to provide hemostatic coverage [4].

Hemophilia patients with hemarthrosis should be managed using the PRICE (protection, rest, ice, compression, and elevation) approach. Complete rest is not recommended; instead, patients are encouraged to mobilize the joint within the limits of pain. In the acute setting, the use of compressive bandaging and unloading of the joint is advised until a medical check-up in the following hours. The application of local cold is controversial [5].

Whenever possible, in acute major hemarthrosis or when infection is suspected, intra-articular blood should be evacuated by arthrocentesis (joint aspiration). This joint drainage should always be done under hemostatic coverage and aseptic conditions, once it has been verified with imaging that the bleeding is in the liquid phase [6].

Acute hemarthrosis can be extremely painful, and prompt administration of effective analgesia in addition to clotting factor concentrate replacement is a key aspect of pain management [4]. The use of anti-inflammatory drugs with a safety profile and analgesics may be helpful (see Sect. 12.2.6).

As soon as the pain ceases, the patient should be encouraged to mobilize the joint, trying to regain its natural range of motion. Active assisted exercises should be indicated at the level of the affected joint to avoid soft tissue retractions, as well as in the adjacent joints. In addition, isometric exercises can generally be started early; they allow joint rest to be respected and are effective in avoiding reflex muscle inhibition secondary to pain. These exercises should be performed in short periods of time and serial repetitions at the patient's home and, if necessary, supervised in the physiotherapy room. A dynamic orthosis can be used to protect the joint and promote the recovery of its joint balance. Subsequently, isotonic concentric and eccentric muscle strengthening exercises (preferably in open kinetic chain) and proprioceptive, balance and functional exercises should be introduced [4]. Once the resolution of the bleeding is confirmed by imaging tests, joint weight bearing, i.e., walking without canes in case of hemarthrosis of the knee or ankle, is authorized. Whether the patient would benefit from other treatment techniques will be assessed on an individual basis. Physical therapy should be continued until joint function is restored to the pre-hemorrhage state [1]. More on the treatment of hemarthrosis can be read in Chap. 14 of this book.

12.2.2 Chronic Synovitis

If hemarthroses have not been prevented, synovitis usually appears in the first two decades of life. With recurrent hemarthroses, the synovial membrane becomes inflamed and undergoes hypertrophic changes, resulting in hypervascularization that in turn increases the risk of rebleeding. In addition, the inflammatory molecules released (IL-1beta, TNF-alpha, IL-6, and RANK-L) have a damaging effect on chondrocyte and subchondral bone metabolism [7]. Therefore, early diagnosis of synovitis is essential to prevent progression of damage and to make an adjustment of hematological treatment as early as possible.

In very hypertrophic synovitis, the appearance on inspection is a swollen, inflamed and enlarged joint. It is important not to confuse hemarthrosis and synovitis; the differentiating clinical features shown in Table 12.3 should be taken into account.

However, in its early stages, synovitis is usually asymptomatic and may go unnoticed. This is also common when synovitis is mild, which is often in patients treated with effective prophylactic agents. Detection of synovial proliferation is an important step in the suspicion of subclinical joint bleeding in asymptomatic patients [8]. Detection of synovial proliferation should be encouraged, as it is the best biomarker of subclinical bleeding and a predictor of worsening joint function and health. Fortunately, we now have simple tools that allow accurate diagnosis of synovitis such as ultrasonography (US) or magnetic resonance imaging (MRI). It is of great value to add the sensitivity of point-of-care ultrasound for early detection of subclinical hemorrhages and synovial proliferation as markers of disease activity [9].

When the synovial membrane becomes hypertrophied and hypervascular, the tendency to hemarthrosis increases, creating a vicious cycle. Since synovitis is a reflection of inadequate hemostasis, the initial treatment will be clotting factor replacement therapy, which should be

Table 12.3 Differentiating clinical features between hemarthrosis and synovitis

Hemarthrosis	Synovitis
• Acute onset • Severe or moderate pain • Antalgic attitude in flexion • Liquid content • Absent or limited joint mobility • Loss of strength • Immediate response to substitutive treatment	• Insidious onset • Mild or absent pain • Normal postural attitude • Solid content • Normal joint mobility • Mild muscular insufficiency • No immediate response to treatment

administered for at least 6–8 weeks on a prophylactic or intermittent basis, with sufficient frequency and dosage to prevent recurrent bleeding. The use of selective COX-2 inhibitor anti-inflammatory drugs may reduce pain and inflammation. If a functional deficit in the joint is associated, a program of physiotherapy and/or occupational therapy may help to recover it [4]. If after 3–6 months of hematologic replacement therapy synovitis persists or there are recurrent hemarthroses, synoviorthesis is indicated. Radiosynovectomy is of choice in this scenario. More on this technique can be read in Chap. 15 of this book.

12.2.3 Osteochondral Damage: Hemophilic Arthropathy

The repeated exposure of joint structures to blood produces histopathological changes that eventually deteriorate the joint. This damage begins early, after only a small number of hemarthroses [10]. Experimental studies show that cartilage and subchondral bone are damaged by well-defined pathophysiological mechanisms, related to the presence of free blood in the joint [7]. Chondrocyte metabolism is altered by a dual mechanism. On the one hand, through the interaction between inflammatory molecules and metalloproteases; and on the other hand, by the direct action of blood iron through redox reactions and release of free radicals. This chondrocytic apoptosis will not be repairable. At the bone level, the imbalance between osteoprotegerin and RANK-L, in favor of the latter, causes it to bind to its receptor, increasing the action of osteoclasts and thus bone resorption [7]. All this would explain why patients with hemophilia end up developing osteochondral damage, known as hemophilic arthropathy. Secondarily, loss of joint mobility, muscle wasting, loss of proprioception, malalignment, and deformity can also appear. In the most severe cases, the structural changes generated by the arthropathy can end up damaging the joint capsule, ligaments, nerves, and tendons. The composite effect of this process in multiple joints (ankles, knees, elbows most frequently) generates major biomechanical disorders that condition a greater or lesser degree of disability [1]. We must not forget the chronic pain component that this generates and that we must also treat (see Sect. 12.2.6).

The early diagnosis of osteochondral damage should be made before it becomes symptomatic, with routine assessments using sensitive techniques. Around 14% of hemophiliac patients with no history of bleeding and normal physical examination have subclinical joint damage when assessed with US [11, 12]. Plain radiography is useful for assessing established hemophilic arthropathy, as it can determine decreased joint space, cysts, and bony erosions. However, its sensitivity is poor for detecting early changes in arthropathy, so its use is best suited to assessment of adult patients with advanced joint disease [13]. MRI has great advantages over radiography; these include better visualization of all intra- and extra-articular elements, as well as the absence of exposure to ionizing radiation. However, the need to perform polyarticular studies repeatedly decreases its practical usefulness.

For the treatment of osteochondral damage, a combination of regular replacement therapy to reduce the frequency of bleeding and rehabilitation therapy is recommended. The goal of rehabilitative treatment of hemophilic arthropathy is generally to improve function and relieve pain [1]. Treatment options will depend on the stage of the disease, symptomatology, and available resources. In addition to pain management with different drugs, such as paracetamol, metamizole, cox-2 inhibitors or opioids, we can also resort to physical techniques such as transcutaneous electrical nerve stimulation (TENS). Physiotherapy sessions are useful to work on tissue flexibility, joint mobility, muscle strengthening, proprioception, and gait re-education. Hydrokinesitherapy (water therapy) is of great interest because it allows improvements in flexibility and tone of large body segments (very useful in hemophilic polyarthropathy) [14]. Functional exercises should also be incorporated. Physical therapy can be performed with or without factor coverage, depending on availability and the patient's response to therapy. Other modes of therapy such as exercise therapy, manual therapy, magnet therapy, or electrotherapy have also been used. Occupational therapy sessions are very useful for training ADLs and upper limb management in case of elbow arthropathy. Home and workplace adaptations to encourage participation and facilitate ADLs are essential [1].

Intra-articular injections of hyaluronic acid can be helpful with effect on pain and function extending to more than 3 months [15]. Intra-articular injections of corticosteroids have a shorter effect over time and are also not routinely recommended [16].

In order to unload the arthropathic joint, valgus knee orthoses may be useful in knees with varus deformity and plantar orthoses with internal varus wedges may be useful in ankles with hindfoot valgus. Gait aids can be introduced to decrease the degree of stress on weight-bearing joints. Many patients require a detailed report from their rehabilitation physician detailing their physical and functional condition in order to request the degree of disability. Collaboration with social workers is essential. If conservative treatment fails, surgical treatment should be considered. In this case the orthopedic surgeon with experience in the management of patients with hemophilia will determine the most indicated technique in each case [17].

12.2.4 Muscle Hematomas

Muscle hematomas represent the second most common cause of bleeding in the musculoskeletal system in patients with hemophilia. The clinical manifestation of hematoma depends on the location and intensity of the bleeding, and is generally more insidious than hemarthrosis. It is defined as an episode of muscle hemorrhage determined clinically and/or by imaging studies, generally associated with great functional limitation. The clinical features usually include an antalgic gait, local induration, and muscle pain that is aggravated by muscle elongation. The most critical sites are those where neurovascular function may be compromised; bleeding in the iliopsoas muscle may lead to femoral nerve palsy; a hematoma in the gastrocnemius may affect the posterior tibial nerve. In addition, they can be complicated by acute compartment syndromes, which would have serious functional consequences if an emergency surgical fasciotomy is not performed.

Early identification and proper management of muscle hematomas are critical to avoid permanent contractures, rebleeding, and the formation of hemophilic pseudotumors [18]. Iliopsoas muscle hemorrhage has a special presentation; its signs may include pain in the hypogastrium, groin and/or lower lumbar area, pain with hip extension and paresthesias in the medial thigh area or other signs of nerve compression (such as decreased patellar reflex and quadriceps motor deficit). It is important to make a differential diagnosis with other entities such as hip hemarthrosis, avascular necrosis of the hip, and appendicitis (if on the right side).

The diagnosis of muscular hematoma should be confirmed with imaging techniques, among which ultrasound has the advantage of immediacy, capacity to determine the size, shape, location and evolution. In less accessible locations, as in the case of the iliopsoas muscle, MRI or computed tomography (CT) scan may be necessary to clarify the diagnosis.

Administration of clotting factor should be initiated immediately, ideally at home when the patient identifies the first signs of discomfort or after the trauma and maintained until resolution of the trauma. General measures to control bleeding and pain include rest in a comfortable position, and analgesic/anti-inflammatory treatment. Close follow-up is important to ensure that the hematoma is not complicated by compartment syndrome or neuropathy. In case of clear blood collections, evacuation should be considered in the acute phase, with ultrasound guidance [19].

If the patient responds well to hematologic treatment, rehabilitation treatment is then initiated. Therapeutic ultrasound in pulsed form could improve hematoma resorption, although its efficacy has not been demonstrated.

Kinesitherapy is particularly useful for the recovery of articular range of motion by applying it in an assisted and progressive manner. Physical therapy sessions should be done under coagulation factor coverage, as long as the bleeding is not resolved. Sometimes it is necessary to resort to the use of soft traction or dynamic orthoses, to avoid muscle shortening and bring the limb to its natural alignment. Imaging tests should verify the progressive resorption of the bleeding. Gradual progressive muscular exercises (isometric and isotonic exercises, preferably concentric) can be introduced to improve muscle activation, while respecting pain. If the hematoma is accompanied by paresis due to compressive neuropathy, a treatment aimed at this lesion should be applied. These are usually neurapraxias or axonotmesis due to compression, in which case the long-term prognosis is usually favorable.

12.2.5 Hemophilic Pseudotumor

It is a potentially serious condition for the affected limb. It is more frequent in long bones and pelvis. It is the result of inadequate management of soft tissue bleeding, especially muscles adjacent to the bone, which can be affected secondarily. Its diagnosis is made by clinical examination with the finding of tumor-like masses. Radiographically a soft tissue mass can be seen adjacent to bone destruction. A better assessment can be made by CT scan or MRI.

If left untreated, the pseudotumor can reach an enormous size capable of compressing neurovascular structures and causing pathologic fractures [18]. Its management will depend on the site, size and speed of growth, as well as its effects on adjacent structures. A 6–8-week course of treatment with clotting factor is usually performed, with MRI monitoring, and if the pseudotumor shrinks, 3 more cycles are repeated [4]. In many cases surgery becomes necessary, with the aim of resecting the pseudotumor. In some cases, aspiration followed by fibrin injection, arterial embolization, or radiotherapy may be effective.

12.2.6 Pain Management

Acute and chronic pain are common in people with hemophilia (PWH), so it is essential to evaluate it properly to determine its cause and guide the appropriate management. PWH may suffer from different types of pain (neuropathic or nociceptive) [20], so assessing its characteristics, location, and intensity, among other parameters, will help in its proper management.

Adequate treatment of pain improves joint function, prevents immobility and increases quality of life. The approach should be multimodal and establish a therapeutic plan agreed with the patient, through shared decision making [21].

12.2.6.1 Painkillers

Ninety-five percent of pain syndromes are treatable with painkillers [22]. The World Health Organization (WHO) analgesic ladder is still valid and has been adapted for PWH [4]. It includes different drugs according to pain intensity, and recommends the use of adjuvant drugs (Table 12.4). The analgesic prescription should be made according to the intensity and type of pain, with the simplest and most effective dosage and administration. Pain, drug response, and side effects should be evaluated periodically [21]. In PWH with mild/moderate hepatic or renal insufficiency, dose and dosage adjustment should be made. Rescue medication should be included and the intramuscular route is not advised [4]. Due to opioids abuse crises, it has been published that minimally invasive procedures could be considered in the third step, leaving major opioids as a last option [23].

12.2.6.2 Minimally Invasive Interventional Procedures

Intra-articular injections are useful for pain relief in PWH. They should always be done with controlled hemostasis and asepsis [21]. Hyaluronic acid can relieve joint pain for 6–12 months. Corticosteroids produce benefit for weeks, although they are not routinely recommended. Local anesthetics can be added. The efficacy of platelet-rich plasma (PRP) and mesenchymal stem cells (MSCs) in hemophilic arthropathy is still under study [17]. In this context, in addition to

Table 12.4 Painkillers recommended in hemophilia based on the World Health Organization (WHO) analgesic ladder

	Pain intensity	Recommendation	Painkillers
1	Mild pain	Non-opioid ± Adjuvant	Acetaminophen (paracetamol) Metamizol COX-2 inhibitors
2	Mild to moderate pain	Weak opioid + Non-opioid ± Adjuvant	Tramadol Codeine[a]
3	Moderate to severe pain	Strong opioid + Non-opioid ± Adjuvant	Morphine Buprenorfine Fentanyl Oxycodone (±naloxone) Hidromorphone Tapentadol

Adjuvants: steroids, antidepressants (amitriptyline, serotonin and norepinephrine reuptake inhibitor—SNRI), anticonvulsivants (gabapentine, pregabaline), duloxetine, lidocaine, capsaicine
Opioids from second and third steps cannot be associated
An approach using combinations of drugs that target different metabolic pathways may improve analgesia and reduce side effects
[a] Avoid use of codeine in children under 12 years of age

intra-articular injections, nerve blocks or radiofrequency ablation are options to be considered, provided they are performed by pain specialists [23].

12.2.6.3 Physical Exercise

The physical, psychological, and socio-affective benefits of physical exercise are multiple and well known and can reduce pain through central neurobiological mechanisms [24]. Although the actual effects of physical exercise on chronic pain in PWH are not fully known, we know that it is fundamental in the optimal management of hemophilia [25]. We should therefore recommend physical exercise at moderate intensities and avoiding contusion to prevent the risk of bleeding [26]. Aquatic exercise may be more analgesic than dry exercise [14]. Although there is little experience in hemophilia, mind-body therapies are recommended as complementary techniques [4].

12.2.6.4 External Devices

Immobilization of the joint in a position of comfort may be useful in the early stages to relieve the pain of joint or muscle bleeding, although this period should end when the pain begins to subside [4]. Other orthoses may be useful for chronic pain due to hemophilic arthropathy, especially when there is associated malalignment. Knee valgus orthoses seem to improve short-term pain in patients with osteoarthritis, or custom-made insoles seem to improve joint pain and ankle function in hemophilic arthropathy of the ankle when there is hindfoot malalignment. Athletic footwear may provide better comfort and support for the foot, and therefore may improve pain in patients with ankle arthropathy. The use of crutches, by reducing the load, can alleviate pain in different joints of the lower limbs [27].

12.2.6.5 Other Modalities

For PWH with chronic pain, it is recommended to add the use of complementary pain management techniques. This requires a care team that integrates all points of view [21]. These include lifestyle changes and educational/psychological approaches, and simple techniques such as meditation, distraction, mindfulness, or music therapy can be incorporated [4]. Some techniques such as mindfulness have been shown to improve chronic pain, depressive symptoms, and quality of life [28]. Some other rehabilitation techniques such as manual therapy, electrotherapy, and thermotherapy may be useful, although published studies are of low quality and their usefulness is unclear [29]. People with persistent pain should be referred to a specialized pain management team for interventional techniques. When pain is disabling and not controlled by non-surgical therapies, we should also consider the benefits of different orthopedic surgical techniques for pain relief (see Chaps. 16, 17, and 18 of this book). For patients with hemophilia and postoperative pain, proportional pain management in coordination with the anesthesiologist or pain specialist is advised. Management should be similar to that used in patients without hemophilia, avoiding nonsteroidal anti-inflammatory drugs (NSAIDs, although selective cyclooxygenase-2 (COX-2) inhibitors can be used) and the intramuscular route for analgesic administration [4].

12.2.7 Osteoporosis

Lower bone mineral density (BMD) has been demonstrated in people with hemophilia. The direct effects of intra-articular blood derivatives on bone remodeling and inactivity associated with polyarthropathy are associated with lower BMD [30]. In addition to good hemostatic coverage to prevent hemarthroses, weight-bearing activities that promote the development and maintenance of good bone quality should be encouraged. This is especially important in younger patients, so that during growth they build bone mass and reduce the risk of subsequent osteoporosis. All patients with hemophilia should be encouraged to engage in regular physical activity and to have adequate calcium and vitamin D intake. When low BMD is suspected, accurate diagnosis should be made by bone densitometry. Osteoporosis increases the risk of fragility fractures. To avoid this increased risk of fracture in patients with hemophilia and osteoporosis, treatment with calcium and vitamin D supplements as well as bisphosphonates should be considered [31].

12.2.8 Age-Related Musculoskeletal (MSK) Comorbidities

Due to improvements in hemophilia treatment and care, the life expectancy of people with hemophilia has approached that of the general population. Although arthropathy remains the main comorbidity, with increasing age, other orthopedic comorbidities such as osteoarthritis, sarcopenia, muscle weakness, and gait and balance disturbances are superimposed. This leads to an increased risk of falls and fractures [32].

It appears that age-related effects on the MSK system can be reduced by exercise. Multicomponent programs, including weight-bearing exercise, gait and balance training, functional tasks, muscle strengthening, and three-dimensional exercise, performed two to three times per week for at least 12 weeks, appear to be most effective in the older person [33]. It also appears that orthopedic surgery in this group of patients is safe and effective, with outcomes close to those of the general population. However, establishing whether exercise programs and orthopedic surgery offer good results in older people with hemophilia is a priority for future research [32].

12.3 Conclusions

Knowledge of the MSK and functional manifestations of hemophilia is essential when applying an adequate and individualized treatment. Acute MSK hemorrhages should be treated with on-demand administration of the deficient factor until adequate levels are reached to stop the bleeding event. The role of MSK Medicine includes the prevention, diagnosis, and treatment of MSK bleeds and their consequences, as well as the management of pain and related biomechanical disorders. The ultimate goal in the management of hemophilia is to prevent the development of disability and impairment of quality of life often associated with hemophilia. In patients with hemophilia, physical activity should be promoted to achieve better joint protection, and impact and collision activities should be avoided.

References

1. De la Corte-Rodriguez H, Rodriguez-Merchan EC. The role of physical medicine and rehabilitation in haemophiliac patients. Blood Coagul Fibrinolysis. 2013;24:1–9.

2. Blanchette VS, Key NS, Ljung LR, Manco-Johnson MJ, van den Berg HM, Srivastava A. Definitions in hemophilia: communication from the SSC of the ISTH. J Thromb Haemost. 2014;12:1935–9.
3. Lafeber FP, Miossec P, Valentino LA. Physiopathology of haemophilic arthropathy. Haemophilia. 2008;14(4):3–9.
4. Srivastava A, Santagostino E, Dougall A, Kitchen S, Sutherland M, Pipe SW, et al. WFH guidelines for the management of hemophilia. Haemophilia. 2020;26(6):1–158.
5. Rodriguez-Merchan EC, De la Corte-Rodriguez H. Acute hemophilic hemarthrosis: is local cryotherapy recommended? Expert Rev Hematol. 2017;10:1029–32.
6. De la Corte-Rodriguez H, Rodriguez-Merchan EC, Alvarez-Roman MT, Martin-Salces M, Romero-Garrido JA, Jimenez-Yuste V. Accelerating recovery from acute hemarthrosis in patients with hemophilia: the role of joint aspiration. Blood Coagul Fibrinolysis. 2019;30:111–9.
7. Pulles AE, Mastbergen SC, Schutgens RE, Lafeber FP, van Vulpen LF. Pathophysiology of hemophilic arthropathy and potential targets for therapy. Pharmacol Res. 2017;115:192–9.
8. Foppen W, Fischer K, van der Schaaf IC. Imaging of haemophilic arthropathy: awareness of pitfalls and need for standardization. Haemophilia. 2017;23:645–7.
9. Nguyen S, Lu X, Ma Y, Du J, Chang EY, von Drygalski A. Musculoskeletal ultrasound for intra-articular bleed detection: a highly sensitive imaging modality compared with conventional magnetic resonance imaging. J Thromb Haemost. 2018;16:490–9.
10. Gringeri A, Ewenstein B, Reininger A. The burden of bleeding in haemophilia: is one bleed too many? Haemophilia. 2014;20:459–63.
11. Martinoli C, Casa D, Di Minno G, Graziano E, Molinari AC, Pasta G, et al. Development and definition of a simplified scanning procedure and scoring method for haemophilia early arthropathy detection with ultrasound. Thromb Haemost. 2013;109:1170–9.
12. De la Corte-Rodriguez H, Rodriguez-Merchan EC, Alvarez-Roman MT, Martin-Salces M, Martinoli C, Jimenez-Yuste V. The value of HEAD-US system in detecting subclinicalabnormalities in joints of patients with hemophilia. Expert Rev Hematol. 2018;11:253–61.
13. Poonnoose PM, Hilliard P, Doria AS, Keshava SN, Gibikote S, Kavitha ML, et al. Correlating clinical and radiological assessment of joints in haemophilia: results of a cross sectional study. Haemophilia. 2016;22:925–33.
14. Strike K, Mulder K, Michael R. Exercise for haemophilia. Cochrane Database Syst Rev. 2016;12:CD011180. https://doi.org/10.1002/14651858.CD011180.pub2.
15. Buccheri E, Avola M, Vitale N, Pavone P, Vecchio M. Haemophilic arthropathy: a narrative review on the use of intra-articular drugs for arthritis. Haemophilia. 2019;25:919–27.
16. McAlindon TE, LaValley MP, Harvey WF, Price LL, Driban JB, Zhang M, et al. Effect of intra-articular triamcinolone vs saline on knee cartilage volume and pain in patients with knee osteoarthritis. JAMA. 2017;317:1967–75.
17. Rodriguez-Merchan EC. Musculo-skeletal manifestations of haemophilia. Blood Rev. 2016;30:401–9.
18. Rodriguez-Merchan EC. The role of orthopedic surgery in haemophiia: current rationale, indications and results. EFORT Open Rev. 2019;4:165–73.
19. De la Corte-Rodriguez H, Rodriguez-Merchan EC. Treatment of muscle haematomas in haemophiliacs with special emphasis on percutaneous drainage. Blood Coagul Fibrinolysis. 2014;25:787–94.
20. Roussel NA. Gaining insight into the complexity of pain in patients with haemophilia: State-of-the-art review on pain processing. Haemophilia. 2018;24(6):3–8.
21. Rodriguez-Merchan EC. Treatment of musculo-skeletal pain in haemophilia. Blood Rev. 2018;32:116–21.
22. WHO guidelines for the pharmacological treatment of persisting pain in adults with medical illnesses. 2012. Available at: https://www.who.int/medicines/areas/quality_safety/Scoping_WHO_GLs_PersistPainAdults_webversion.pdf?ua=1.
23. Yang J, Bauer BA, Wahner-Roedler DL, Chon TY, Xiao L. The modified WHO analgesic ladder: is it appropriate for chronic non-cancer pain? J Pain Res. 2020;13:411–7.
24. de Zoete RMJ, Chen K, Sterling M. Central neurobiological effects of physical exercise in individuals with chronic musculoskeletal pain: a systematic review. BMJ Open. 2020;10(7):e036151.
25. Siqueira TC, Dominski FH, Andrade A. Effects of exercise in people with haemophilia: an umbrella review of systematic reviews and meta-analyses. Haemophilia. 2019;25:928–37.
26. Broderick CR, Herbert RD, Latimer J, Barnes C, Curtin JA, Mathieu E, et al. Association between physical activity and risk of bleeding in children with hemophilia. JAMA. 2012;308:1452–9.
27. De la Corte-Rodriguez H, Rodriguez-Merchan EC. The current role of orthoses in treating haemophilic arthropathy. Haemophilia. 2015;21:723–30.
28. Hilton L, Hempel S, Ewing BA, Apaydin E, Xenakis L, Newberry S, et al. Mindfulness meditation for chronic pain: systematic review and meta-analysis. Ann Behav Med. 2017;51:199–213.
29. McLaughlin P, Hurley M, Chowdary P, Khair K, Stephensen D. Physiotherapy interventions for pain management in haemophilia: a systematic review. Haemophilia. 2020;26:667–84.
30. Iorio A, Fabbriciani G, Marcucci M, Brozzetti M, Filipponi P. Bone mineral density in haemophilia patients: a meta-analysis. Thromb Haemost. 2010;103:596–603.

31. Kovacs CS. Hemophilia, low bone mass, and osteopenia/osteoporosis. Transfus Apher Sci. 2008;38:33–40.
32. Stephensen D, Rodriguez-Merchan EC. Orthopaedic co-morbidities in the elderly haemophilia population: a review. Haemophilia. 2013;19:166–73.
33. Liu CJ, Latham NK. Progressive resistance strength training for improving physical function in older adults. Cochrane Database Syst Rev. 2009;3:CD002759.

13 Management of Acute Hemarthrosis in Hemophilia (Including Joint Aspiration)

E. Carlos Rodríguez-Merchán and Hortensia De la Corte-Rodríguez

13.1 Introduction

About 90% of bleeds in hemophilia happen in the joints (hemarthroses), mainly the knees, ankles, and elbows. Such hemarthroses cause severe disability and reduced health-related quality of life (HRQoL) to hemophilic patients [1–3]. When hemarthroses are frequent, the synovium will be unable to reabsorb all the intra-articular blood. Then it will become hypertrophic, causing chronic hemophilic synovitis [4–10]. Therefore, it is paramount not only to avoid acute joint bleeds, but also to manage them as efficiently as possible. Intra-articular bleeding also causes cartilage damage (chondrocyte apoptosis). Such damage will destroy the joint eventually (hemophilic arthropathy) [11].

Primary hematologic prophylaxis from the age of two to the end of skeletal maturity is the gold standard of current treatment of hemophilia. Such prophylaxis will decrease the frequency of joint hemorrhages in hemophilic patients [12, 13]. However, problems may be caused by the permanent intravenous infusion of factor concentrates. Two bypassing agents, FEIBA, factor eight inhibitor bypassing agent (Baxter AG, Vienna, Austria) and NovoSeven [recombinant factor VIIa (rFVIIa), NovoNordisk, Denmark] are available for prophylaxis in people with hemophilia (PWH) who have developed inhibitors (antibodies against factor VIII and IX that make patients not to respond to intravenous infusion of factor VIII or factor IX (FVIII or FIX) [14].

The early management of intra-articular bleeding will prevent cartilage and joint destruction [15]. Unfortunately, most developing countries have limited resources and only use on-demand treatment, which consists of the administration of the deficient coagulation factor when a joint bleed occurs. The aim of this chapter is to review the current management of acute hemarthroses in PWH.

13.2 Clinical Manifestations of Acute Bleeding

The typical symptoms of joint bleed are pain, swelling, and limited range of motion. Intra-articular blood causes cartilage cell apoptosis and also hemophilic synovitis. It seems that one or more of the many components of blood are responsible for the inflammatory and synovial/vascular cell proliferation response associated with recurrent intra-articular bleeds [16]. The exact mechanisms related to blood-induced joint disease are not known yet. It is likely that iron deposition in the synovium induces an inflamma-

E. C. Rodríguez-Merchán (✉)
Department of Orthopedic Surgery, La Paz University Hospital, Madrid, Spain

H. De la Corte-Rodríguez
Department of Physical and Rehabilitation Medicine, La Paz University Hospital, Madrid, Spain

E. C. Rodríguez-Merchán (ed.), *Advances in Hemophilia Treatment*,
https://doi.org/10.1007/978-3-030-93990-8_13

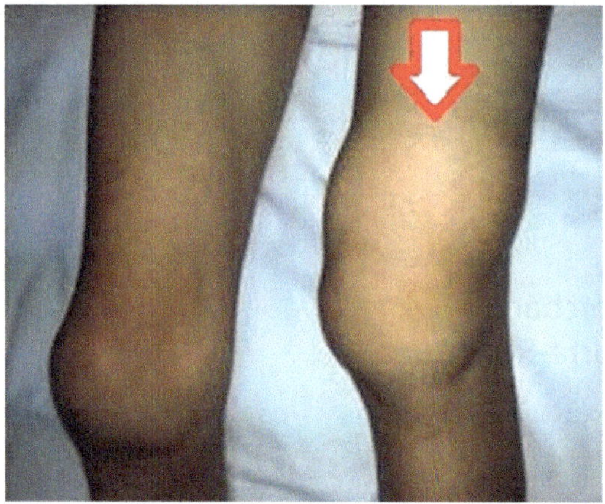

Fig. 13.1 Clinical view of acute bleeding in the knee joint (arrow)

tory response that causes not only immune system activation but also stimulates angiogenesis. This process will lead to cartilage destruction. Three cellular regulators (p53, p21, and TRAIL) that are important for iron metabolism seem to be induced in the synovium [17].

Acute bleeding is usually felt by the hemophilic patient as a burning sensation in the joint. Hemarthrosis develops within a few hours; in clinical examination the joint is inflamed, tense, warm, and the skin becomes red (Fig. 13.1). The affected joint is always held in an antalgic flexion position, and the range of motion is very limited (Fig. 13.2).

Ideally, the clinical diagnosis of hemarthrosis must be confirmed by means of ultrasonography (US), and hematologic treatment must be continued until full disappearance of blood into the joint [18, 19] (Fig. 13.3). This can be confirmed by a new US performed 1–2 weeks later. Otherwise, there will be a tendency to recurrent hemarthroses, chronic synovitis, and joint degeneration [11].

An experimental study showed that hemarthrosis induces synovial urokinase-type plasminogen activator (uPA) expression and results in an increase in synovial plasmin levels, making the joint more vulnerable to recurrent bleedings [20]. Another report demonstrated alterations in monocyte/macrophage polarization following hemarthrosis resulting in a blood monocyte M1 phenotype and a combined M1-M2 monocyte/macrophage phenotype in the joint [21]. A third experimental study showed detrimental effects of the blood on the overall cartilage function under loading. That is why non-weight bearing (rest) and early joint aspiration were recommended [22]. Finally, this has been proved that more than two to three bleeding into the same joint may cause irreversible joint damage that will compromise HRQoL [23].

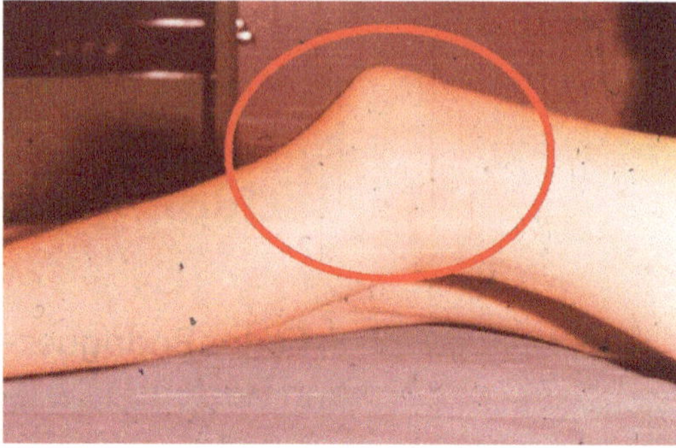

Fig. 13.2 Clinical view of knee flexion contracture (circle)

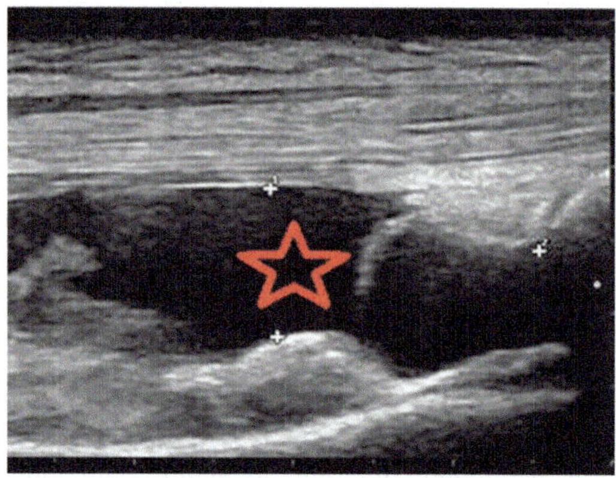

Fig. 13.3 Confirmation of acute articular bleeding (star) by means of ultrasonography (US)

13.3 Treatment of Acute Hemarthrosis

13.3.1 Hematologic Treatment

On-demand therapy with a plasma-derived or recombinant FVIII or FIX concentrate is the first-line treatment for acute bleeding episodes in hemophilic patients [1, 3, 13]. Dosing ranges from 20 to 40 IU/kg administered until bleeding stops. Infusion of FVIII 40 IU/kg at the time of joint hemorrhage and 20 IU/kg at 24 and 72 h after the first dose is recommended. Then we must continue infusions of 20 IU/kg every other day, until joint pain and impairment of mobility had completely resolved. US is very important in acute hemarthroses. US can identify the presence of blood in the joints and confirm its complete disappearance [18].

In patients with inhibitors, bypassing agents must be used [24]. Smejkal et al. found that the median cumulative dose of FEIBA per bleeding episode was 205 U kg^{-1}. Although bleeding stopped in 97% of events, re-bleeding occurred in 5% of events within 48 h after cessation of bleeding [25]. Regarding rFVIIa, the recommended dose is 90 mcg kg^{-1} [26].

A study evaluated and compared one to three doses of vatreptacog alfa at 5, 10, 20, 40, and 80 lg kg^{-1} with one to three doses of rFVIIa at 90 lg kg^{-1} in the treatment of acute joint bleeds in PWH with inhibitors [27]. 98% of bleeds were controlled within 9 h of the initial dose in a combined evaluation of 20–80 lg kg^{-1} vatreptacog alfa.

After the administration of the appropriate hematologic treatment, pain will rapidly diminish, although inflammation and limitation of range of motion commonly disappear more slowly.

13.3.2 Rest and Splinting

In lower limb bleeding episodes bed rest for one day is recommended. In the following 3–5 days, weight-bearing is contraindicated. Crutches must be used when ambulating and elevation when sitting. For the knee a compressive bandage is adequate. For the ankle, a short-leg posterior plaster splint is recommended. For the upper limb, usually a sling (for the shoulder) or a long-arm posterior plaster splint (for the elbow) will provide sufficient rest. Lifting and carrying heavy items is contraindicated until the bleeding has resolved (3–5 days).

13.3.3 Ice

Ice therapy could help to relieve pain and reduce the extent of bleeding, although its current role in hemophilia remains controversial. Experimental cooling of blood and/or tissue can significantly impair coagulation and prolong bleeding [28].

13.3.4 Analgesia

For pain, analgesic medication should be administered, including paracetamol in mild pain, metamizole for more intense pain, and in a few precise patients, soft opioids such as codeine or tramadol [29]. In the circumstance of intolerable pain we should use morphine hydrochloride either by continual infusion or a patient-controlled analgesia (PCA) pump, determined by the age, mental condition, and grade of observance of the patient. Epidural blocks utilizing bupivacaine and fentanyl may be very efficacious as well [29].

13.3.5 Joint Aspiration (Arthrocentesis)

In cases of severe bleeding arthrocentesis may relieve the patient's pain and speed up rehabilitation. There is a great deal of controversy on the role of arthrocentesis in hemophilia. Arthrocentesis should be performed in major hemarthrosis (very tense and painful joints) (Fig. 13.4). Joint aspiration should always be done under factor coverage and in aseptic conditions. In immunodepressed patients, septic arthritis can mimic hemarthrosis [30].

It is important to emphasize that while arthrocentesis of the elbow, knee, and ankle (Fig. 13.5) are quite simple procedures that can be done at the outpatient clinic, both shoulder and hip joint aspirations require sedation and radiographic control by an image intensifier, that is to say, they are surgical procedures done in an operating room, with an anesthesiologist and by an orthopedic surgeon [31].

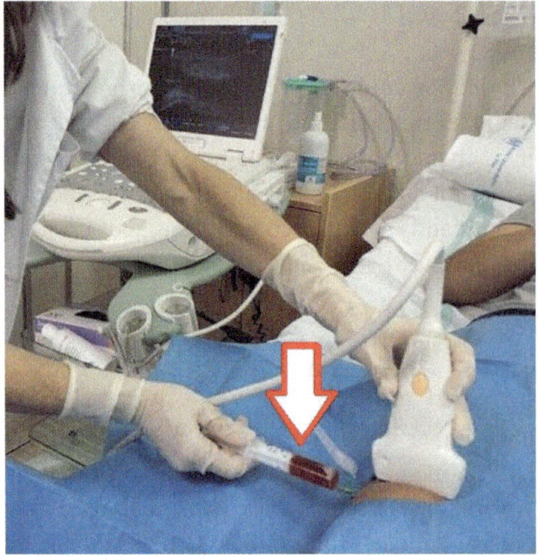

Fig. 13.4 Joint aspiration (arrow) of acute knee hemarthrosis guided by ultrasonography (US)

Our study published in 2019 showed that early aspiration of an acute hemarthrosis, combined with appropriate hematologic treatment, may result in a shorter time to recovery as compared with conventional treatment (without joint aspiration) [19]. Indeed, aspiration reduced the number of days during which the joint was exposed to blood; the number of days of additional hematologic therapy; the number of days of pain and decreased joint range of motion; and the number of days away from school/work. Moreover, joint aspiration proved to be a safe procedure with no short- or long-term complications. We consider that arthrocentesis, performed under hemostatic cover and in aseptic conditions, can safely and effectively contribute to faster recovery in patients with hemophilia following an acute hemarthrosis.

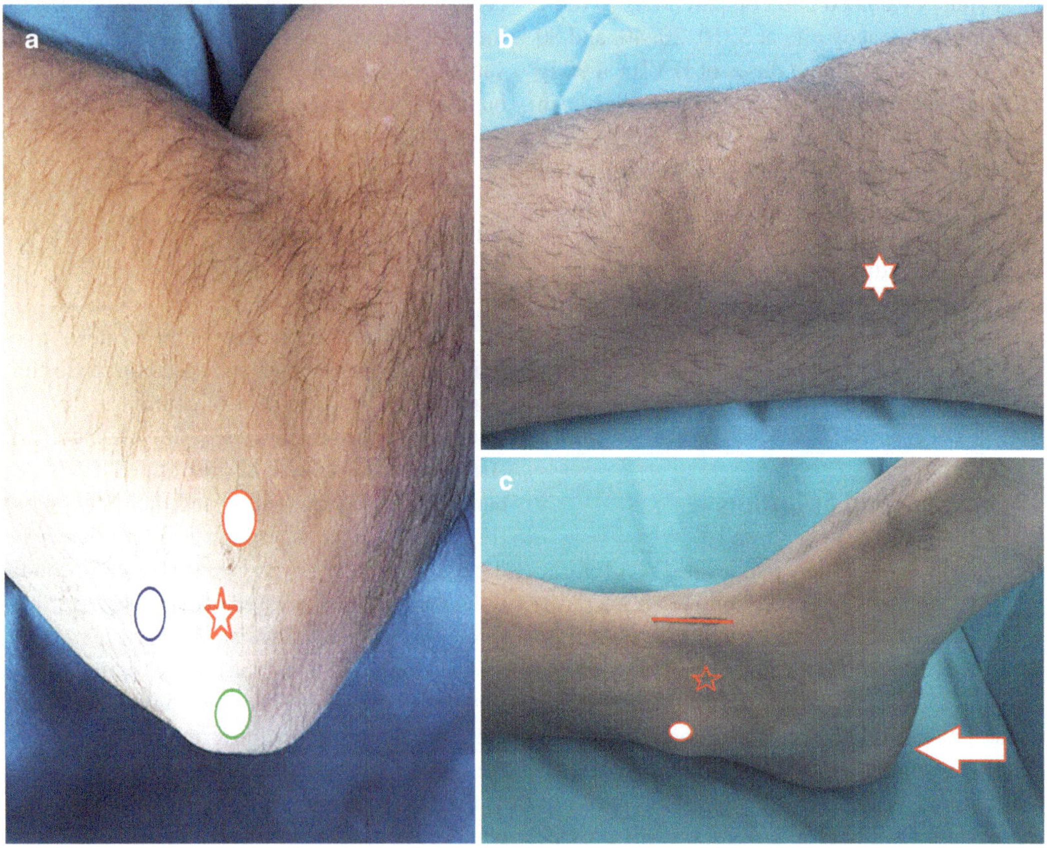

Fig. 13.5 (**a**–**c**) Joint aspiration technique: Sites for needle insertion into the intra-articular space for the different joints. (**a**) Elbow: at the center of the triangle (star) formed by the olecranon (green circle), the lateral epicondyle (red circle), and the radial head (blue circle). (**b**) Knee: 2 cm proximal and 2 cm lateral to the superolateral angle of the patella (star). (**c**) Ankle: at the depression (star) that lies between the anterior tibial tendon (line) and the medial malleolus (circle). The heel is marked with an arrow

13.3.6 Arterial Embolization

Arterial embolization must be taken into account in recurrent massive bleeds. To avoid recurrent articular bleeds. This way, consumption of factor concentrate can decrease to one-third of the amount consumed before embolization [32–35].

To sum up, diagnosis and treatment of intra-articular hemorrhages must be carried out as early as possible. Treatment must be administered intensively (enhanced on-demand treatment) until the resolution of symptoms. Joint aspiration plays an important role in acute and profuse hemarthroses. US is paramount to assess the evolution of acute hemarthroses in hemophilic patients [36].

13.4 Conclusions

Treatment of acute hemarthroses is a combination of adequate factor replacement, joint aspiration, rest, ice therapy, analgesia, and physical medicine and rehabilitation. The objectives of treatment are to avoid recurrent hemarthroses and muscular atrophy and maintain an adequate articular range of motion. The joints treated with joint aspiration exhibit a significantly faster resolution of bleeding (fewer days). The joints treated with joint aspiration require fewer days of hematological treatment. In joints treated with joint aspiration faster achievement of functional recovery and resumption of school/work are observed. Joint aspiration under hemostatic cover and in strictly aseptic conditions is the most effective and safest route to recovery in hemophilic patients with acute hemarthrosis.

References

1. Simpson ML, Valentino LA. Management of joint bleeding in hemophilia. Expert Rev Hematol. 2012;5:459–68.
2. Rodriguez-Merchan EC, De la Corte-Garcia H. Musculoskeletal manifestations of hemophilia. In: Rodríguez-Merchan EC, editor. Joint surgery in the adult patient with hemophilia. Cham: Springer; 2015. p. 1–12.
3. Rodriguez-Merchan EC. Articular bleeding in hemophilia. Cardiovasc Hematol Disord Drug Targets. 2016;16:21–4.
4. Rodriguez-Merchan EC. Pathogenesis, early diagnosis, and prophylaxis for chronic hemophilic synovitis. Clin Orthop Relat Res. 1997;343:6–11.
5. Rodriguez-Merchan EC. Management of musculoskeletal complications of hemophilia. Semin Thromb Hemost. 2003;29:87–96.
6. Rodriguez-Merchan EC. Effects of hemophilia on articulations of children and adults. Clin Orthop Relat Res. 1996;328:7–13.
7. Rodriguez-Merchan EC, Magallon M, Galindo E, Lopez-Cabarcos C. Hemophilic synovitis of the knee and elbow. Clin Orthop Relat Res. 1997;343:47–53.
8. Dunn AL. Pathophysiology, diagnosis and prevention of arthropathy in patients with haemophilia. Haemophilia. 2011;17:571–8.
9. Valentino LA, Hakobyan N, Enockson C, Simpson ML, Kakodkar NC, Cong L, et al. Exploring the biological basis of haemophilic joint disease: experimental studies. Haemophilia. 2012;18:310–8.
10. Roosendaal G, Lafeber FP. Pathogenesis of haemophilic arthropathy. Haemophilia. 2006;12(3):117–21.
11. Rodriguez-Merchan EC, Jimenez-Yuste V, Aznar JA, Hedner U, Knobe K, Lee CA, et al. Joint protection in haemophilia. Haemophilia. 2011;17(2):1–23.
12. Manco-Johnson MJ, Abshire TC, Shapiro AD, Riske B, Hacker MR, Kilcoyne R, et al. Prophylaxis versus episodic treatment to prevent joint disease in boys with severe hemophilia. N Engl J Med. 2007;357:535–44.
13. Srivastava A, Brewer AK, Mauser-Bunschoten EP, Key NS, Kitchen S, Llinas A, et al. Treatment Guidelines Working Group on Behalf of The World Federation of Hemophilia. Guidelines for the management of hemophilia. Haemophilia. 2013;19:1–47.
14. Carcao M, Lambert T. Prophylaxis in haemophilia with inhibitors: update from international experience. Haemophilia. 2010;16(2):16–23.
15. Hermans C, De Moerloose P, Fischer K, Holstein K, Klamroth R, Lambert T, et al. Management of acute haemarthrosis in haemophilia A without inhibitors: literature review, European survey and recommendations. Haemophilia. 2011;17:383–92.
16. Valentino LA, Hakobyan N, Enockson C. Blood-induced joint disease: the confluence of dysregulated oncogenes, inflammatory signals, and angiogenic cues. Semin Hematol. 2008;45(2):S50–7.
17. Valentino LA, Hakobyan N, Rodriguez N, Hoots WK. Pathogenesis of haemophilic synovitis: experimental studies on blood-induced joint damage. Haemophilia. 2007;13(3):10–3.
18. Querol F, Rodriguez-Merchan EC. The role of ultrasonography in the diagnosis of the musculo-skeletal problems of haemophilia. Haemophilia. 2012;18:e215–26.
19. De la Corte-Rodriguez H, Rodriguez-Merchan EC, Alvarez-Roman MT, Martin-Salces M, Romero-Garrido JA, Jimenez-Yuste V. Accelerating recovery from acute hemarthrosis in patients with hemophilia:

the role of joint aspiration. Blood Coagul Fibrinolysis. 2019;30:111–9.
20. Nieuwenhuizen L, Roosendaal G, Coeleveld K, Lubberts E, Biesma DH, Lafeber FP, et al. Haemarthrosis stimulates the synovial fibrinolytic system in haemophilic mice. Thromb Haemost. 2013;110:173–83.
21. Nieuwenhuizen L, Schutgens RE, Coeleveld K, Mastbergen SC, Roosendaal G, Biesma DH, et al. Hemarthrosis in hemophilic mice results in alterations in M1-M2 monocyte/macrophage polarization. Thromb Res. 2014;133:390–5.
22. Ravanbod R, Torkaman G, Esteki A. Biotribological and biomechanical changes after experimental haemarthrosis in the rabbit knee. Haemophilia. 2011;17:124–33.
23. Gringeri A, Ewenstein B, Reininger A. The burden of bleeding in haemophilia: is one bleed too many? Haemophilia. 2014;20:459–63.
24. Berntorp E. Importance of rapid bleeding control in haemophilia complicated by inhibitors. Haemophilia. 2011;17:11–6.
25. Smejkal P, Brabec P, Matyskova M, Bulikova A, Slechtova M, Kissova J, et al. FEIBA in treatment of acute bleeding episodes in patients with haemophilia A and factor VIII inhibitors: a retrospective survey in regional haemophilia centre. Haemophilia. 2009;15:743–51.
26. Young G, Auerswald G, Jimenez-Yuste V, Konkle BA, Lambert T, Morfini M, et al. When should prophylaxis therapy in inhibitor patients be considered? Haemophilia. 2011;17:849–57.
27. de Paula EV, Kavakli K, Mahlangu J, Ayob Y, Lentz SR, Morfini M, et al. Recombinant factor VIIa analog (vatreptacog alfa [activated]) for treatment of joint bleeds in hemophilia patients with inhibitors: a randomized controlled trial. J Thromb Haemost. 2012;10:81–9.
28. Forsyth AL, Zourikian N, Valentino LA, Rivard GE. The effect of cooling on coagulation and haemostasis: should "Ice" be part of treatment of acute haemarthrosis in haemophilia? Haemophilia. 2012;18:843–50.
29. Rodriguez-Merchan EC. Treatment of musculoskeletal pain in haemophilia. Blood Rev. 2018;32:116–21.
30. Rodriguez-Merchan EC, Magallon M, Manso F, Martin-Villar J. Septic arthritis in HIV positive haemophiliacs. Four cases and a literature review. Int Orthop. 1992;16:302–6.
31. Heim M, Varon D, Strauss S, Martinowitz U. The management of a person with haemophilia who has a fixed flexed hip and intractable pain. Haemophilia. 1998;4:842–4.
32. Klamroth R, Gottstein S, Essers E, Landgraf H, Wilaschek M, Oldenburg J. Successful angiographic embolization of recurrent elbow and knee joint bleeds in seven patients with severe haemophilia. Haemophilia. 2009;15:247–52.
33. Mauser-Bunschoten EP, Zijl JA, Mali W, van Rinsum AC, van den Berg HM, Roosendaal G. Successful treatment of severe bleeding in hemophilic target joints by selective angiographic embolization. Blood. 2005;105:2654–7.
34. Rodriguez-Merchan EC. Methods to treat chronic haemophilic synovitis. Haemophilia. 2001;7:1–5.
35. Galli E, Baques A, Moretti N, Candela M, Caviglia H. Hemophilic chronic synovitis: therapy of hemarthrosis using endovascular embolization of knee and elbow arteries. Cardiovasc Intervent Radiol. 2013;36:964–9.
36. Rodriguez-Merchan EC, Jimenez-Yuste V. The role of selective angiographic embolization of the musculoskeletal system in haemophilia. Haemophilia. 2009;15:864–8.

Hemophilic Arthropathy: Radiosynovectomy

14

E. Carlos Rodríguez-Merchán and Hortensia De la Corte-Rodríguez

14.1 Introduction

Hemophilic arthropathy takes place due to repeated hemorrhages into articulations leading to swelling, destruction of cartilage and bone, and development of osteoarthritis [1]. Although prophylactic replacement therapy helps in precluding arthropathy, it is not at all times appropriate (due to patient's lack of adherence) or affordable [2–8]. Early primary prophylaxis is the only approach for precluding arthropathy in hemophilia patients without inhibitors, admitting that it is not invariably totally effective in eluding joint complications [2–5].

In children with inhibitors, bypassing agents (aPCCs and/or rFVIIa) prophylaxis is also advised to hinder musculoskeletal impairment [2–5, 9]. Consequently, early primary prophylaxis is the gold standard of management of hemophilia to preclude articular damage due to the effect of blood on the synovium and the chondrocytes.

Hemarthrosis produces chondrocyte apoptosis and synovitis leading to a vicious cycle of synovitis-hemarthrosis-synovitis. Such a cycle must be ruptured as soon as possible to arrest or decelerate the development of hemophilic arthropathy. The hypertrophic synovial membrane can be palpated as a solid tissue in clinical examination.

Extirpation of the hypertrophic synovium can be carried out by means of radioactive materials [10–23]. The objective is to decrease the risk of chronic synovitis and repeated hemarthroses that in the end will cause joint degeneration (hemophilic arthropathy) (Fig. 14.1).

Hemophilia is a polyarticular illness (affecting principally ankles, knees, and elbows). Accordingly, therapeutic indications must take into consideration that we always treat a multiarticular problem. Ratification of diagnosis must be achieved by means of magnetic resonance imaging (MRI) and/or ultrasonography (US) [24–28]. The aim of this chapter is to review the contemporary role of radiosynovectomy (RS) in the management of chronic hemophilic synovitis, both in patients with inhibitors and patients without inhibitors.

14.2 Indications for Radiosynovectomy

RS consists of the extirpation of the hypertrophic synovial membrane by means of the intraarticular injection of a radioactive material. Our indications for RS are the following [16–21]: (1) Two or more incidents of hemarthrosis in the preceding

E. C. Rodríguez-Merchán (✉)
Department of Orthopedic Surgery, La Paz University Hospital, Madrid, Spain

H. De la Corte-Rodríguez
Department of Physical and Rehabilitation Medicine, La Paz University Hospital, Madrid, Spain

E. C. Rodríguez-Merchán (ed.), *Advances in Hemophilia Treatment*,
https://doi.org/10.1007/978-3-030-93990-8_14

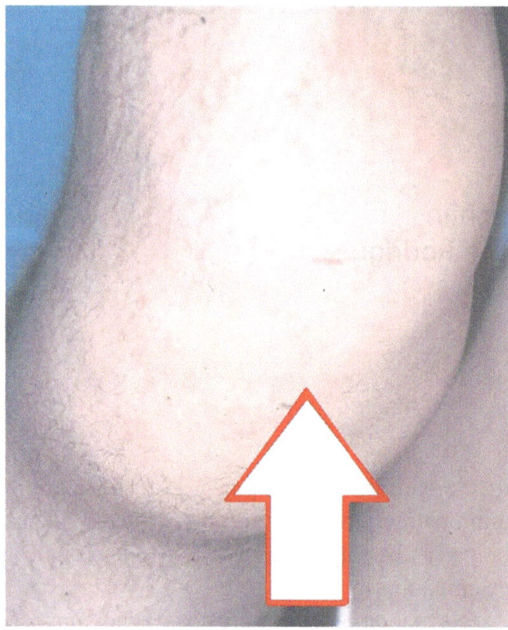

Fig. 14.1 Severe degree of chronic synovitis in a young hemophilia patient (arrow)

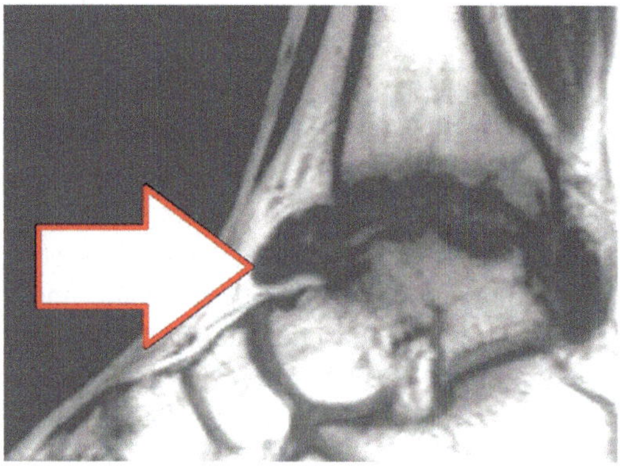

Fig. 14.2 Magnetic resonance imaging (MRI) image showing severe synovitis of the ankle (arrow)

6 months; synovitis must be proved by MRI (Fig. 14.2) and/or US (Fig. 14.3). (2) A new RS must be carried out in patients with two or more incidents of hemarthrosis in the subsequent 6 months. RS must only be performed in a hemophilia treatment center setting.

MRI (which is the gold standard) and/or US may augment our early discovery of synovial hypertrophy. RS can be carried out at any age. According to Doria et al. [29], although MRI

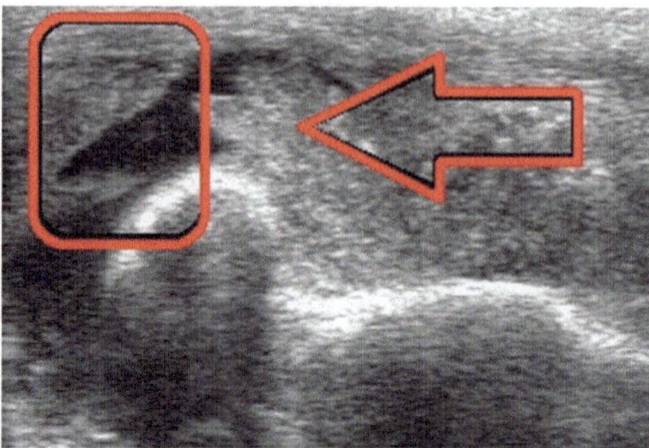

Fig. 14.3 Ultrasonography (US) longitudinal view of a hemophilic elbow with joint effusion (square) and severe synovial thickening (arrow)

is the gold standard, US is extremely sensitive (>92%) for evaluating synovial hypertrophy. MRI can be carried out every 6–12 months whereas US can be performed as many times as required (from once a week to once a month).

In a study Sierra-Aisa et al. [30] compared the outcomes of US imaging for the diagnosis of musculoskeletal injuries in hemophilia patients with scores obtained utilizing MRI. Sierra-Aisa et al. concluded that US is valuable in identifying hemarthroses, synovitis and articular erosions, with results equivalent to those of MRI.

When RS needs to be redone, the technique is equal to that carried out for the first injection. The outcome parameters must be taken 6 months following each RS and then every 6 months till the end of the follow-up. The most significant outcome parameters are the number of hemarthroses per month (diminution in joint bleeding), factor consumption, and the clinical result (range of motion of the affected articulation).

For us arthroscopic synovectomy is the second-line therapy being advised after the failure of three RSs with 6-month intervals. In a report 28 (6.3%) articulations ultimately required arthroscopic synovectomy or total knee arthroplasty (TKA) [21]. It is important to underline that RS is tremendously cost-effective. The cost per RS injection in the USA is about $2500 USD, while a surgical synovectomy has a cost estimation of $25,000 USD [21].

14.3 Radiosynovectomy in Patients with Inhibitors

Prophylaxis with bypassing agents has demonstrated its efficacy in many publications. So far aPCC has been utilized in 110 patients and rFVIIa in 29. Both bypassing agents have exhibited diminution of bleeding incidence and amelioration of QoL [31–48].

When repeated hemarthroses cannot be controlled in patients with inhibitors by means of prophylaxis with bypassing agents, a RS should be advised. In 1982 Rivard et al. [49] reported four patients (6 RSs) aged 13 to 17 years. Subjective and objective improvement was encountered in all the patients. During a follow-up period of 22 to 34 weeks the number of bleeding episodes per year ranged from 1 to 5, a significant decrease.

In five patients under the age of 15 with hemophilia and inhibitors, 13 joints underwent RS (radioactive gold) [50]. Of the 13 joints treated, a bleeding-free interval of more than 6 months was achieved in nine of which six remained free from hemarthroses for more than a year.

In nine patients with hemophilia and factor inhibitor, 19 articulations were managed with RS utilizing radioactive gold by Lofqvist et al. [51]. Ages ranged from 3 to 40 years. RS was carried out when the antibody titer was low (<10 Bethesda units), thus making hemostasis feasible by factor administration for 2 to 4 days. On five occasions, RS was carried out at the same time with tolerance induction according to the Malmö protocol. A bleeding-free interval of more than 6 months was achieved in 11 articulations, six of which remained bleeding free for more than a year. At long run follow-up (range, 18–182 months) five articulations were rated good, one joint was fair, and 11 articulations were poor. The outcomes were worse to those for patients with hemophilia without inhibitor.

In 2007, Rodríguez-Merchán et al. [52] reported that prophylaxis is paramount to try to elude the development of hemophilic synovitis. The best management for synovitis in patients with inhibitors is RS (rhenium-186 for ankle and elbows, yttrium-90 for knees). With both treatments (prophylaxis and RS), the development of severe hemophilic arthropathy can be postponed.

According to Pasta et al. [53], in hemophilia patients with inhibitors, a more severe grade of synovitis is commonly seen owing to the fact that management is more problematic in this setting. For them, the first treatment alternative of repeated hemarthroses and/or chronic synovitis is represented by chemical synovectomy (several weekly injections) and RS, with a success rate of about 80% for both. Nevertheless, RS should be preferred in inhibitor patients because it makes it feasible to achieve full synovial fibrosis commonly in one session, without the need for repeated injections, thus diminishing the risk of bleeding complications and concentrate consumption.

14.4 Technique of Radiosynovectomy

Figure 14.4 shows the procedure for ankle RS. Technetium-99 scintigraphy is carried out following the technique to demonstrate the normal distribution of the radioactive material into the articulation.

RS should be carried out under factor coverage to elude the risk of re-bleeding during the

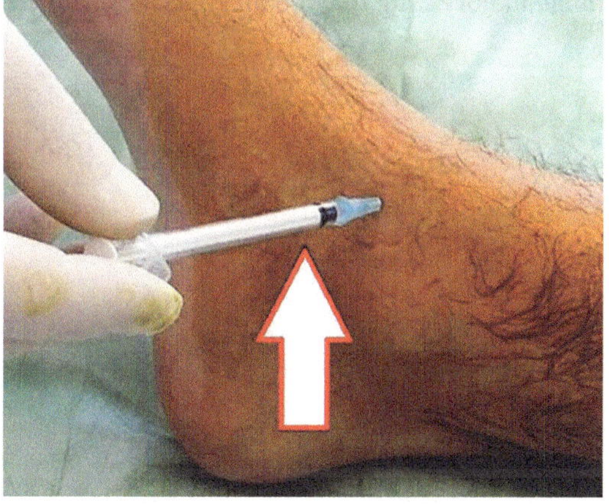

Fig. 14.4 Radiosynovectomy (RS) of the ankle with Rhenium-186 (arrow). The needle must be then withdrawn very slowly while at the same time injecting an anti-inflammatory drug

technique. Our protocol is the following [16–21]: In hemophilia A patients, we attain factor coverage by means of the intravenous infusion of 50 UI/kg of factor VIII every 24 h for 4 days, starting 30 min prior to the technique. In patients with hemophilia B, we infuse factor IX at a dose of 60 UI/kg every 24 h for 4 days, also starting 30 min prior to the RS. In patients with inhibitors we utilize aPCCs (75 UI/kg every 12 h for 4 days) or rFVIIa (90 μg/kg every 2 h for 1 day). An informed consent is needed.

The principal radioactive materials utilized in the literature and their characteristics are yttrium-90, rhenium-186, and phosphorus-32. All of them emit beta radiation and their therapeutic penetration powers (TPP) in millimeters are 2.8 mm, 1 mm, and 2.2 mm, apiece. For the knee we utilize yttrium-90 at a dose of 185 Megabecquerels (MBq). Rhenium-186 is utilized for elbows (56–74 MBq) and ankles (74 MBq). A little amount of technetium-99 is added to carry out joint scintigraphy following the technique (to check the correct distribution of the radioactive material into the articulation) (Fig. 14.5) [16–21].

We do not utilize local anesthetic. A common needle is enough. Once the articulation has been entered all the liquid content (blood or synovial fluid) is aspirated, and only then the radioactive material is injected. The needle should be retired very slowly as at the same time injecting an anti-inflammatory drug (e.g. betamethasone) in order to elude the risk of radioactive burn of the needle track or even worse, a contiguous skin burn.

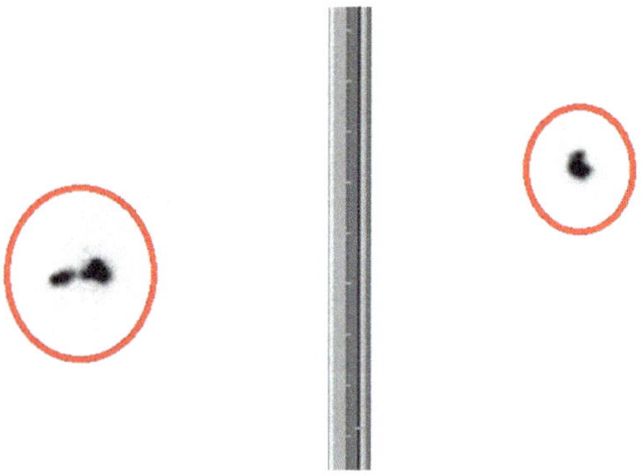

Fig. 14.5 Joint scintigraphy following radiosynovectomy to check the correct distribution of the radioactive material into the articulation (circles)

14.5 Effect of the Radioactive Material on the Synovium

The diameter of the colloid particle is between 2 and 5 μm, which is small enough to be phagocytized, but big enough not to enter bloodstream via capillary fenestrations [54]. Immediately after the injection, most of the radiocolloid is phagocytized by type 2 synoviocytes (synovial macrophages) and captured in the external cell layers of the synovial membrane.

High energy β-radiation induces water hydrolysis, production of reactive oxygen species, and cell apoptosis due to oxidative stress. Emission of radiation continues for several weeks. In time, this leads to necrosis and subsequent fibrosis of the synovial membrane, and, clinically, reduction of inflammation symptoms. β-radiation has very limited tissue penetration, depositing more than 90% of energy within 10 mm from the point of origin, thus affecting almost exclusively the joint cavity.

Most of the radiation is absorbed by the synovium, synovial fluid, superficial layers of cartilage, and articular capsule. Subchondral bone and other paraarticular tissues, in turn, receive negligible doses of radiation [54].

14.6 Efficacy of Radiosynovectomy

In the literature, between 40% and 85% of joints accomplish good clinical results; 30 to 80% of articulations show a diminution in articular bleeding; and between 35% and 85% of patients show a diminution in factor consumption; that is to say, the number of hemarthroses per month diminish from 3 to 6 on average prior to the technique to 1 following the technique [10–22]. In a 38-year period (1976–2013), we have carried out 500 RSs in 443 articulations of 345 patients with hemophilia diagnosed with chronic synovitis [21]. The mean patient age was 23 years (range,

6–53). The mean follow-up was 18 years (range: 6 months-38 years). The RS was performed with either yttrium-90 or rhenium-186. We carried out 1 to 3 injections (RS-1, RS-2, RS-3), with a 6-month interval between them. Bleeding incidence diminished 64% on average. In another study we observed that mean reduction of joint bleeding following RS was 68% when RS-1 was utilized, 62% with RS-2, and 61% with RS-3 [17]. Synovial size (clinical, imaging) diminished 31%. World Federation of Hemophilia (WFH) clinical score ameliorated 19%. WFH radiological score did not ameliorate [15, 17]. In one of our studies we observed that the knee needed more injections than the elbow or the ankle and that the more severe hypertrophic synovitis needed a higher number of RS techniques [16]. In another study we encountered that RS is efficacious in all patient groups, independently of the existence of circulating inhibitor antibody, the type of articulation involved, the grade of synovitis and the existence of radiographic findings of articular degeneration (arthropathy) [18]. In our group we have also observed that each consecutive RS behaves independently [19]. In another report we encountered that the parameters studied ameliorated to an equal degree in joints with articular degeneration in simple radiography (ADSR) and without ADSR. No articulation without ADSR needed RS-3; this was the only difference our study encountered between articulations without ADSR and those with ADSR at the time of the RS [20].

In 2001, Silva et al. [10] analyzed 130 RSs utilizing phosphorus 32 with an average follow-up of 36 months. For primary techniques, excellent and good results (hemarthrosis reduction from 75% to 100%) were achieved in 79% of cases at 6 months to 8 years. For repeat techniques a combination of excellent and good results was achieved in 62.4% of cases at 6 months to 3 years. Regression analysis demonstrated no correlation between outcomes and age or grade of arthropathy. Radiation was well contained within the articulation. No complications were reported.

In another study published by Siegel et al. [11] in 2001, 125 RSs in 81 patients were performed. Two- to 10-year follow-up by age and articulation included joint bleeding and quality-of-life evaluation. Besides, a relative cost comparison, scintigraphic imaging, and assessment of biodistribution of the radionuclide were done. Of 125 techniques, 54% resulted in complete cessation of bleeding into the treated articulation following the technique, and 73% of patients experienced improved motion of the treated joint. Of patients 18 years old and younger, 79% had a greater than 75% diminution in bleeding rate, and of patients older than 40 years, only 56% had a similar reduction. Seventy-nine percent of patients analyzed had a significant amelioration in QoL attributable to the treated joint. No evidence of significant leakage was found.

The outcomes of RS with Yttrium-90 in 163 articulations were reported by Heim et al. [12] in 2001. The median age at the time of the initial technique was between 11 and 15 years and the median follow-up period 11 years. Over 80% of the patients with hemophilia experienced a diminution in the number of hemarthroses and 15% stopped bleeding altogether in the injected joint.

In 2007, Mortazavi et al. [13] published the treatments outcomes of RS with phosphorus-32. Forty-six patients were followed for an average of 31 months. The mean age of patients at the time of RS was 16 years. There were three repeat injections. In latest follow-up, 77% of patients reported at least a 50% diminution in bleeding frequency after treatment. The need for antihemophilic factor consumption decreased by about 74% post-RS. In most of the treated articulations, the ROM remained stable or ameliorated. A trend was encountered for the number of hemarthrosis to augment following a period of considerable amelioration. RS utilizing phosphorus-32 effectively diminished the intraarticular bleeding frequency and factor concentrate use.

In 2009, Calegaro et al. [14] assessed the efficiency of RS with 153-Sm-HA (Samarium-153 hydroxyapatite) in hemophilic arthropathy. Thirty-one patients (30 males) with ages ranging from 8 to 34 years (average age 20.6 years) were managed with fixed intraarticular dose of 185 MBq and divided into two groups: infantile-juvenile (13 patients with up to 18 years of age, an average age of 12 years and arthropathy evolution of 7 years) and adult (18 patients older than 18 years, an average age of 24 years and arthropathy evolution of 18 years). The outcomes were classified as: 1, good (remission from 70% to 100% of manifestations); 2, moderate (remission from 40% to 69%); and 3, poor (remission from 0% to 39%). Seventy-eight articulations were analyzed: 15 knees, 36 elbows, 24 ankles, 1 shoulder, and 2 hips. No significant difference in the RS result between groups was found. The outcomes were good for 75% of elbows, 87.5% of ankles, and 40% of knees; the reduction in hemarthrosis and use of the coagulation factor was, respectively, 78% and 80% for elbows, 82% and 85% for ankles, and 30% and 35% for knees. Four cases of reactional synovitis were found in the 31 patients. The use of 153 Sm-HA in the management of the hemophilic arthropathy was efficacious for intermediate-size articulations (elbows and ankles), but less effective for knees. Besides, this treatment showed an excellent safety profile and accessible cost.

In 2010, Cho et al. [15] analyzed clinical outcomes and radiologic assessment of RS using Holmium-166-chitosan complex in hemophilic arthropathy. From 2001 to 2003, 58 RSs were carried out in 53 hemophiliacs. The average age at procedure was 13 years. Holmium-166-chitosan complex was injected in 31 ankle joints, 19 elbow joints, and 8 knee joints. Average follow-up was 33 months since primary technique. The ROM of each joint, frequency of intraarticular bleeding and factor dose utilized were analyzed for clinical evaluation. There was no significant amelioration of ROM in affected articulations. Following RS, the average frequency of bleeding of the elbow decreased from 3.76 to 0.47 times per month, the knee from 5.87 to 1.12 times per month, and the ankle from 3.62 to 0.73 times per month, respectively. After RS, the average coagulation factor dose injected was significantly diminished to 779.3 units per month from 2814.8 units per month prior to RS.

In 2014, Turkmen et al. [22] analyzed their 10-year experience with yttrium-90 RS. Eighty-two knee joints of 67 patients with hemophilic synovitis were treated with yttrium-90 RS. The mean age was 16 years (range: 5–39 years). The mean follow-up was 39 months (range: 12–95 months). Failure of treatment represented re-bleeding after a RS was utilized as an endpoint in patient time to progression (TTP) analysis. The median TTP was calculated as 72 months in Kaplan–Meier analysis. The 1-, 3-, and 5-year survival rates were 89%, 73%, and 63%, respectively. Longer TTP was obvious in patients who have greater reduction in bleeding rate within 6 months after RS [22].

In 2016 Rodríguez-Merchán and De la Corte-Rodríguez found that yttrium-90 RS and rhenium-186 RS were equally effective in reducing the number of hemarthroses and the size of the synovium in ankles and elbows in the short-run (6 months) [55]. This year Zhang et al. reported that phosphorus-32 was effective in the short-run [56]. In 2017 Wang et al. published that RS with phosphorus-32 colloid on 6 hemophilic synovitis was a safe and effective procedure [57]. Patients with inhibitors suffer more hemarthroses (in frequency and intensity). Therefore, they experience greater range of motion (ROM) restriction, more mobility handicaps, more severe orthopedic problems, and worse quality-of-life (QoL) [58–61].

14.7 Complications of Radiosynovectomy

Our rate of complications is 1%. The complications that we have observed are the following [16–21]: (1) Small cutaneous burns cured in 1–2 weeks just by cleaning the wound. They happen when the isotope is accidentally injected out of the articulation; (2) infection (septic arthritis) which needs surgical treatment (arthrotomy and joint debridement) together with intravenous antibiotic treatment; and (3) inflammatory reaction after RSs resolved by means of rest and NSAIDS (nonsteroidal anti-inflammatory drugs). We especially advise cyclooxigenase-2 (COX-2) inhibitor inhibitors. Moreover, COX-2 inhibitors entail a lower risk of gastrointestinal complications than traditional NSAIDs [62].

14.8 Safety of Radiosynovectomy

Many pediatric patients with hemophilia who might benefit from RS for the control of synovitis do not undergo the technique since there is controversy in the literature regarding the safety of radiation exposure after two cases of acute lymphocytic leukemia in children with hemophilia treated with phosphorus-32 RS were reported [63].

In 2007 Turkmen et al. [64] investigated the genotoxic effect on the peripheral blood lymphocytes potentially induced by yttrium-90 in children who were undergoing RS for hemophilic synovitis, using chromosomal aberration analysis and the micronuclei assay for detecting chromosomal aberrations, as well as the sister chromatid exchanges technique for assessed DNA damage. The findings of this study indicated that high radiation doses were not obtained by peripheral lymphocytes of children who undergo yttrium-90 RS and, consequently, they contradict a high cancer risk.

No increase in the risk of cancer has been found by Infante-Rivard et al. [65]. Besides, they encounter no dose–response relationship with the amount of isotope injected or number of RSs. The study of Infante-Rivard et al. provided some indication for the safety of RS but homogenous diagnostic groups of younger hemophilic patients receiving RS require more evaluation.

Children undergoing knee RS receive a radiation dose of about 0.74 millisieverts-mSv (90 megabecquerels-MBq) and elbow and ankle RSs a dose of around 0.32 mSv (30–40 MBq). The radiation dose from natural sources is about 2 mSv and the advised limit for patients (apart from natural sources) is 1 mSv per year. The lifetime cancer risk augments about 0.5% per 100 mSv per year [66–68].

14.9 Conclusions

The indication for radiosynovectomy (RS) is the presence of repeated hemarthroses associated with synovitis (confirmed clinically and by imaging techniques) that cannot be controlled by means of hematological treatment. RS can be carried out at any age, ideally in teenagers (>13–14 years). Intraarticular injection in a very young child may be difficult because it needs patient co-operation and this may require general anesthesia. RS is our first alternative for treatment of chronic synovitis. We recommend yttrium-90 for the knees and rhenium-186 for elbows and ankles (1 to 3 injections with 6-month interval). The technique is highly cost-effective in comparison to arthroscopic synovectomy (that must be the second option). Surgery must be indicated after the failure of three RSs with 6-month intervals. RS is an efficacious minimally invasive procedure for management of recurrent hemarthroses due to chronic synovitis in hemophilic articulations.

No increase in the risk of cancer has been published and the dose of radiation utilized in RS is minimal. In hemophilic patients with recurrent hemarthrosis, RS should be performed under factor coverage as soon as possible, once the existence of synovitis has been confirmed by ultrasonography (US). In relation to this topic it is necessary to remember that an acute hemarthrosis must be treated immediately by intense hematological treatment and arthrocentesis (evacuation of the articular blood). Also, that synovitis usually presents as a hard joint inflammation on palpation, little or nothing painful.

RS should really be considered as a useful adjunctive procedure to the primary intervention, which is intensive replacement therapy. Its role is to control synovitis due to recurrent hemarthroses in order to get a decrease in the intensity and frequency of such hemarthroses. It is well-known that effective prophylaxis is even becoming more feasible for inhibitor patients, with the recent and anticipated introduction of new treatments such as bispecific antibodies and antagonists to natural anticoagulants. However, prophylaxis is not 100% effective even in patients treated in specialized hemophilia centers, like ours.

A potential limitation to the use of RS in developing countries is access to radionuclides. This problem should not exist in specialized hemophilia centers of developed countries that usually have Departments of Nuclear Medicine.

We hope that as childhood and adult prophylaxis is more universal this technique may become unnecessary in the long run (although we are afraid that it will take many years to be achieved all over the world).

References

1. Rodriguez-Merchan EC. Musculo-skeletal manifestations of haemophilia. Blood Rev. 2016;30:401–9.
2. Astermark J. When to start and when to stop primary prophylaxis in patients with severe haemophilia. Haemophilia. 2003;9(Suppl 1):32–6.
3. Manco-Johnson MJ, Abshire TC, Shapiro AD, Riske B, Hacker MR, Kilcoyne R, et al. Prophylaxis versus episodic treatment to prevent joint disease in boys with severe hemophilia. N Engl J Med. 2007;357:535–44.
4. Berntorp E, Fischer K, Miners A. Models of prophylaxis. Haemophilia. 2012;18(Suppl 4):136–40.
5. Ljung R. Hemophilia and prophylaxis. Pediatr Blood Cancer. 2013;60(Suppl 1):S23–6.
6. Carcao MD, Aledort L. Prophylactic factor replacement in hemophilia. Blood Rev. 2004;18:101–13.
7. Ljung R. Prophylactic therapy in haemophilia. Blood Rev. 2009;23:267–74.
8. Teitel JM, Sholzberg M. Current status and future prospects for the prophylactic management of hemophilia patients with inhibitor antibodies. Blood Rev. 2013;27:103–9.
9. Gomperts ED, Astermark J, Gringeri A, Teitel J. From theory to practice: applying current clinical knowledge and treatment strategies to the care of hemophilia a patients with inhibitors. Blood Rev. 2008;22(Suppl 1):S1–11.
10. Silva M, Luck JV Jr, Siegel ME. 32P chromic phosphate radiosynovectomy for chronic haemophilic synovitis. Haemophilia. 2001;7(Suppl 2):40–9.
11. Siegel HJ, Luck JV Jr, Siegel ME, Quinones C. Phosphate-32 colloid radiosynovectomy in hemophilia: outcome of 125 procedures. Clin Orthop Relat Res. 2001:409–17.
12. Heim M, Goshen E, Amit Y, Martinowitz U. Synoviorthesis with radioactive Yttrium in haemophilia: Israel experience. Haemophilia. 2001;7(Suppl 2):36–9.
13. Mortazavi SM, Asadollahi S, Farzan M, Shahriaran S, Aghili M, Izadyar S, et al. (32)P colloid radiosynovectomy in treatment of chronic haemophilic synovitis: Iran experience. Haemophilia. 2007;13:182–8.
14. Calegaro JU, Machado J, DE Paula JC, DE Almeida JS, Casulari LA. Clinical evaluation after 1 year of 153-samarium hydroxyapatite synovectomy in patients with haemophilic arthropathy. Haemophilia. 2009;15:240–6.
15. Cho YJ, Kim KI, Chun YS, Rhyu KH, Kwon BK, Kim DY, et al. Radioisotope synoviorthesis with Holmium-166-chitosan complex in haemophilic arthropathy. Haemophilia. 2010;16:640–6.
16. De la Corte-Rodriguez H, Rodriguez-Merchan EC, Jimenez-Yuste V. Radiosynovectomy in patients with chronic haemophilic synovitis: when is more than one injection necessary? Eur J Haematol. 2011;86:430–5.
17. De la Corte-Rodriguez H, Rodriguez-Merchan EC, Jimenez-Yuste V. Radiosynovectomy in hemophilia: quantification of its effectiveness through the assessment of 10 articular parameters. J Thromb Haemost. 2011;9:928–35.
18. De la Corte-Rodriguez H, Rodriguez-Merchan EC, Jimenez-Yuste V. What patient, joint and isotope characteristics influence the response to radiosynovectomy in patients with haemophilia? Haemophilia. 2011;17:e990–8.
19. De la Corte-Rodriguez H, Rodriguez-Merchan EC, Jimenez-Yuste V. Consecutive radiosynovectomy procedures at 6-monthly intervals behave independently in haemophilic synovitis. Blood Transfus. 2013;11:254–9.
20. Rodriguez-Merchan EC, De la Corte-Rodriguez H, Jimenez-Yuste V. Is radiosynovectomy (RS) effective for joints damaged by haemophilia with articular degeneration in simple radiography (ADSR)? Thromb Res. 2014;133:875–9.
21. Rodriguez-Merchan EC, De la Corte-Rodriguez H, Jimenez-Yuste V. Radiosynovectomy in haemophilia: long-term results of 500 procedures performed in a 38-year period. Thromb Res. 2014;134:985–90.
22. Turkmen C, Kilicoglu O, Dikici F, Bezgal F, Kuyumcu S, Gorgun O, et al. Survival analysis of Y-90 radiosynovectomy in the treatment of haemophilic synovitis of the knee: a 10-year retrospective review. Haemophilia. 2014;20:e45–50.
23. Pasta G, Mancuso ME, Perfetto OS, Solimeno LP. Radiosynoviorthesis in children with haemophilia. Hamostaseologie. 2009;29(Suppl 1):S62–4.
24. Merchan ECR, De Orbe A, Gago J. Ultrasound in the diagnosis of the early stages of hemophilic arthropathy of the knee. Acta Orthop Belg. 1992;58:122–5.
25. Martinoli C, Della Casa Alberighi O, Di Minno G, Graziano E, Molinari AC, Pasta G, et al. Development and definition of a simplified scanning procedure and scoring method for Haemophilia Early Arthropathy Detection with Ultrasound (HEAD-US). Thromb Haemost. 2013;109:1170–9.
26. De la Corte-Rodriguez H, Rodriguez-Merchan EC, Alvarez-Roman MT, Martin-Salces M, Martinoli C, Jimenez-Yuste V. The value of HEAD-US system in detecting subclinical abnormalities in joints of patients with hemophilia. Expert Rev Hematol. 2018;11:253–61.
27. Foppen W, van der Schaaf IC, Beek FJA, Mali WPTM, Fischer K. Diagnostic accuracy of point-of-care ultrasound for evaluation of early blood-induced joint changes: comparison with MRI. Haemophilia. 2018;24(6):971–9. https://doi.org/10.1111/hae.13524.

28. Di Minno A, Sparadella G, Nardone A, Mormile M, Ventre I, Morfini M, et al. Attempting to remedy suboptimal medication adherence in haemophilia: the rationale for repeated ultrasound visualisations of the patient's joint status. Blood Rev. 2018;33:106–16. https://doi.org/10.1016/j.blre.2018.08.003.
29. Doria AS, Keshava SN, Mohanta A, Jarrin J, Blanchette V, Srivastava A, et al. Diagnostic accuracy of ultrasound for assessment of hemophilic arthropathy: MRI correlation. AJR Am J Roentgenol. 2015;204:W336–47.
30. Sierra Aisa C, Lucía Cuesta JF, Rubio Martínez A, Fernández Mosteirín N, Iborra Muñoz A, Abío Calvete M, et al. Comparison of ultrasound and magnetic resonance imaging for diagnosis and follow-up of joint lesions in patients with haemophilia. Haemophilia. 2014;20:e51–7.
31. Hilgartner MW, Makipernaa A, Dimichele DM. Long-term FEIBA prophylaxis does not prevent progression of existing joint disease. Haemophilia. 2003;9:261–8.
32. Young G, McDaniel M, Nugent DJ. Prophylactic recombinant factor VIIa in haemophilia patients with inhibitors. Haemophilia. 2005;11:203–7.
33. Leissinger CA, Becton DL, Ewing NP, Valentino LA. Prophylactic treatment with activated prothrombin complex concentrate (FEIBA) reduces the frequency of bleeding episodes in paediatric patients with haemophilia A and inhibitors. Haemophilia. 2007;13:249–55.
34. Rodriguez-Merchan EC. Some recent developments regarding arthropathy and inhibitors in haemophilia. Haemophilia. 2008;14:242–7.
35. Fischer K, Valentino L, Ljung R, Blanchette V. Prophylaxis for severe haemophilia: clinical challenges in the absence as well as in the presence of inhibitors. Haemophilia. 2008;14(Suppl 3):196–201.
36. Jimenez-Yuste V, Quintana M, Alvarez MT, Martin-Salces M, Hernandez-Navarro F. "Primary prophylaxis" with rFVIIa in a patient with severe haemophilia A and inhibitor. Blood Coagul Fibrinolysis. 2008;19:719–20.
37. Rodriguez-Merchan EC. Prevention of haemophilic arthropathy in haemophilic children with inhibitors. Haemophilia. 2008;14(Suppl 6):1–3.
38. Jimenez-Yuste V, Rodriguez-Merchan EC, Alvarez MT, Quintana M, Martin-Salces M, Hernandez-Navarro F. Experiences in the prevention of arthropathy in haemophila patients with inhibitors. Haemophilia. 2008;14(Suppl 6):28–35.
39. Jimenez-Yuste V, Alvarez MT, Martín-Salces M, Quintana M, Rodriguez-Merchan C, Lopez-Cabarcos C, et al. Prophylaxis in 10 patients with severe haemophilia A and inhibitor: different approaches for different clinical situations. Haemophilia. 2009;15:203–9.
40. Valentino LA. The benefits of prophylactic treatment with APCC in patients with haemophilia and high-titre inhibitors: a retrospective case series. Haemophilia. 2009;15:733–42.
41. Franchini M, Manzato F, Salvagno GL, Montagnana M, Zaffanello M, Lippi G. Prophylaxis in congenital hemophilia with inhibitors: the role of recombinant activated factor VII. Semin Thromb Hemost. 2009;35:814–9.
42. Perry D, Berntorp E, Tait C, Dolan G, Holme PA, Laffan M, et al. FEIBA prophylaxis in haemophilia patients: a clinical update and treatment recommendations. Haemophilia. 2010;16:80–9.
43. Ettingshausen CE, Kreuz W. Early long-term FEIBA prophylaxis in haemophilia A patients with inhibitor after failing immune tolerance induction: a prospective clinical case series. Haemophilia. 2010;16:90–100.
44. Valentino LA. Assessing the benefits of FEIBA prophylaxis in haemophilia patients with inhibitors. Haemophilia. 2010;16:263–71.
45. Young G, Auerswald G, Jimenez-Yuste V, Konkle BA, Lambert T, Morfini M, et al. When should prophylaxis therapy in inhibitor patients be considered? Haemophilia. 2011;17:e849–57.
46. Rodriguez-Merchan EC, Jimenez-Yuste V, Aznar JA, Hedner U, Knobe K, Lee CA, et al. Joint protection in haemophilia. Haemophilia. 2011;17(Suppl 2):1–23.
47. Gringeri A, Leissinger C, Cortesi PA, Jo H, Fusco F, Riva S, et al. Health-related quality of life in patients with haemophilia and inhibitors on prophylaxis with anti-inhibitor complex concentrate: results from the pro-FEIBA study. Haemophilia. 2013;19:736–43.
48. Stasyshyn O, Antunes S, Mamonov V, Ye X, Epstein J, Xiong Y, et al. Prophylaxis with anti-inhibitor coagulant complex improves health-related quality of life inhaemophilia patients with inhibitors: results from FEIBA NF. Haemophilia. 2014;20:644–50.
49. Rivard GE, Girard M, Cliche CL, Guay JP, Bélanger R, Besner R. Synoviorthesis in patients with hemophilia and inhibitors. Can Med Assoc J. 1982;127:41–2.
50. Löfqvist T, Petersson C. Synoviorthesis in young patients with hemophilia and inhibitory antibodies. Pediatr Hematol Oncol. 1992;9:167–70.
51. Löfqvist T, Petersson C, Nilsson IM. Radioactive synoviorthesis in patients with hemophilia with factor inhibitor. Clin Orthop Relat Res. 1997;343:37–41.
52. Rodriguez-Merchan EC, Valentino L, Quintana M. Prophylaxis and treatment of chronic synovitis in haemophilia patients with inhibitors. Haemophilia. 2007;13(Suppl 3):45–8.
53. Pasta G, Mancuso ME, Perfetto OS, Solimeno LP. Synoviorthesis in haemophilia patients with inhibitors. Haemophilia. 2008;14(Suppl 6):52–5.
54. Chojnowski MM, Felis-Giemza A, Kobylecka M. Radionuclide synovectomy - essentials for rheumatologists. Reumatologia. 2016;54:108–16.
55. Rodriguez-Merchan EC, De la Corte-Rodriguez H. Radiosynovectomy in haemophilic synovitis of elbows and ankles: is the effectiveness of yttrium-90 and rhenium-186 different? Thromb Res. 2016;140:41–5.
56. Zhang WQ, Han SQ, Yuan Z, He YT, Zhang H, Zhang M. Effects of intraarticular (32)P colloid in the treatment of hemophilic synovitis of the knee: a short term clinical study. Indian J Orthop. 2016;50:55–8.

57. Wang Z, Zhang Y, Ge YH, Liu HJ, Liu YH, Zhao JJ, Dou YC, Lei PC. [Therapeutic response of radiosynovectomy with p-32 colloid in 326 patients with hemophilic arthropathy].[Article in Chinese; Abstract available in Chinese from the publisher]. Zhonghua Xue Ye Xue Za Zhi. 2017;38:39–43.
58. Soucie JM, Cianfrini C, Janco RL, Kulkarni R, Hambleton J, Evatt B, et al. Joint range-of-motion limitations among young males with hemophilia: prevalence and risk factors. Blood. 2004;103:2467–73.
59. Leissinger CA. Prophylaxis in haemophilia patients with inhibitors. Haemophilia. 2006;12(Suppl 6):67–72.
60. Morfini M. Articular status of haemophilia patients with inhibitors. Haemophilia. 2008;14(Suppl 6):20–2.
61. Brown TM, Lee WC, Joshi AV, Pashos CL. Health-related quality of life and productivity impact in haemophilia patients with inhibitors. Haemophilia. 2009;15:911–7.
62. Rodriguez-Merchan EC, de la Corte-Rodriguez H, Jimenez-Yuste V. Efficacy of celecoxib in the treatment of joint pain caused by advanced haemophilic arthropathy in adult patients with haemophilia A. Haemophilia. 2014;20:e225–7.
63. Dunn AL, Busch MT, Wyly JB, Abshire TC. Radionuclide synovectomy for hemophilic arthropathy: a comprehensive review of safety and efficacy and recommendation for a standardized treatment protocol. Thromb Haemost. 2002;87:383–93.
64. Turkmen C, Ozturk S, Unal SN, Zulfikar B, Taser O, Sanli Y, Cefle K, Kilicoglu O, Palanduz S. The genotoxic effects in lymphocyte cultures of children treated with radiosynovectomy by using yttrium-90 citrate colloid. Cancer Biother Radiopharm. 2007;22:393–9.
65. Infante-Rivard C, Rivard GE, Derome F, Cusson A, Winikoff R, Chartrand R, et al. A retrospective cohort study of cancer incidence among patients treated with radiosynoviorthesis. Haemophilia. 2012;18:805–9.
66. Rodriguez-Merchan EC. Radiosynovectomy in haemophilia. Blood Rev. 2019;35:1–6.
67. Rodriguez-Merchan EC. The role of orthopaedic surgery in haemophilia: current rationale, indications and results. EFORT Open Rev. 2019;4:165–73.
68. Rodríguez-Merchan EC, De la Corte-Garcia H. Musculoskeletal manifestations of hemophilia. In: Rodriguez-Merchan EC, editor. Joint surgery in the adult patient with hemophilia. Springer; 2015. p. 1–12.

Hemophilic Arthropathy: Arthroscopic Joint Debridement

15

E. Carlos Rodríguez-Merchán, Primitivo Gómez-Cardero, and Carlos A. Encinas-Ullán

15.1 Introduction

Open or arthroscopic surgical knee and ankle debridement in the treatment of hemophilic arthropathy has been reported to give the patient years of life without pain [1–4]. Other authors, however, have reported that arthroscopic knee debridement (AKD) and arthroscopic ankle debridement (AAK) have a limited benefit for undiscriminated degenerative osteoarthritis (mechanical or inflammatory causes) [5].

According to Ogilvie-Harris and Sekyi-Otu arthroscopic ankle debridement (AAD) can offer relief to about two-thirds of patients with ankle osteoarthritis, but the degree of improvement is limited [6]. Fitzgibbons stated that AAD should only be used in patients with minimal to no degenerative ankle osteoarthritis [7]. Some authors have reported that arthroscopically treated impingement ankles have an excellent prognosis, while osteoarthritic ankles had a less favored prognosis, with a high percentage requiring further surgery [8]. Other authors, however, have reported that lesions associated with ankle osteoarthritis, such as impinging osteophytes and loose bodies, can be treated effectively with arthroscopy [9].

E. C. Rodríguez-Merchán (✉) · P. Gómez-Cardero
C. A. Encinas-Ullán
Department of Orthopedic Surgery, La Paz University Hospital, Madrid, Spain

In the later stages of ankle hemophilic arthropathy AAD can help to improve the joint function, even in the presence of articular cartilage damage (loose pieces of cartilage or anterior osteophytes) [10–12].

The purpose of this chapter is to describe the results of AKD and AAD with the aim of determining whether it is possible to delay TKR and ankle fusion or total ankle replacement (TAR) for painful moderate hemophilic arthropathy of the knee and ankle in adult patients.

15.2 Arthroscopic Knee Debridement

In a14-year period (1998–2011) 27 patients (27 knees) affected with severe hemophilia A (less than 1% of coagulation factor VIII) were treated by AKD because of knee joint involvement (hemophilic arthropathy) [13]. No patient developed an inhibitor against the deficient coagulation factor. Their average age at operation was 28.6 years (range 26–39 years) and the average follow-up 7.5 years (range 2–14 years).

Indications for AKD (inclusion criteria) were: more than 90° of knee flexion, flexion deformity <30°, good axial alignment of the knee, good patellar alignment, and pain >60 points in a visual analogue scale (0-no pain to 100 points). The axial alignment of the knee was assessed before surgery by means of long-length standing AP

E. C. Rodríguez-Merchán (ed.), *Advances in Hemophilia Treatment*,
https://doi.org/10.1007/978-3-030-93990-8_15

radiographs; more than 5° of varus or more than 10° of valgus was considered as malalignment in this study. In order to get bleeding control, secondary hematological prophylaxis was given for 3 months before operation. If there was increasing pain and disability and this conservative treatment failed, an AKD was indicated despite radiological involvement [13].

Each patient was admitted to hospital for 4 days and given factor VIII as summarized in Table 15.1. All the procedures were performed under general anesthesia. At operation, menisci tears were trimmed to a stable rim. Using a thermal ablation device on a low-intensity setting, we brushed the surface to remove the inflamed portion of the synovium (that was always inflamed and hypertrophic). Infrapatellar plica and suprapatellar plica were also removed. Chondroplasty was performed as needed, and loose bodies were removed. Anterior osteophytes often blocked full knee extension, so they were removed with a burr or shaver. That means that all components of the arthroscopic debridement procedure were performed in a combined fashion at surgery. Portals used were anteromedial and anterolateral. A tourniquet was used with tourniquet time being 64.5 min on average (range 55–75 min) [13].

The patients were mobilized on the second day after operation and were allowed partial weight-bearing (two crutches). On the third week after operation patients were allowed full weight-bearing. Rehabilitation (physiotherapy) was started on the second day after operation and then given during a 3-month period under hematological secondary prophylaxis. The principal goals of the rehabilitation program included the maintenance of joint volume and the prevention of scar reformation while preserving joint mobility.

Table 15.1 Recommended plasma factor trough levels and duration of administration in patients with hemophilia A undergoing arthroscopic knee debridement (AKD) and arthroscopic ankle debridement (AAD) [13, 14]

	Level (IU/dl)	Duration (days)
Preoperative	80–100	
Postoperative	60–80	1–3
	40–60	4–6
	30–50	7–14

Regaining strength was a secondary goal. The rehabilitation program excluded exercises that elicit significant pain, and postoperative regimens are specifically tailored to each patient. Full activity was resumed after 12 weeks [13].

We assessed the clinical outcome before surgery and at the time of latest follow-up using the Knee Society Score (KSS), pain (100 points maximum—excellent, 0 points minimum—worst result) and function (100 points maximum—excellent, 0 points minimum—worst result), and the range of motion (ROM) in degrees. Radiographic assessment was undertaken before operation and at follow-up as recommended by the World Federation of Hemophilia (WFH), with the minimum score of 0 (normal joint) and a maximum of 13 points (fully deteriorated joint) [15]. All patients had between 4 and 7 points (4.5 on average). That means that arthroscopic debridement was performed only for patients with moderate radiographic changes. Statistical analysis was conducted using the SPSS 11 program. All comparisons between variables at the end follow-up were made by means of McNemar test. A value of $p < 0.05$ was considered statistically significant [13].

Mean length of follow-up was 7.5 years (range: 2–14 years). Knee Society pain scores improved from 39 preoperatively to 66 postoperatively ($p < 0.05$), and function scores improved from 36 to 52 ($p < 0.05$). ROM improved on average from −15° of extension and 90° of flexion before surgery to −5° of extension and 110° of flexion at the last follow-up ($p = 0.03$). Radiographic deterioration was 2.8 on average (range 3–5). There were two cases (7.4%) of postoperative hemarthrosis resolved by means of joint aspiration. Only one patient (3.7%) required a TKR after 12.5 years [13].

The efficacy of AKD is a controversial topic in current literature. A report published by the Cochrane Library on AKD in osteoarthritis in 2008 stated that the procedure has no benefit for undiscriminated osteoarthritis (mechanical or inflammatory causes) [5]. However, a recent systematic review of the literature showed that AKD results in an excellent or good outcome in approximately 60% of patients in approximately

5 years [16]. Another recent report found that most patients with knee osteoarthritis associated with unstable cartilage or meniscal injuries reported good-to-excellent symptomatic results at the short- and mid-term follow-ups [17]. It has been reported that in hemophilia, open surgical knee debridement gives years of life without pain [1, 2].

TKR is an operation frequently needed by hemophilia patients which greatly improves their quality of life. TKR, however, carries a higher risk of bleeding and infection for hemophiliacs than it does for osteoarthritis sufferers. The life span of TKA in hemophilic patients is shorter than in patients with osteoarthritis because of the increased infection rate [14].

AKD does not jeopardize the possibility of subsequent surgery and can delay the need for TKR. Although our series is small, the results suggest that AKD should be considered as worthwhile treatment which may give the patient years of life without intense pain. In conclusion, AKD should be considered in the adult hemophiliac to delay TKR.

15.3 Arthroscopic Ankle Debridement

In a 12-year period (2000–2011) 23 patients (24 ankles) affected with hemophilic arthropathy were treated by AAD [18]. Twenty-two were suffering from hemophilia A (deficit of factor VIII) and one had hemophilia B (deficit of factor IX). No patient developed an inhibitor against the deficient coagulation factor. Their average age at operation was 25.3 years (range 21 to 36 years) and the average follow-up 5.4 years (range 2–14 years). All were severely affected, with a level of factor VIII <1%. Inclusion criteria were: pain >6 points (VAS-visual analogue scale from 0 to 10 points), more than 90° of ankle motion, and good axial alignment of the ankle (increased varus or valgus angulation was a contraindication for AAD) (Fig. 15.1).

Medical treatment, including secondary hematological prophylaxis and rehabilitation (physiotherapy), was given for 3 months before operation. If there was increasing pain and disability and this conservative treatment failed, the possibilities considered were AAD, ankle fusion, or TAR. We preferred not to consider ankle fusion or TAR without attempting AAD.

Radiographic assessment was undertaken before operation and at follow-up as recommended by the Orthopedic Advisory Committee of the World Federation of Hemophilia, with the minimum score of 0 and a maximum of 13 points [15]. All patients had >7 points. Each patient was admitted to hospital for 4 days and given factor VIII or IX as summarized in Table 15.1.

All the procedures were performed under general anesthesia. At operation, arthroscopic synovectomy, debridement, removal of loose bodies, and resection of anterior osteophytes were carried out.

The patients were mobilized on the second day after operation and were allowed partial weight-bearing (two crutches). On the third week after operation patients were allowed full weight-bearing. Rehabilitation (physiotherapy) was started on the second day after operation and then given during a 6-week period under hematological secondary prophylaxis. The principal goals of the rehabilitation program included the maintenance of joint volume and the prevention of scar reformation while preserving joint mobility. Regaining strength was a secondary goal. The rehabilitation program excluded exercises that elicit significant pain, and postoperative regimens are specifically tailored to each patient. Full activity was resumed after 8 or 10 weeks.

The American Orthopedic Foot and Ankle Society (AOFAS) Ankle-Hindfoot Scale was used evaluation [19]; an excellent result scored 85–100 points, good 70–84, fair 60–74, and poor less than 60. The average score in our patients was 35.4 before and 79.2 after operation. The average range pain score was 6.6 (range 6–9) before and 2.3 (range 1–3) after operation.

Clinical results in patients were excellent in 13 (54.2%), good in 9 (37.5%), and fair in 2 (8.3%). Radiographic deterioration was 1.7 on average (range 1–3). There were two cases

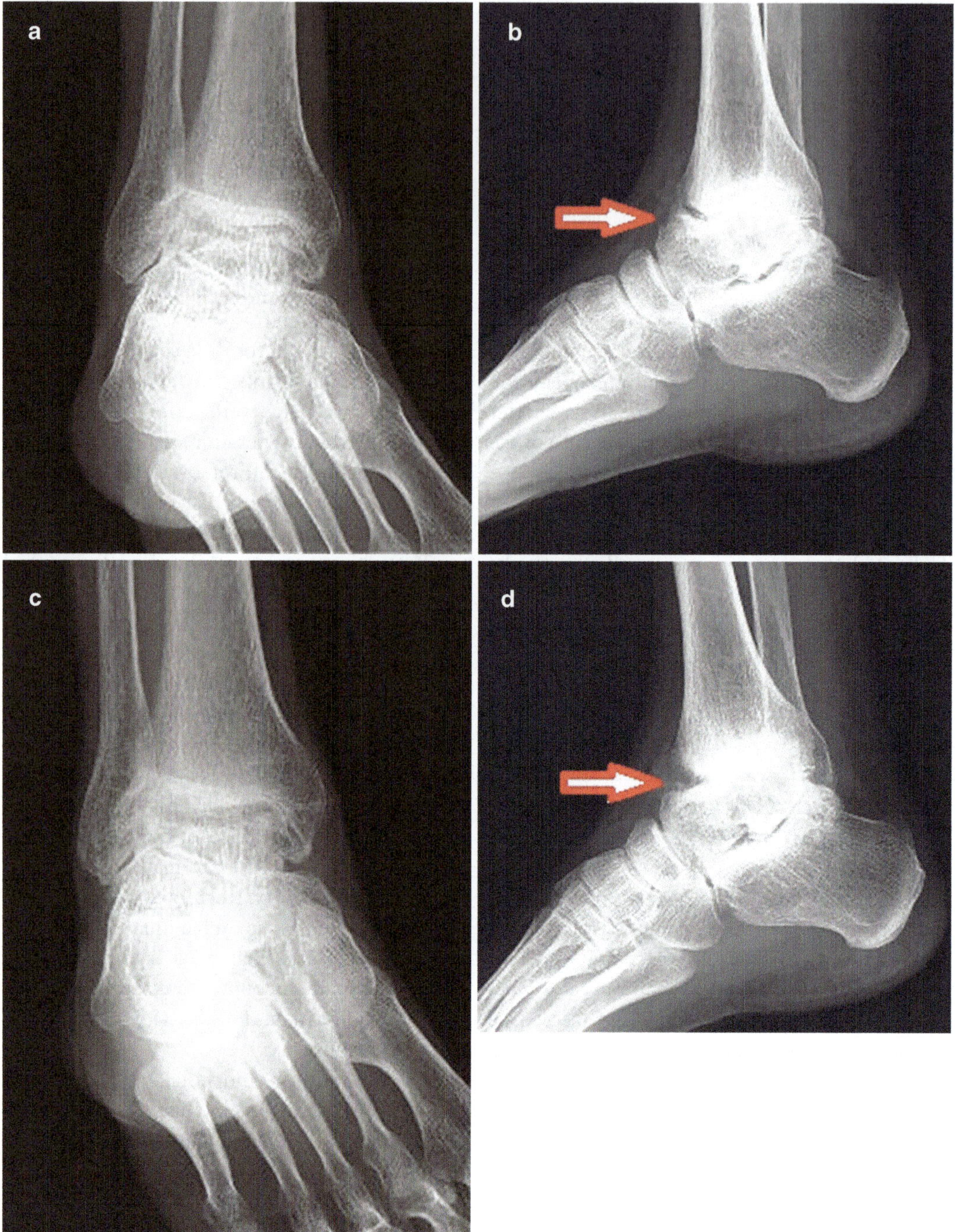

Fig. 15.1 Radiographs showing hemophilic arthropathy before arthroscopic ankle debridement (AAD) and 7 years later: (**a**) Anteroposterior preoperative view. (**b**) Preoperative lateral radiograph of the ankle. Note the anterior osteophyte (arrow) to be removed. (**c**) Anteroposterior view 7 years after operation. (**d**) Lateral radiograph 7 years after AAD. Note that the anterior osteophyte was removed in a satisfactory way (arrow). The clinical result was excellent

(8.3%) of postoperative hemarthrosis resolved by means of joint aspiration. Three patients (12.5%) required an ankle fusion.

The efficacy of AAD is a controversial topic in current literature. In a report AAD offered relief to approximately two-thirds of patients with ankle osteoarthritis, but the degree of improvement was limited [6]. Some authors have stated that AAD should only be used on those patients with minimal to no degenerative osteoarthritis [7]. Hassouna et al. reported that arthroscopically treated impingement ankles have an excellent prognosis, while osteoarthritic ankles had a less favored prognosis, with a high percentage requiring further surgical procedures [8]. Other authors have reported that lesions associated with ankle osteoarthritis, such as impinging osteophytes and loose bodies, can be treated effectively with arthroscopy [9].

Regarding ankle hemophilic arthropathy, some authors have reported that advanced ankle hemophilic arthropathy AAD can help to improve the joint function, even in the presence of articular cartilage damage [10–12].

Ankle fusion and TAR are surgical procedures frequently needed by hemophiliacs which greatly improve their quality of life. TAR, however, carries a higher risk of bleeding and infection for hemophiliacs than it does for osteoarthritis patients. The life span of TAR in hemophilic patients is shorter than in patients with osteoarthritis because of the higher risk of infection [20].

AAD does not jeopardize the possibility of subsequent surgery and can delay the need for ankle fusion or TAR. Our results suggest that AAD should be considered as worthwhile treatment which may give the patient years of life without pain [18].

In conclusion, when advanced ankle hemophilic arthropathy is present, AAD appears to be an effective method and is an alternative to ankle fusion or TAR, but when AAD fails to relieve pain ankle fusion or TAR must be considered. However, we have shown that the benefits of AAD are lasting.

15.4 Conclusions

In hemophilia, AKD gives years of life without pain. AKD does not jeopardize the possibility of subsequent surgery and can delay the need for TKR. AKD should be considered as worthwhile treatment which may give the patient years of life without intense pain.

Regarding ankle hemophilic arthropathy, some authors have reported that AAD can help to improve the joint function, even in the presence of articular cartilage damage. AAD does not jeopardize the possibility of subsequent surgery and can delay the need for ankle fusion or TAR. Our results suggest that AAD should be considered as worthwhile treatment which may give the patient years of life without pain.

In conclusion, when advanced knee and ankle hemophilic arthropathy is present, AKD and AAD appear to be an effective method and are an alternative to TKR and ankle fusion or TAR, but when AKD and AAD fail to relieve pain TKR, ankle fusion or TAR must be considered.

References

1. Soreff J. Joint debridement in the treatment of advanced haemophilic arthropathy. Clin Orthop Relat Res. 1984;191:179–84.
2. Rodriguez-Merchan EC, Magallon M, Galindo E. Joint debridement for haemophilic arthropathy of the knee. Int Orthop. 1994;18:135–8.
3. Rodriguez-Merchan EC, De la Corte-Garcia H. Musculoskeletal manifestations of hemophilia. In: Rodriguez-Merchan EC, editor. Joint surgery in the adult patient with hemophilia. Springer; 2015. p. 1–12.
4. Rodriguez-Merchan EC, Gomez-Cardero P, Martinez-Lloreda A. Knee surgery in hemophilia. In: Rodriguez-Merchan EC, editor. Joint surgery in the adult patient with hemophilia. Springer; 2015. p. 57–65.
5. Laupattarakasem W, Laopaiboon M, Laupattarakasem P, Sumananont C. Arthroscopic debridement for knee osteoarthritis. Editorial Group: Cochrane Musculoskeletal Group; 2008. https://doi.org/10.1002/14651858.CD005118.pub2.
6. Ogilvie-Harris DJ, Sekyi-Otu A. Arthroscopic debridement for the osteoarthritic ankle. Arthroscopy. 1995;11:433–6.

7. Fitzgibbons TC. Arthroscopic ankle debridement and fusion: indications, techniques, and results. Instr Course Lect. 1999;48:243–8.
8. Hassouna H, Kumar S, Bendall S. Arthroscopic ankle debridement: 5-year survival analysis. Acta Orthop Belg. 2007;73:737–40.
9. Cheng JC, Ferkel RD. The role of arthroscopy in ankle and subtalar degenerative joint disease. Clin Orthop Relat Res. 1998;349:65–72.
10. Rodriguez-Merchan EC. The haemophilic ankle. Haemophilia. 2006;12:337–44.
11. Pasta G, Forsyth A, Merchan CR, Mortazavi SM, Silva M, Mulder K, et al. Orthopaedic management of haemophilia arthropathy of the ankle. Haemophilia. 2008;14(Suppl 3):170–6.
12. Rodriguez-Merchan EC. Ankle surgery in haemophilia with special emphasis on arthroscopic debridement. Haemophilia. 2008;14:913–9.
13. Rodriguez-Merchan EC, Gomez-Cardero P. Arthroscopic knee debridement (AKD) can delay total knee replacement (TKR) in painful moderate hemophilic arthropathy of the knee in adult patients. Blood Coagul Fibrynol. 2016;27:645–7.
14. Rodriguez-Merchan EC. Special features of total knee replacement in hemophilia. Experts Rev Hematol. 2013;6:637–42.
15. Pettersson H, Ahlberg A, Nilsson IM. A radiologic classification of hemophilic arthropathy. Clin Orthop Relat Res. 1980;149:153–9.
16. Spahn G, Hofmann GO, Klinger HM. The effects of arthroscopic joint debridement in the knee osteoarthritis: results of a meta-analysis. Knee Surg Sports Traumatol Arthrosc. 2013;21:1553–61.
17. Figueroa D, Calvo R, Villalón IE, Meleán P, Novoa F, Vaisman A. Clinical outcomes after arthroscopic treatment of knee osteoarthritis. Knee. 2013;20:591–4.
18. Rodriguez-Merchan EC, Gomez-Cardero P, Martinez-Lloreda A, De la Corte-Rodriguez H, Jimenez-Yuste V. Arthroscopic debridement for ankle hemophilic arthropathy. Blood Coagul Fibrinolysis. 2015;26:279–81.
19. Kitaoka HB, Alexander IJ, Adelaar RS, Nunley JA, Myerson MS, Sanders M. Clinical rating systems for the ankle-hindfoot, midfoot, hallux, and lesser toes. Foot Ankle Int. 1994;15:349–53.
20. Rodriguez-Merchan EC. End-stage haemophilic arthropathy of the ankle: ankle fusion or total ankle replacement (TAR). Haemophilia. 2014;20:e106–7.

Hemophilic Arthropathy: Total Joint Arthroplasty

16

E. Carlos Rodríguez-Merchán, Primitivo Gómez-Cardero, and Carlos A. Encinas-Ullán

16.1 Introduction

About 90% of bleeding episodes in hemophilic patients occur within the musculoskeletal system and, of these, 80% occur with the joints (mainly elbows, knees, and ankles). Planning and undertaking elective orthopedic surgery in hemophilic patients is most effective with the involvement of an experienced multidisciplinary team at a specialized hemophilia treatment center [1]. The team at least requires a hematologist, whose function is to control hemostasis, an orthopedic surgeon, and a physical medicine and rehabilitation physician. At all stages the patient should be informed to ensure that their expectations and functional goals are realistic and can be accomplished. The planning phase should ensure that surgery proceeds without complication, but the surgical team should be ready to handle unanticipated problems. Postoperative rehabilitation should begin soon after surgery, with attention paid to treatment of hemostasis and pain. Surgery in patients with inhibitor requires even more careful preparation [1]. The orthopedic complications of hemophilia are patient-specific and treatment protocols often need to be altered to suit the individual.

E. C. Rodríguez-Merchán (✉) · P. Gómez-Cardero
C. A. Encinas-Ullán
Department of Orthopedic Surgery, La Paz University Hospital, Madrid, Spain

16.2 Total Knee Arthroplasty

Reported results of primary total knee arthroplasty (TKA) in hemophilia are satisfactory [2–6]. The reported rate of survival after TKA at 10 years is between 83% and 92% [7–9]. However, the high risk of infection (7% on average) is a concern [2–6].

In a meta-analysis reported in 2016 by Moore et al., a total of 336 TKAs in 254 hemophilic patients were analyzed with mean follow-up of 6.3 years [10]. Statistically significant ROM improvements were found with 9.72° improvement of flexion contracture, and 15.69°increase into flexion. Knee scores showed statistically significant improvements: clinically, 37.9 point increase and functionally, 13.50 point increase. Moore et al. concluded that TKA was an effective procedure for improving ROM and decreasing functional deficits resulting from hemophilic arthropathy. Knee score data showed TKA improves overall function. However, a 31.5% complication rate was calculated with 106 reported in 336 TKAs [10].

It is paramount today to use a multimodal blood loss prevention approach (MBLPA) including intraarticular tranexamic acid (TXA) in primary and revision TKA for patients with hemophilia (Figs. 16.1 and 16.2).

In a reported study, a MBLPA-TXA in TKA for hemophilic patients was effective, with a zero transfusion rate (compared with 40% in the

E. C. Rodríguez-Merchán (ed.), *Advances in Hemophilia Treatment*,
https://doi.org/10.1007/978-3-030-93990-8_16

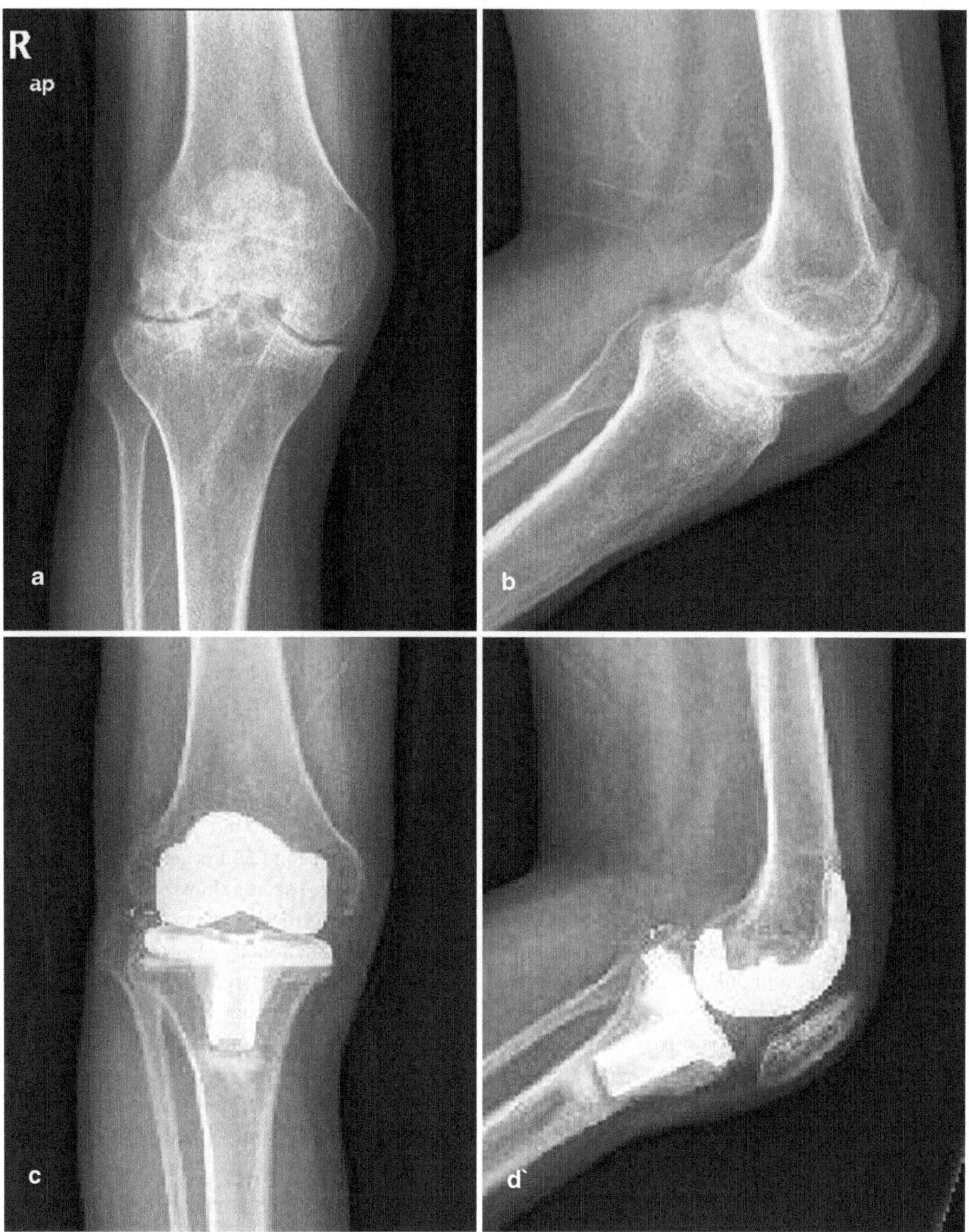

Fig. 16.1 Total knee arthroplasty (TKA) in a patient with inhibitor: (**a**) Anteroposterior preoperative radiograph; (**b**) lateral preoperative view; (**c**) anteroposterior postoperative radiograph; (**d**) lateral postoperative view. The result was excellent

non-MBLPA-TXA group) [7]. The MBLPA-TXA group had less postoperative blood loss than the non-MBLPA-TXA group. The MBLPA-TXA group included the following: (a) Tourniquet with 100 mmHg above systolic pressure, released after skin closure; (b) Surgical blood saving protocol,

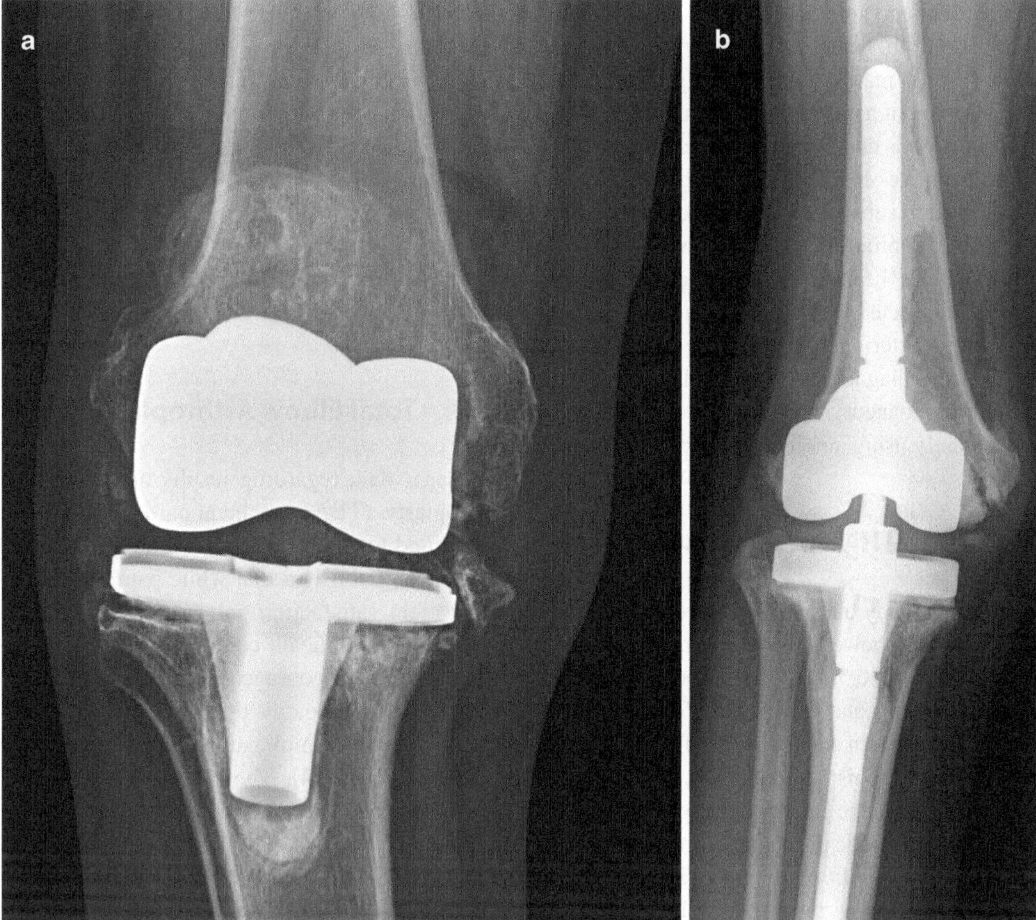

Fig. 16.2 Aseptic loosening of a primary total knee arthroplasty (TKA) 18 years after implantation that required revision arthroplasty with a CCK (constrained condylar knee) implant: (**a**) Anteroposterior preoperative view; (**b**) anteroposterior postoperative radiograph. The result was excellent

including: femoral canal obturation with bone graft and intraarticular infiltration of posterior capsule, medial and lateral capsule, and ligaments, before closure, of 80 cc saline with adrenalin 300 mcg, morphic chloride 10 mg, tobramycin 100 mg, betamethasone sodium phosphate 6 mg, betamethasone acetate 6 mg, and ropivacaine 200 mg; (c) An intraarticular injection of a combination of TXA (25 mL, 2500 mg) and sodium chloride (10 mL, 18 mg) [7].

In the non-MBLPA-TXA group, the standard procedure was used, without any particular blood saving technique (tourniquet with 350 mmHg, released before skin closure for electrocoagulation of bleeding; no limits or treatment to preoperative hemoglobin; no femoral canal obturation, 24–48 h vacuum drain, opened with skin closure, no intraarticular infiltration; and no TXA administration) [7].

The reported rate of survival after TKA at 10 years is between 83% and 92% [8, 9, 11, 12]. Late periprosthetic infections are a major concern, and precautions aimed to avoid hematogenous spread of infections during factor concentrate infusions should be strongly encouraged (Fig. 16.3).

Pseudoaneurysms after TKA may happen (Fig. 16.4). In hemophilia, the most common cause of a hemarthrosis following TKA is the development of a pseudoaneurysm [13–17]. This complication is due to unrecognized injury of the periarticular vessels. Failure to diagnose and treat it may lead to subsequent recurrence of bleeding. Following aspiration of the hemarthrosis via arthrocentesis the existence of a pseudoaneurysm must be suspected. A CT angiogram and a digital subtraction arteriography must be performed to confirm the diagnosis. An arterial embolization of the pseudoaneurysm must then be performed immediately using a helical microcoil [15].

16.3 Total Hip Arthroplasty

In 2008 our study on total hip arthroplasty (THA) in hemophilia showed significant improvement in function (Figs. 16.5 and 16.6). The incidence of aseptic loosening and significant infection remains a cause for concern and long-term follow-up must continue [18]. This suggests that the improvements in knowledge of arthroplasty fixation techniques and antibiotic prophylaxis are giving rise to a reduction in significant complications for hemophilia sufferers requiring THA. Following consideration of the risks and benefits, with age, functional demands, life expectancy and concurrent immunological compromise and all factors, the patient with disabling hip arthropathy may very well benefit from hip replacement.

In 2017 Strauss et al. reported that THA in hemophilic patients leads to a significant increase of function, reduction of pain, and a high satisfaction. They stated that due to the relatively high complication rate (6% infections and 10% aseptic loosening) compared to patients without hemophilia, an individual assessment of the risk–benefit ratio from surgical and hematological point of view is needed [19].

In 2019 Wang et al. found that hemophilia patients have higher rates of postoperative transfusion, hospital costs, and increased length of stay than patients without hemophilia [20]. There was an appreciable clinical difference in 1-year infection rates following THA (8.11% versus 3.38%). Other postoperative complications and mortality rates were comparable. Patients with hemophilia should be counseled that infection rate may be as high as 8% following THA.

16.4 Total Elbow Arthroplasty

The scant data regarding results of total elbow arthroplasty (TEA) for hemophilic arthropathy are limited to small case series and case reports. It has been published that while pain alleviation and patient satisfaction are promising, variable results with significant complications and infection rates may discourage routine use of TEA for hemophilic arthropathy of the elbow [21]. The rate of reported complications is between 12.5% and 85% [8, 22–24]. The rate of reported revisions is between 12.5% and 37.5% [25, 26].

While patients with severe hemophilic arthropathy of the elbow are likely to make gains in terms of pain control and range of motion following TEA, there is insufficient data to routinely recommend its use. Complication and infection rates are concerning, and the lack of survival analysis data makes it difficult to quantify the benefit to the patient in light of the risks and resources involved in the procedure [21].

16.5 Total Ankle Arthroplasty

While patients with severe hemophilic arthropathy of the ankle are likely to improve pain and range of motion after total ankle arthroplasty (TAA), there is insufficient information to rou-

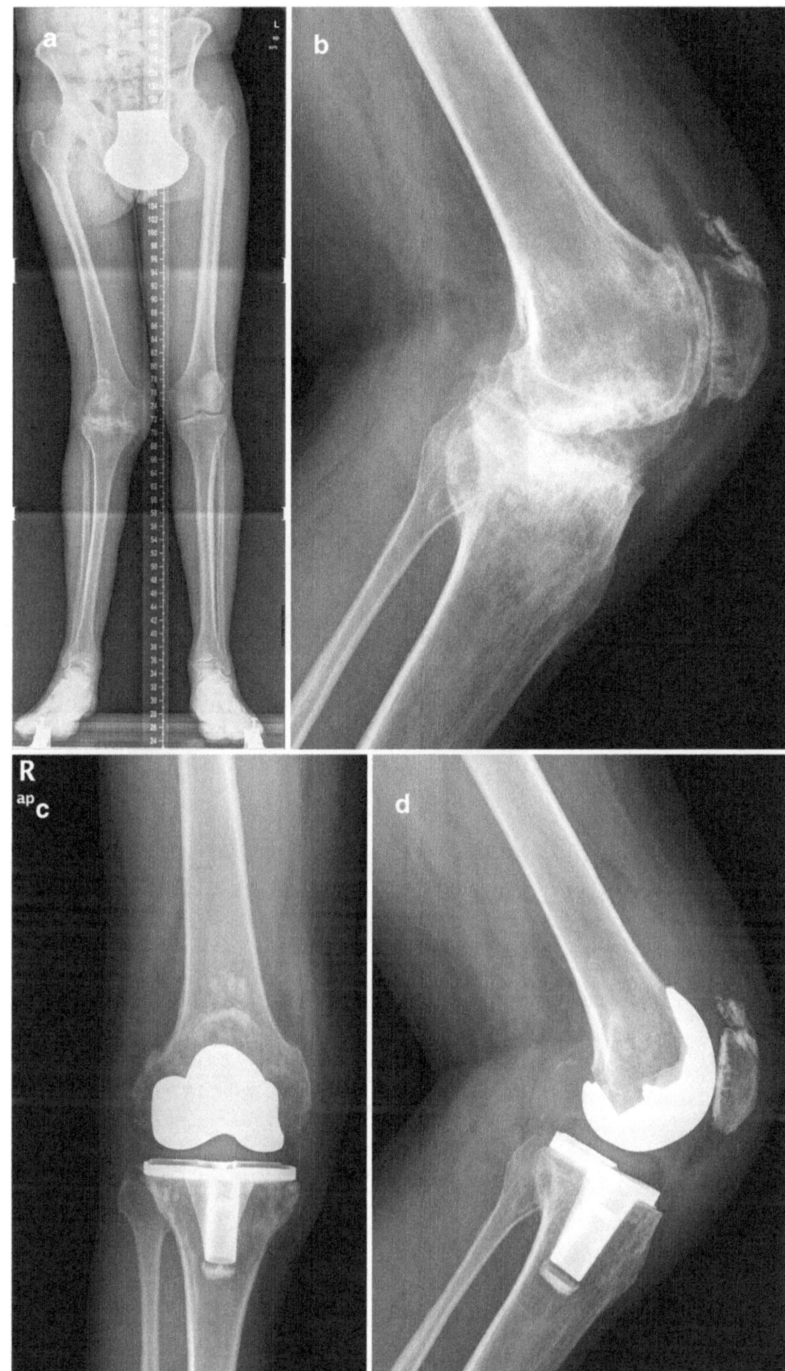

Fig. 16.3 Two-stage revision total knee arthroplasty (TKA) in a periprosthetic infection: (**a**) Anteroposterior view of the knee before TKA; (**b**) lateral radiograph of the knee prior to TKA; (**c**) anteroposterior view of the knee after TKA; (**d**) lateral view of the knee after TKA; (**e**) articulated spacer implanted in the first stage of the two-stage revision arthroplasty performed (anteroposterior view); (**f**) lateral radiograph of the articulated spacer; (**g**) anteroposterior view of the revised implant (constrained condylar knee, CCK design) after the second stage of the two-stage revision arthroplasty; (**h**) lateral radiograph of the revised implant (CCK design) after the second stage of the two-stage revision arthroplasty. The result was excellent

Fig. 16.3 (continued)

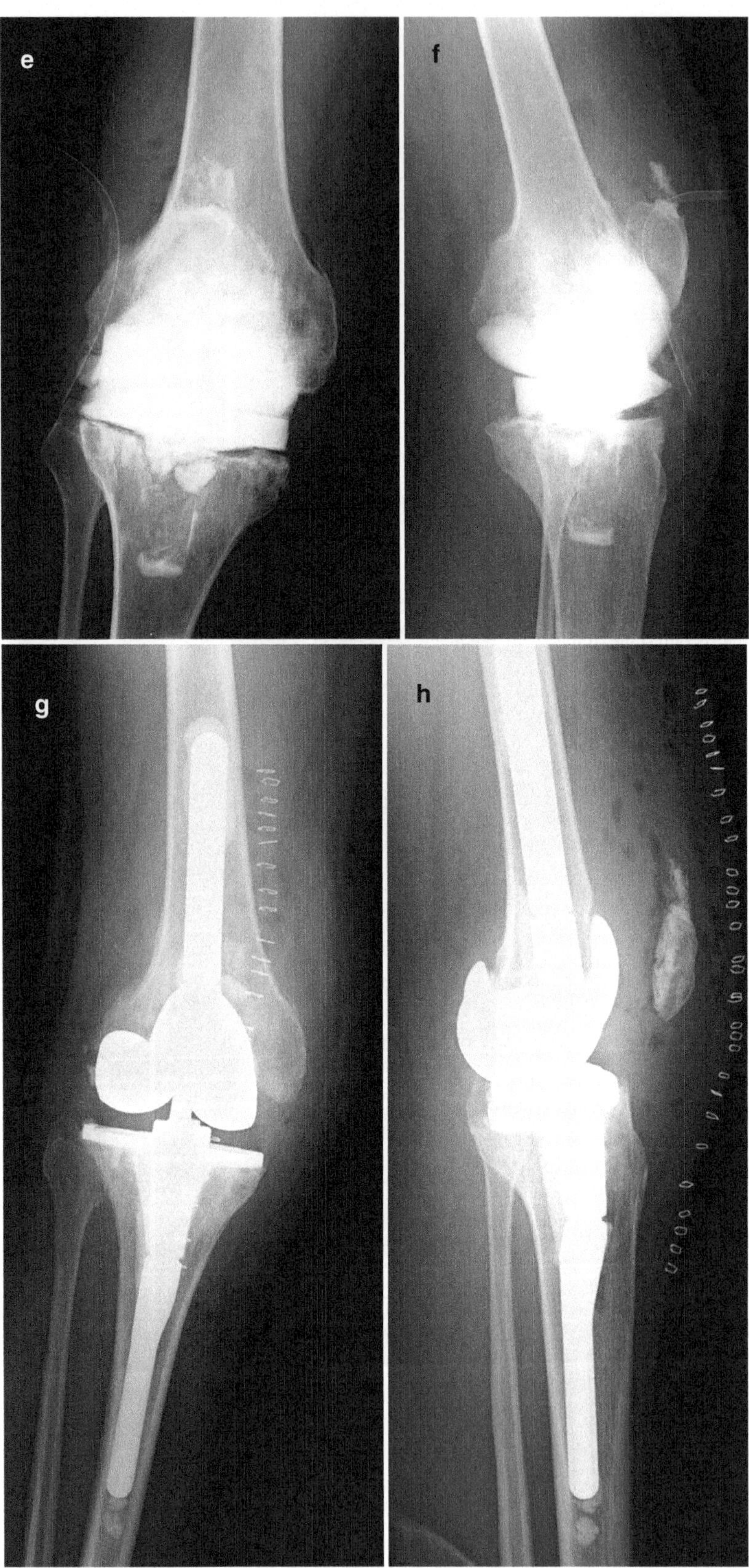

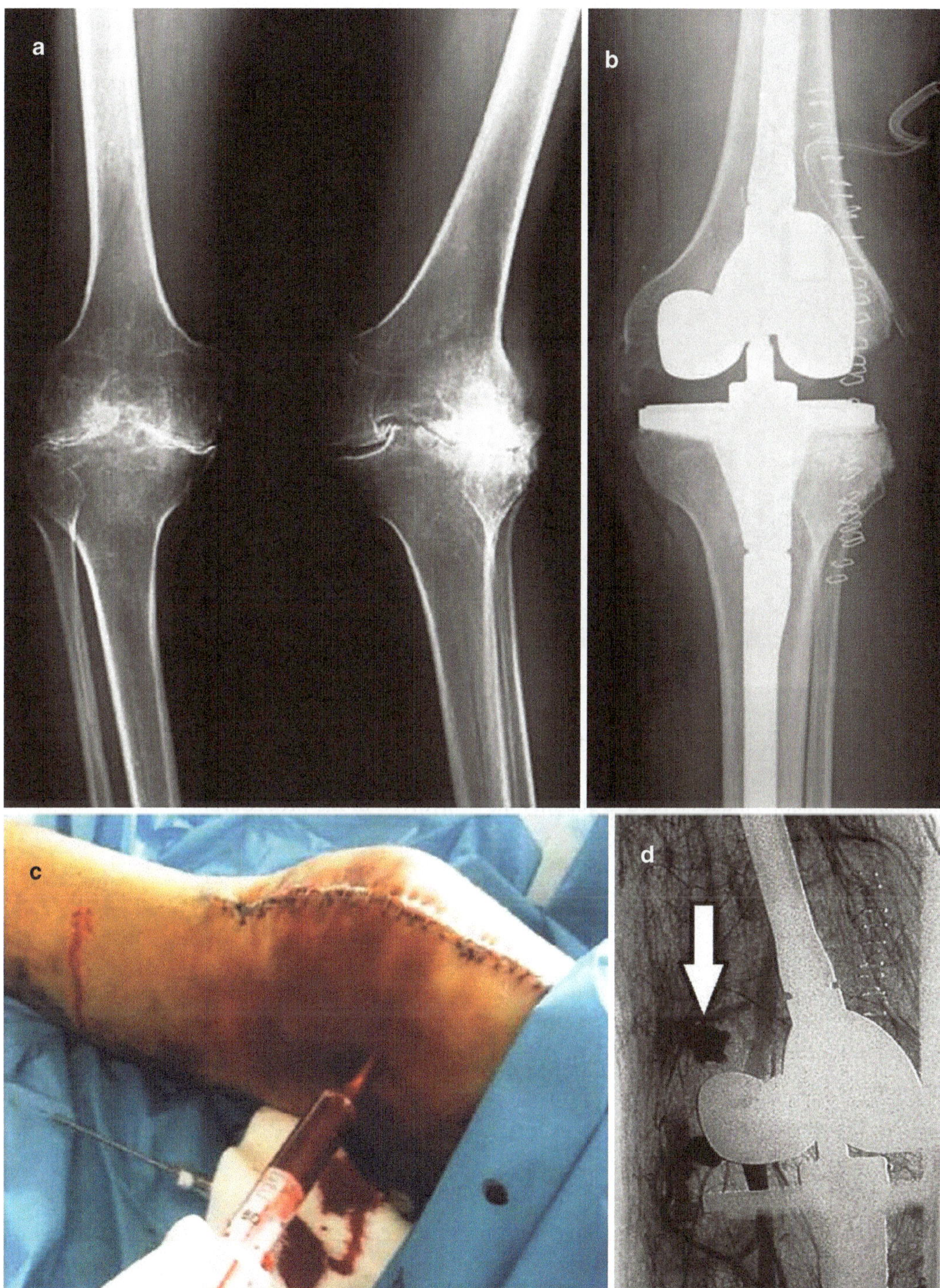

Fig. 16.4 Pseudoaneurysm after primary total knee arthroplasty (TKA) with a constrained condylar knee (CCK) design due to severe varus deformity and muscular atrophy: (**a**) Anteroposterior view of the knee before TKA; (**b**) lateral radiograph prior to TKA; (**c**) severe post-operative hemarthroses 5 days after surgery was treated with joint aspiration; (**d**) angiogram demonstrated the existence of an arterial pseudoaneurysm (arrow); (**e**) arterial embolization (arrow) solved the problem

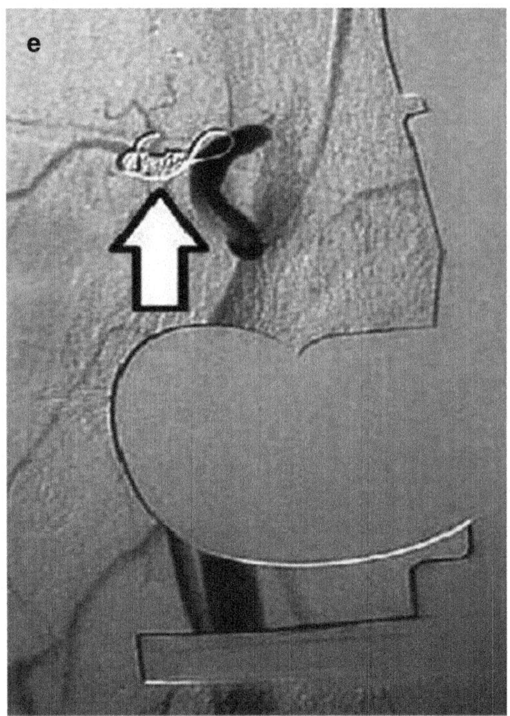

Fig. 16.4 (continued)

tinely advise its use. Complication and infection rates are concerning, and the absence of survival analysis information makes it hard to quantify the profit to the patient in light of the dangers and resources implicated in the procedure [27]. A study found a total rate of intraoperative and postoperative complications of 33% [28]. In other report the predicted implant survival of TAA was 94% at 5, 85% at 10, and 70% at 15 years, respectively [29].

16.6 Conclusions

Reported results of primary THA and TKA in hemophilia are satisfactory. It is paramount today to use a multimodal blood loss prevention approach (MBLPA) including intraarticular tranexamic acid (TXA) in primary and revision TKA for patients with hemophilia. While patients with severe hemophilic arthropathy of the elbow and ankle are likely to make gains in terms of pain control and range of motion following TEA and TAA, there is insufficient data to routinely recommend its use. Complication and infection rates are concerning, and the lack of survival analysis data makes it difficult to quantify the benefit to the patient in light of the risks and resources involved in the procedure.

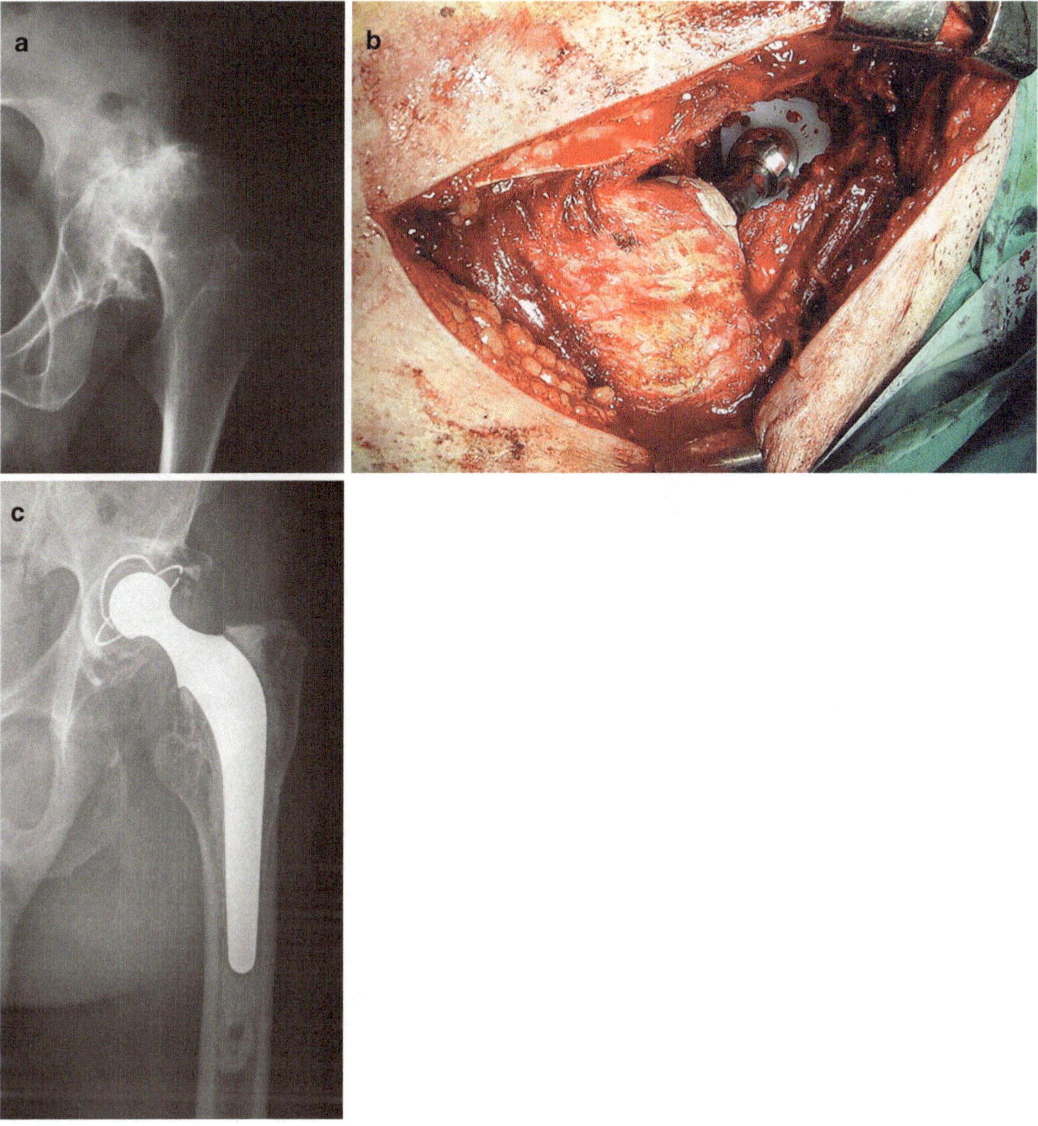

Fig. 16.5 Total hip arthroplasty (THA) in a patient with hemophilia: (**a**) Anteroposterior preoperative radiograph; (**b**) intraoperative view; (**c**) anteroposterior postoperative radiograph. The result was excellent

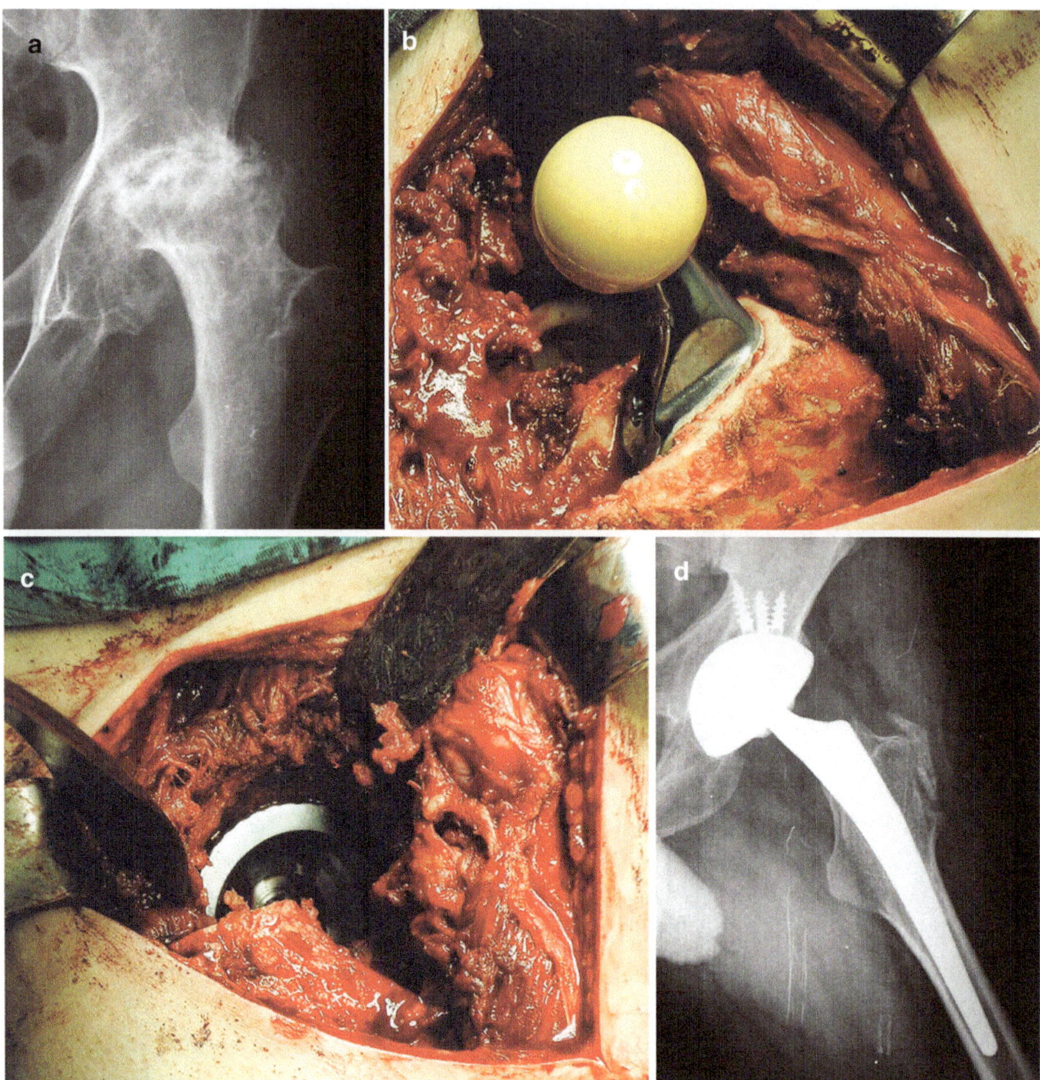

Fig. 16.6 Total hip arthroplasty (THA) in a patient with hemophilia: (**a**) Anteroposterior preoperative radiograph; (**b**) intraoperative view of the artificial femoral head; (**c**) intraoperative view of the acetabular components; (**d**) anteroposterior postoperative radiograph The result was excellent

References

1. Escobar MA, Brewer A, Caviglia H, Forsyth A, Jimenez-Yuste V, Laudenbach L, et al. Recommendations on multidisciplinary management of elective surgery in people with haemophilia. Haemophilia. 2018;24:693–702.
2. Rodriguez-Merchan EC. Total knee replacement in haemophilic arthropathy. J Bone Joint Surg Br. 2007;89:186–8.
3. Goddard NJ, Mann HA, Lee CA. Total knee replacement in patients with end-stage haemophilic arthropathy: 25-year results. J Bone Joint Surg Br. 2010;92:1085–9.
4. Solimeno LP, Mancuso ME, Pasta G, Santagostino E, Perfetto S, Mannucci PM. Factors influencing the long-term outcome of primary total knee replacement in haemophiliacs: a review of 116 procedures at a single institution. Br J Haematol. 2009;145:227–34.
5. Goddard NJ, Rodriguez-Merchan EC, Wiedel JD. Total knee replacement in haemophilia. Haemophilia. 2002;8:382–6.
6. Rodriguez-Merchan EC. Total knee arthroplasty in hemophilic arthropathy. Am J Orthop (Belle Mead NJ). 2015;44:E503–7.

7. Rodriguez-Merchan EC, Romero-Garrido JA, Gomez-Cardero P. Multimodal blood loss prevention approach including intra-articular tranexamic acid in primary total knee arthroplasty for patients with severe haemophilia A. Haemophilia. 2016;22:e318–20.
8. Wang K, Street A, Dowrick A, Liew S. Clinical outcomes and patient satisfaction following total joint replacement in haemophilia--23-year experience in knees, hips and elbows. Haemophilia. 2012;18:86–93.
9. Chevalier Y, Dargaud Y, Lienhart A, Chamouard V, Negrier C. Seventy-two total knee arthroplasties performed in patients with haemophilia using continuous infusion. Vox Sang. 2013;104:135–43.
10. Moore MF, Tobase P, Allen DD. Meta-analysis: outcomes of total knee arthroplasty in the haemophilia population. Haemophilia. 2016;22:e275–85.
11. Silva M, Luck JV Jr. Long-term results of primary total knee replacement in patients with hemophilia. J Bone Joint Surg Am. 2005;87:85–91.
12. Zingg PO, Fucentese SF, Lutz W, Brand B, Mamisch N, Koch PP. Haemophilic knee arthropathy: long-term outcome after total knee replacement. Knee Surg Sports Traumatol Arthrosc. 2012;20:2465–70.
13. Scoles PV, King D. Traumatic aneurysm of the descending geniculate artery: a complication of suction drainage in synovectomy for hemophilic arthropathy. Clin Orthop Relat Res. 1980;150:245–6.
14. Kickuth R, Anderson S, Peter-Salonen K, Lämmle B, Eggli S, Triller J. Hemophilia a pseudoaneurysm in a patient with high responding inhibitors complicating total knee arthroplasty: embolization: a cost-reducing alternative to medical therapy. Cardiovasc Intervent Radiol. 2006;29:1132–5.
15. Rodriguez-Merchan EC, Jimenez-Yuste V, Gomez-Cardero P, Rodriguez T. Severe postoperative haemarthrosis following a total knee replacement in a haemophiliac patient caused by a pseudoaneurysm: early treatment with arterial embolization. Haemophilia. 2014;20:e86–9.
16. Park JJ, Slover JD, Stuchin SA. Recurrent hemarthrosis in a hemophilic patient after revision total knee arthroplasty. Orthopedics. 2010;33:771.
17. Saarela MS, Tiitola M, Lappalainen K, Vikatmaa P, Pinomäki A, Alberty A, et al. Pseudoaneurysm in association with a knee endoprothesis operation in an inhibitor-positive haemophilia A patient - treatment with local thrombin. Haemophilia. 2010;16:686–8.
18. Miles J, Rodriguez-Merchan EC, Goddard NJ. The impact of haemophilia on the success of total hip arthroplasty. Haemophilia. 2008;14:81–4.
19. Strauss AC, Rommelspacher Y, Nouri B, Bornemann R, Wimmer MD, Oldenburg J, et al. Long-term outcome of total hip arthroplasty in patients with haemophilia. Haemophilia. 2017;23:129–34.
20. Wang SH, Chung CH, Chen YC, Cooper AM, Chien WC, Pan RY. Does hemophilia increase risk of adverse outcomes following total hip and knee arthroplasty? A propensity score-matched analysis of a nationwide, population-based study. J Arthroplast. 2019;34:2329–2336.e1.
21. Dale TM, Saucedo JM, Rodriguez-Merchan EC. Total elbow arthroplasty in haemophilia. Haemophilia. 2018;24:548–56.
22. Marshall Brooks M, Tobase P, Karp S, Francis D, Fogarty PF. Outcomes in total elbow arthroplasty in patients with haemophilia at the University of California, San Francisco: a retrospective review. Haemophilia. 2011;17:118–23.
23. Kamineni S, Adams RA, O'Driscoll SW, Morrey BF. Hemophilic arthropathy of the elbow treated by total elbow replacement. A case series. J Bone Joint Surg Am. 2004;86-A:584–9.
24. Chapman-Sheath PJ, Giangrande P, Carr AJ. Arthroplasty of the elbow in haemophilia. J Bone Joint Surg Br. 2003;85:1138–40.
25. Sorbie C, Saunders G, Carson P, Hopman WM, Olney SJ, Sorbie J. Long-term effectiveness of Sorbie-QUESTOR elbow arthroplasty: single surgeon's series of 15 years. Orthopedics. 2011;34:e561–9.
26. Vochteloo AJ, Roche SJ, Dachs RP, Vrettos BC. Total elbow arthroplasty in bleeding disorders: an additional series of 8 cases. J Shoulder Elb Surg. 2015;24:773–8.
27. Rodriguez-Merchan EC. Management of hemophilic arthropathy of the ankle. Cardiovasc Hematol Disord Drug Targets. 2017;17:111–8.
28. Barg A, Elsner A, Hefti D, Hintermann B. Haemophilic arthropathy of the ankle treated by total ankle replacement: a case series. Haemophilia. 2010;16:647–55.
29. Eckers F, Bauer DE, Hingsammer A, Sutter R, Brand B, Viehöfer A, et al. Mid- to long-term results of total ankle replacement in patients with haemophilic arthropathy: a 10-year follow-up. Haemophilia. 2018;24:307–15.

Hemophilic Arthropathy: Other Orthopedic Procedures

17

E. Carlos Rodríguez-Merchán, Primitivo Gómez-Cardero, and Carlos A. Encinas-Ullán

17.1 Introduction

Ninety percent of bleeds in hemophilic patients occur in the musculoskeletal system (80% in joints, 10% in muscles). The role of the orthopedic surgeon is to use invasive and/or surgical methods to treat the musculoskeletal disorders suffered by persons with hemophilia within the context of a multidisciplinary team (hematologists, rehabilitators, physical therapists, nurses, etc.) [1, 2].

A multidisciplinary team makes it possible to safely carry out surgical procedures in persons with hemophilia, even those with inhibitors or infected with the HIV or HCV viruses. Persons with hemophilia have a higher bleeding and infection risk than the rest of patients, i.e. a higher risk of complications and poor results. Institutional support is essential given the high cost associated with the treatment of hemophilia. Close cooperation of the orthopedic surgeon with other specialists makes it possible to significantly improve the quality of life of persons with hemophilia.

E. C. Rodríguez-Merchán (✉) · P. Gómez-Cardero
C. A. Encinas-Ullán
Department of Orthopedic Surgery, La Paz University Hospital, Madrid, Spain

17.2 Orthopedic Surgery of Complications of Intra-Articular Bleeds

The orthopedic complications of hemophilia are patient-specific and treatment protocols often need to be altered to suit the individual.

17.2.1 Excision of the Radial Head and Partial Open Synovectomy

Excision of the radial head and partial open synovectomy is a consistently reliable operation that appears to prolong the functional life of the elbow joint (Fig. 17.1). With proper selection it dramatically reduces the rate of hemarthroses, improves forearm rotation by 20° to 60°, decreases pain, improves function, and does not cause a problem with elbow instability [3, 4].

17.2.2 Surgical Ulnar Nerve Release

In some cases of valgus deformity, ulnar nerve involvement may occur. In this case, surgical ulnar nerve release should be indicated [1].

E. C. Rodríguez-Merchán (ed.), *Advances in Hemophilia Treatment*,
https://doi.org/10.1007/978-3-030-93990-8_17

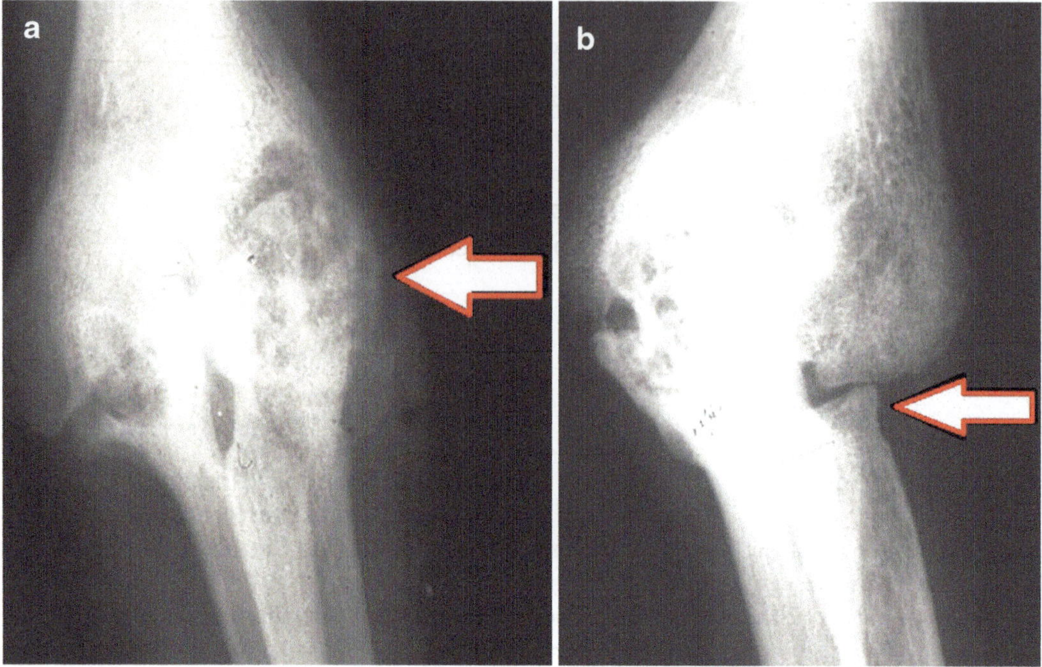

Fig. 17.1 Severe painful elbow hemophilic arthropathy with marked limitation of pronation-supination: (**a**) preoperative anteroposterior view showing radial head hypertrophy (arrow); (**b**) postoperative radiograph after removal of the hypertrophic radial head (arrow)

17.2.3 Ankle Distraction

In 2012 by van Meegeren et al. analyzed three patients with hemophilic ankle arthropathy (one patient with severe hemophilia A, one patient with moderate hemophilia B, one patient with mild hemophilia A) by means of joint distraction using an Ilizarov external fixator [5]. Clinical outcomes (function, participation, and pain) were assessed retrospectively with three questionnaires: the hemophilia activities list, impact on participation and autonomy, and the van Valburg questionnaire. Structural changes on radiographs were blinded and were evaluated using the Pettersson score, ankle images digital analysis (AIDA), and an MRI score. All the patients were satisfied with the clinical outcome of the procedure at the follow-up between 26 and 48 months follow-up. They reported significant improvements in self-perceived functional health, participation in society, autonomy, and pain. Partial ankle motion was preserved in the three patients. The Pettersson score remained the same in one patient and slightly increased in the other two patients, and joint space width measured by AIDA and the MRI score increased in all three patients. This study suggested that ankle joint distraction could be a promising surgical procedure for ankle HA.

For Nguyen et al. [6], positive predictors of ankle survival in patients without hemophilia included a better Ankle Osteoarthritis Scale (AOS) score at 2 years, older age at surgery, and fixed distraction. Radiographs and advanced imaging revealed progression of ankle OA at the time of final follow-up. Adding ankle motion to ankle joint distraction showed an early and sustained beneficial effect on the outcome [6]. In OA, a minimum of 5.8 mm of distraction gap must be achieved because 5 mm of radiographic joint space, as recommended historically, would not prevent contact of the joint surfaces during weight-bearing activities [7].

In conclusion, between 73% and 91% of patients without hemophilia with severe OA of the ankle obtained a clinical benefit from ankle joint distraction, with a minimum 5.8 mm distraction gap. Adding ankle motion to distraction showed an early and sustained beneficial effect on the outcome, although ankle function following joint distraction declines over time. In hemophilia, the only reported study to date (three cases) suggests that ankle joint distraction is a promising surgical procedure for ankle HA.

17.2.4 Ankle Fusion

Hindfoot arthrodesis in patients with hemophilic ankle arthropathy provides a high fusion rate with few complications (Fig. 17.2). In a study arthroscopic tibiotalar fusion did not result in shorter hospital stays [8]. Revision surgery for the hemophilic hindfoot is successful and fusion of the entire hindfoot can be achieved without complications. In conclusion, we believe that hindfoot (tibiotalar and/or subtalar) arthrodesis in hemophilic arthropathy is a successful procedure with comparable outcomes to that of non-hemophiliac populations. The fusion rate of arthroscopic ankle fusion is less promising compared to other methods (minimally access surgery and classical open surgery) and does not afford the benefits of short hospital stays. Minimal access surgery has been shown to provide good outcomes for hemophilic patients and has fewer complications and shorter hospital stays than open and arthroscopic techniques. Revision surgery for the hemophilic ankle is successful and fusion of the entire hemophilic hindfoot can be achieved without complications if indicated [8].

17.2.5 Surgical Lenghtening of the Achilles Tendon Associated with a Posterior Open Capsulotomy

A common deformity associated with tibiotalar and subtalar arthropathy is fixed plantar flexion that can be alleviated by means of the surgical lenghtening of the Achilles tendon associated with a posterior open capsulotomy [9].

17.3 Orthopedic Surgery of Complications of Intramuscular Bleeds

In the majority of cases, bleeds within the muscles are caused by trauma. They are very often associated with direct trauma and the pathology becomes quite evident due to the swelling; pain, local warmth, and bruising that typically appear in the overlying skin. The vast majority of these muscle bleeds resolve spontaneously with adequate factor coverage, leaving no functional loss. It is, however, necessary to examine the patient carefully to ensure that there is no danger to vascular element or neural compromise. Diagnostic US and/or CT scan is paramount to confirm diagnosis [10–12].

The most common and most serious of muscle bleeds occurs in the iliopsoas muscle (Fig. 17.3). Right lower quadrant abdominal pain has mimicked the symptomatology of an acute appendicitis. Compression of the femoral nerve may present as an area of reduced sensation in the anterios aspect of the thigh. Attempts to extend the hip joint cause severe pain and force the patient into hyperlordosis of the lumbar spine. As it is difficult clinically to differentiate between a bleed into the iliopsoas muscle and an intra-articular hemorrhage into the hip joint, one must rely on objective testing. US and/or CT scan is able to differentiate between the largely extended joint capsule with intra-articular hemorrhage and the bleed that is situated within the muscle fibers. The iliopsoas muscle hematoma takes a long time to improve even under hematologcal prophylaxis, and then flexion contracture of the hip joint may persist for weeks. Secondary hemorrhages into the same area are common and hence, prophylactic factor replacement must be continued. Whereas coxhemarthrosis is a problem costing days of extra treatment, an ilipsoas hematoma may require weeks until full disappearance is achieved (to be confirmed with US and/or CT scan) [1].

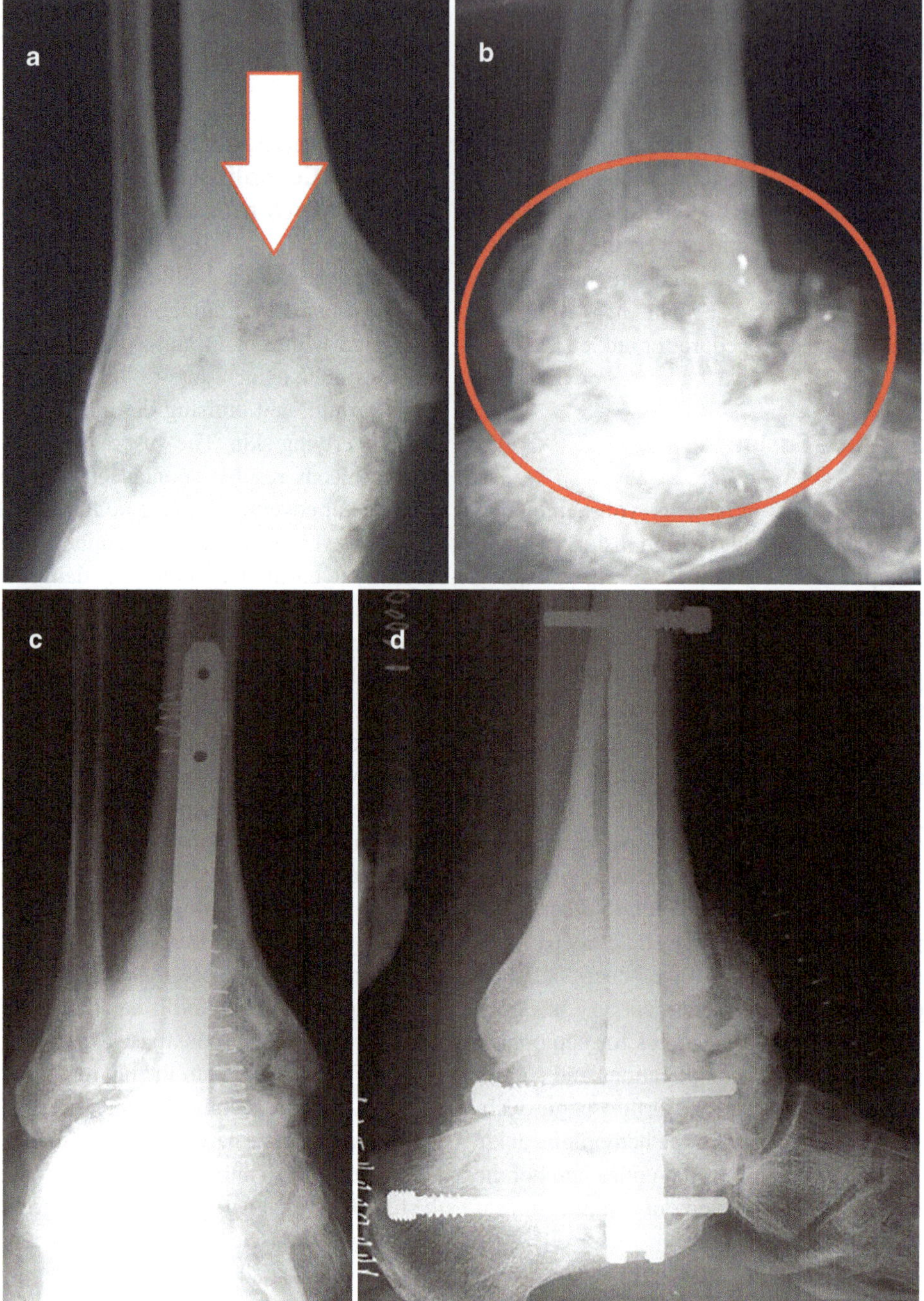

Fig. 17.2 Ankle fusion by means of a retrograde locked intramedullary nail in a case of severe painful ankle hemophilic arthropathy: (**a**) Preoperative anteroposterior view; (**b**) lateral radiograph; (**c**) postoperative anteroposterior view; (**d**) lateral postoperative radiograph

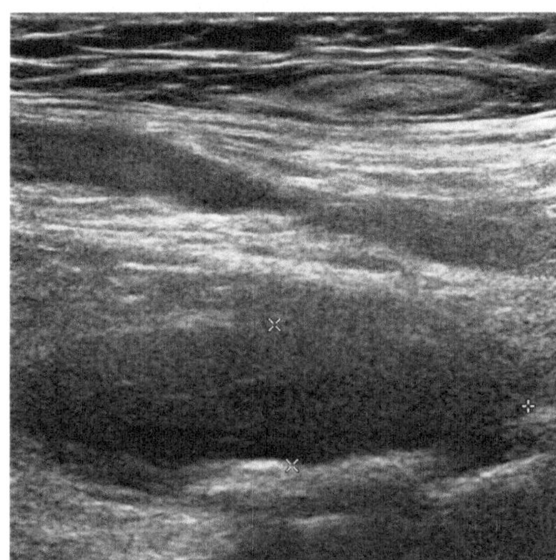

Fig. 17.3 Iliopsoas hematoma confirmed with ultrasonography (US)

17.3.1 Compartment Syndromes

Compartment syndromes (Volkmann's contracture of the hand and foot) have been reported as a result of such bleeding incidences within the closed compartments of the forearm and leg [13]. Compartment syndromes (forearm, leg) are surgical emergencies.

17.3.2 Hemophilic Pseudotumors

The pseudotumor is basically an encapsulated hematoma. A thick fibrous capsule surrounds a hematoma in varying degrees of organization; calcification and ossification may be seen within it.

The management of the patient with a hemophilic pseudotumor is complex and with a high rate of potential complications. There are a number of therapeutic alternatives for this dangerous condition: embolization, radiation, percutaneous management, surgical removal and exeresis and filling of the dead cavity (Fig. 17.4) [14].

Proximal pseudotumors occur in the proximal skeleton, especially around the femur and pelvis. They appear to originate in the soft tissue, erode bone secondarily from outside, and develop slowly over many years. An iliopsoas muscle hematoma may develop a pelvic pseudotumor. Proximal pseudotumors occur in adults and do not respond to conservative treatment. The large proximal pseudotumors in the adults should be removed surgically as soon as they are diagnosed. Distal pseudotumors ocurring distal to the wrist and ankle appear to be secondary to intraosseous hemorrhage and develop rapidly. They are seen mainly in children and adolescents [14].

Distal pseudotumors should be treated primarily with long-term factor replacement and immobilization. In childen, surgical removal or even amputation is indicated when conservative treatment fails to prevent progression. Percutaneous evacuation should be considered in inoperable advanced pseudotumors. Evacuation is carried out with a large trocar under image intensifier control; the cavity is filled with different quantities of fibrin seal or cancellous bone, depending on the size of the pseudotumor [15].

It is hoped that with the advent of widespread maintenance therapy, pseudotumors will be less common in the future. It is important that they are diagnosed early, and prevention of muscular hematomas is key to reducing their incidence. Untreated, proximal pseudotumors will ultimately destroy soft tissues, erode bone, and may produce neurovascular complications. Surgical excision is the treatment of choice but, like all orthopedic procedures in hemophilic patients, should only be carried out in major hemophilia centers by a multidisciplinary surgical team.

17.4 Fractures

In hemophilic patients the fracture can occur anywhere in the long bones but are more prevalent near the joints or in the diaphysis of the long bone. The lower limbs bones, especially femur, are the commonest site of fracture (Figs. 17.5 and 17.6). Fracture hematomas tend to be large in volume and may be the cause of acute compartment syndrome [12, 16].

Poor musculature, osteoporosis, and hemophilic changes in the bone may predispose hemophilic patients to risk of fractures. In patients with hemophilia the fracture can occur after a

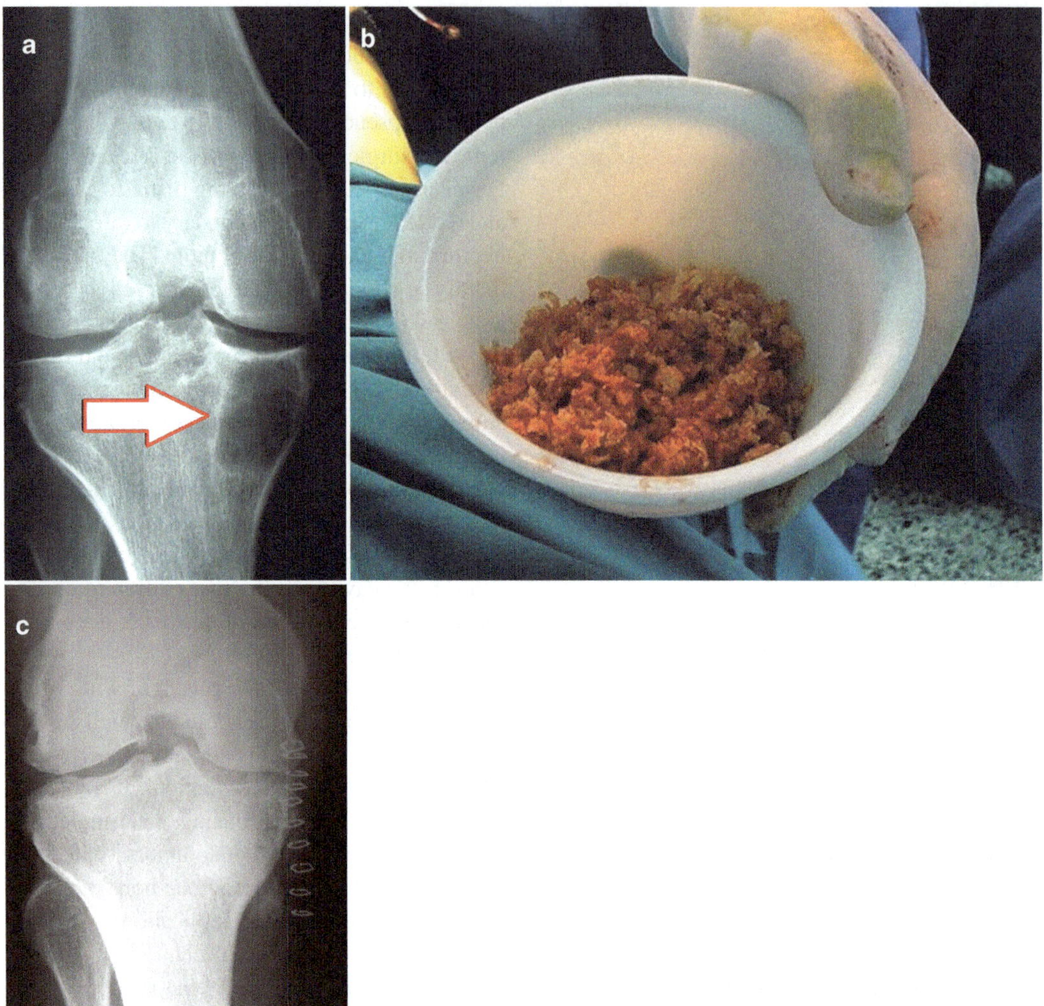

Fig. 17.4 Hemophilic pseudotumor (bone cyst) in proximal tibia (arrow) treated by means of evacuation and filling with cancellous bone taken from the Bone Bank: (**a**) Preoperative anteroporterior radiograph; (**b**) cancellous bone used during surgery to fill the cyst; (**c**) postoperative anteroposterior radiograph

trivial trauma especially if associated factors of hemophilic arthropathy, muscle wasting, and osteoporosis render the bone more fragile and prone to fracture [17].

The goal of modern fracture treatment must be to obtain an optimal outcome with the patient's return to full activity as soon as possible. Today, internal fixation is indicated in most displaced fractures in the adult, whereas external fixation remains the best choice for initial stabilization with severe soft tissue injuries. If a fracture is correctly treated in a hemophilic patient it will progress to consolidation in a similar time frame to those occurring in the general population [12, 16].

17.5 Conclusions

Hemophilia left untreated or treated on demand (only when a hemarthrosis occurs) destroys the joints at a very young age. Primary hematological prophylaxis, currently the gold standard for the management of hemophilia, is not completely efficacious. Moreover, it is only available for 25–30% of patients worldwide. Advances in

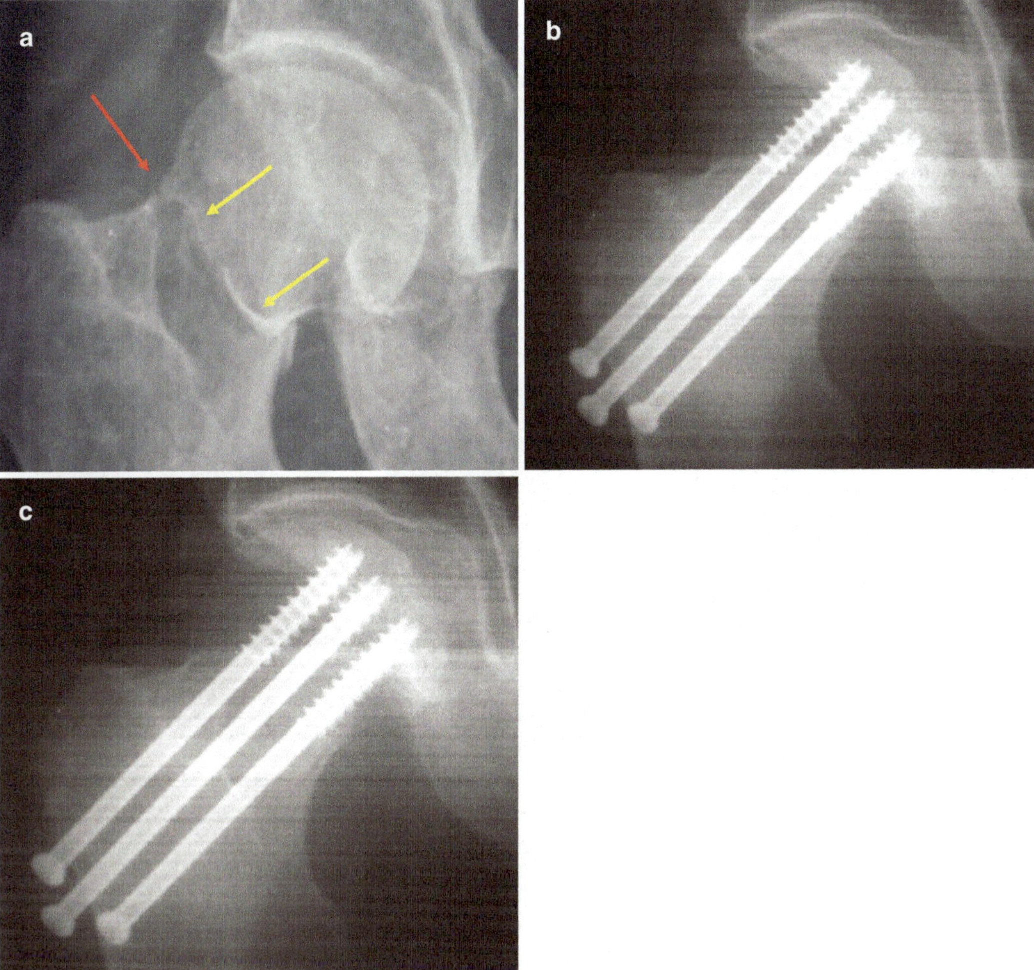

Fig. 17.5 Nondisplaced femoral neck fracture treated with three percutaneous cannulated screws: (**a**) Preoperative anteroposterior radiograph showing the fracture (arrows); (**b**) Immediate postoperative view; (**c**) Postoperative radiograph 1 year later showing bone healing of the fracture

hematology, combined with the advances in orthopedic surgery have made it possible to ameliorate the musculoskeletal complications of hemophilia through orthopedic surgical procedures. These procedures are safe, even in the most complex cases, such as patients with inhibitor. The risk of bleeding in surgical procedures is higher for patients with hemophilia than for the general population and there is also a greater risk of infection. Both these factors augment the risk of a poor result. Whatever the surgical technique, appropriate surgical hemostasis must be achieved by intravenous infusion of concentrate of the deficient factor (factor VIII or factor IX), at the correct doses (ideally for 10–14 days). In patients with inhibitor hemostasis can be achieved with the intravenous infusion of aPCCs and/or rFVIIa. Surgical orthopedic procedures that are usually needed by hemophilic patients include joint aspiration, synovectomy (radiosynovectomy or arthroscopic), arthroscopic joint debridement, Achilles tendon lengthening, removal of ankle osteophytes, arthrodesis of the ankle, TKR, resection or percutaneous treatment of pseudotumors, fasciotomy for compartment syndrome, and neurolysis of the ulnar nerve.

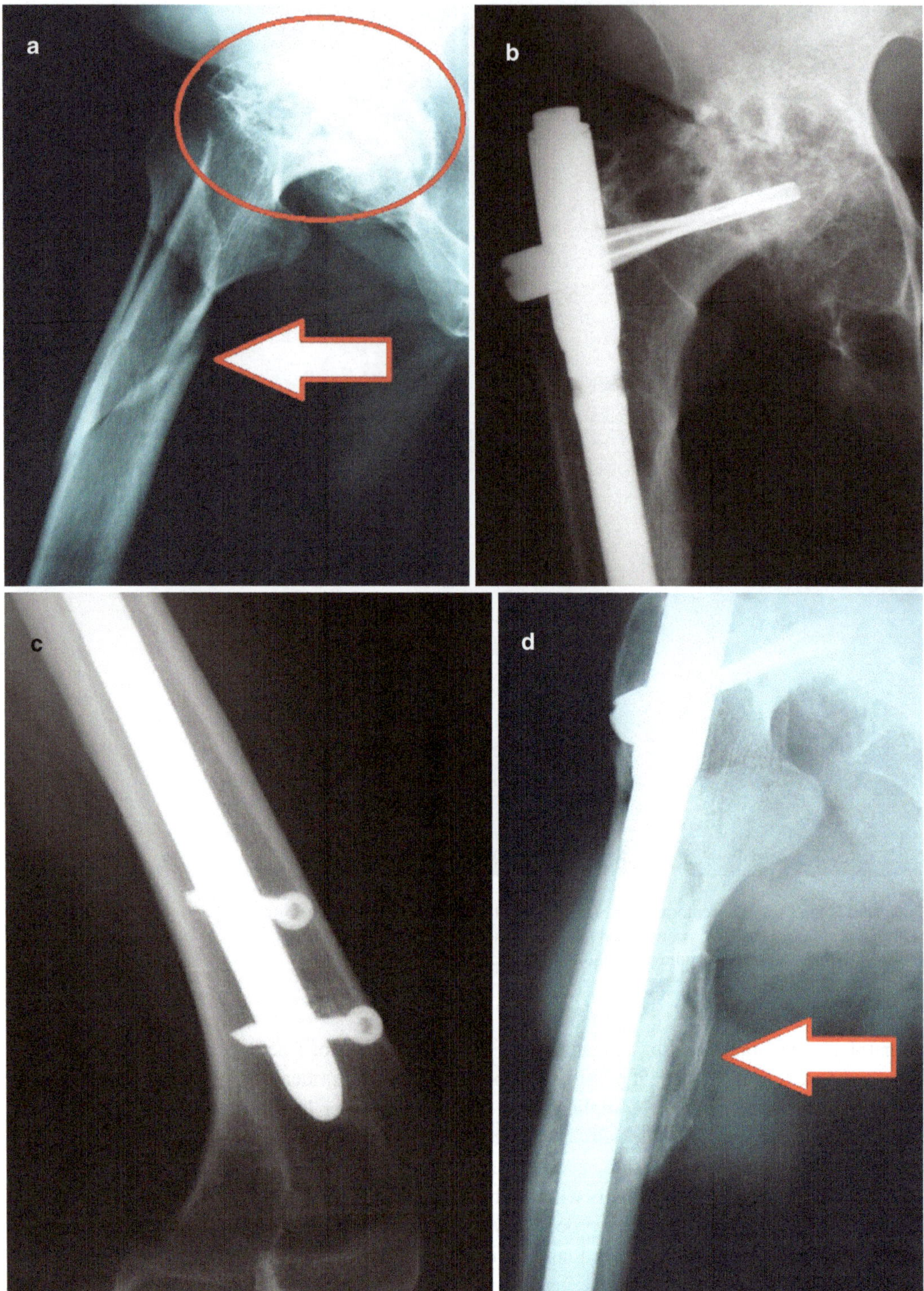

Fig. 17.6 Displaced subtrochanteric fracture treated with anterograde locked reconstruction nail: (**a**) Preoperative anteroposterior radiograph; note previous severe hemophilic arthropathy of the hip (circle) and the fracture site (arrow); (**b**) postoperative view of the proximal part of the femur; (**c**) postoperative radiograph of the distal part of the femur; (**d**) postoperative radiograph 6 months later showing consolidation of the fracture (arrow)

References

1. Rodriguez-Merchan EC. Musculo-skeletal manifestations of haemophilia. Blood Rev. 2016;30:401–19.
2. Rodriguez-Merchan EC. Surgical approaches to hemophilic arthropathy. Blood Coagul Fibrinol. 2019;30(Suppl 1):S11–3.
3. Silva M, Luck JV Jr. Radial head excision and synovectomy in patients with hemophilia. J Bone Joint Surg Am. 2007;89:2156–62.
4. Merchan ECR, Galindo E, Magallon M, Gago J, Villar A, Sanjurjo MJ. Resection of the radial head and partial open synovectomy of the elbow in the young adult with haemophilia: long-term results. Haemophilia. 1995;1:262–6.
5. Van Meegeren ME, Van Veghel K, De Kleijn P, Van Roermund PM, Biesma DH, Lafeber FP, Roosendaal G. Joint distraction results in clinical and structural improvement of haemophilic ankle arthropathy: a series of three cases. Haemophilia. 2012;18:810–7.
6. Nguyen MP, Pedersen DR, Gao Y, Saltzman CL, Amendola A. Intermediate-term follow-up after ankle distraction for treatment of end-stage osteoarthritis. J Bone Joint Surg Am. 2015;97:590–6.
7. Fragomen AT, McCoy TH, Meyers KN, Rozbruch SR. Minimum distraction gap: how much ankle joint space is enough in ankle distraction arthroplasty? HSS J. 2014;10:6–12.
8. Brkljac M, Shah S, Hay C, Rodriguez-Merchan EC. Hindfoot fusion in haemophilic arthropathy: 6-year mean follow-up of 41 procedures performed in 28 adult patients. Haemophilia. 2016;22:e87–98.
9. Rodriguez-Merchan EC. Management of hemophilic arthropathy of the ankle. Cardiovasc Hematol Disord Drug Targets. 2017;17:111–8.
10. Merchan ECR, De Orbe A, Gago J. Ultrasound in the diagnosis of the early stages of hemophilic arthropathy of the knee. Acta Orthop Belg. 1992;58:122–5.
11. De la Corte-Rodriguez H, Rodriguez-Merchan EC, Jimenez-Yuste V. Point-of-care ultrasonography in orthopedic management of hemophilia: multiple uses of an effective tool. HSS J. 2018;14:307–13.
12. Rodriguez-Merchan EC. The role of orthopaedic surgery in haemophilia: current rationale, indications and results. EFORT Open Rev. 2019;4:165–73.
13. Rodriguez-Merchan EC. Acute compartment syndrome in haemophilia. Blood Coagul Fibrinolysis. 2013;24:677–82.
14. Rodriguez-Merchan EC. Haemophilic cysts (pseudotumours). Haemophilia. 2002;8:393–401.
15. Caviglia H, Galatro G, Cambiaggi G, Landro ME, Candela M, Neme D. Treatment of subchondral cysts in patients with haemophilia. Haemophilia. 2016;22:292–7.
16. Rodriguez-Merchan EC. Bone fractures in the haemophilic patient. Haemophilia. 2002;8:104–11.
17. Rodriguez-Merchan EC, Valentino LA. Increased bone resorption in hemophilia. Blood Rev. 2019;33:6–10.

18 Gene Therapy in Hemophilia: Latest Developments

Pedro A. Sanchez-Lara, Joseph Nathanson, and Leonard A. Valentino

18.1 Introduction

18.1.1 History of Gene Therapy

The promise of successful treatment with genetic medicines could positively affect millions of lives globally [1]. With the initiation of the human genome project three decades ago, there was only a dreamers hope and speculation for any form of genetic intervention. Today, there are now thousands of gene therapy clinical trials registered and underway worldwide. When comparing a 2019 search on the clinicaltrials.gov site to a 2021 search today, there were 3836 "gene therapy" trials in 2019 vs 4887 today, Of these, 966 were recruiting vs 1125 today and there were 35 "gene trials," "recruiting" in "hemophilia" in 2019 vs 51 studies today. In one generation, advanced technologies have matured enough to bring hope to many people living with genetic disorders, patient advocacy groups, and to motivate healthcare researchers from all types of academic centers and private industries. With several genetic therapies already approved for clinical use in the USA and Europe, academic health centers, governments, and biopharmaceutical companies are heavily investing their resources into genetic therapy research and development [2, 3].

Gene therapy is typically divided into two main categories: direct in vivo cellular manipulation within the host to a target tissue or ex-vivo genetically engineered stem cells and re-introducing them back to the patient. A therapeutic method can be categorized as gene editing (either replacing the original defective gene or targeting a specific known mutation) or gene transfer (delivery of a manipulated viral vector vehicle that either integrates or stays outside the host DNA).

P. A. Sanchez-Lara
Genetics, Cedars-Sinai Medical Center, David Geffen School of Medicine, UCLA, Los Angeles, CA, USA
e-mail: Pedro.Sanchez@cshs.org

J. Nathanson
Rocky Vista University, Parker, CO, USA
e-mail: joseph.nathanson@rvu.edu

L. A. Valentino (✉)
National Hemophilia Foundation, New York, NY, USA

Rush University, Chicago, IL, USA
e-mail: lvalentino@hemophilia.org

18.1.2 Gene Editing

One of the two mainstays of gene therapy is gene editing. Early methods of gene editing included transcription activator-like effector nucleases (TALENs) and zinc finger nucleases (ZFNs) co-opting the biology of prokaryotic organism nucleases by engineering nonspecific nucleases that are fused to sequence-specific DNA binding domains [4]. These repurposed genome editing tools share one of the central dogmas to genetic

E. C. Rodríguez-Merchán (ed.), *Advances in Hemophilia Treatment*,
https://doi.org/10.1007/978-3-030-93990-8_18

editing: to inducing double stranded DNA breaks (DSBs) in order to tap into the cell's innate DNA repair mechanisms. When these repair mechanisms are activated, efficient edits to the genome can take place [5]. These breaks can be nonspecific and have the risk of disrupting an important gene or induce a second unanticipated effect. There has been much more media coverage and excitement surrounding the discovery and repurposing of a more specific bacterial immune defense mechanism against foreign genetic elements known as clustered regularly interspaced short palindromic repeats (CRISPR) and the adaptative prokaryotic immune system (CRISPR-Cas). The discovery of a more precise genomic editing tool has not only spurred new areas of medical research, but has taken the public by storm and has made "CRISPR" a household name [6].

CRISPRs were first discovered in *Escherichia coli* in 1987; however, the full clinical significance of the discovery was not realized at that time because of the lack of understanding of the information coded within the DNA sequence [7]. Over the next decade CRISPRs were discovered in archaea and bacterial genomes, specifically Haloferax mediterranei [8]. Throughout these discoveries several genes were recognized next to CRISPRs and were named CRISPR-associated genes [9]. To date, there are now six different types of CRISPR systems that are discussed below. Over the last two decades, it has been demonstrated that CRISPRs are transcribed into RNA, which is next cleaved and loaded into CRISPR-Cas proteins, and the RNA–protein complex is sufficient for RNA-guided dsDNA endonuclease activity [10, 11], which is a vital step in genome editing [12]. Table 18.1 (adapted from [12]) depicts available monogenic diseases that have been found to have therapies via CRISPR-Cas utilization.

Types of CRISPR/Cas systems: According to the structure and function of Cas protein, the CRISPR/Cas systems can be categorized into either class I or class II. Both class I class II are further subdivided into six types (type I–VI) [17]. Class I includes type I, III, and IV, and class II includes type II, V, and VI [18]. Type I, II, and V systems recognize and cleave DNA, type VI can edit RNA, and type III edits both DNA and RNA. The effect of type IV system on DNA or RNA is still unknown [19]. Since the structures of type II and V systems are relatively simple, they have been widely used in bacteria. The development of endogenous type I and III systems has expanded the use of CRISPR/Cas technology in bacteria [20].

Table 18.1 Available monogenic diseases that have been encountered to have therapies via CRISPR-Cas utilization

Monogenic disease	Target	Animal model	Delivery system	Strategy	References
Leber congenital amaurosis type 10 (LCA10)	*CEP290*	HuCEP290 IVS26 KI mouse eye	Adeno-associated virus (AAV); (subretinal injection)	Non-homologous end joining (NHEJ) mediated aberrant splicing	[13]
Duchenne muscular dystrophy (DMD)	*Dmd*	mdx mice muscle	AAV; intramuscular injection	NHEJ mediated mutant exon 23 skipping	[14]
Sickle cell disease (SCD)	*BCL11A* erythroid enhancer	CD34+ human hematopoietic stem/progenitor cells (HSPCs) from sickle cell disease patient	Ribonucleoprotein (RNP); electroporation	NHEJ mediated enhancer disruption	[15]
Genetic deafness	*Tmc1*	Beethoven (Bth) mouse ear	AAV; inner ear injections	NHEJ mediated mutant Tmc allele disruption	[16]

18.1.3 Gene Transfer

An alternative therapeutic approach to gene therapy besides direct gene editing as described above is gene transfer. Gene transfer focuses on the avoidance of insertional mutagenesis which is the principal method of gene editing. Optimal vectors for gene delivery should target specific cell types, be biochemically efficient, have little or no geno-and cytotoxicity, and should not trigger an immune response. Two main drawbacks to gene transfer methods are a dilutional effect and the fact that affected cells are prone to epigenetic changes [21].

Gene transfer is dependent upon utilization of viral vectors to deliver the desired therapeutic gene to desired target tissue in the body. There are both integrating and non-integrating vectors that accomplish this task. In the case of integrating vectors, viral DNA translocates into the nucleus and integrates into the host genome. The genetic material of non-integrating vectors, in contrast, remains in the cytoplasm in an episomal form [22].

Major benefits to non-integrating vectors share a reduced risk of genotoxicity and can be retained for long periods of time in post-mitotic tissues. A drawback is that, unless they have been genetically engineered for specific replication and segregation, they will dilute progressively in proliferating cells. Take the monogenic disease, hemophilia A as an example. Imagine a vector transferring a gene that can be transcribed into functional factor VIII protein. Initially this would be an effective therapy for someone without much functional factor VIII of their own. However, after several generations of cell division, there could eventually be a negligible amount of the transferred gene to transcribe functional factor VIII [21]. Moreover, this principle highlights the problems that arise when considering genetic treatments for children. Consider non-integrating vectors delivering a therapeutic gene to a liver to help produce adequate factor VIII or factor IX; the liver is still dividing in children, therefore a profound dilutional effect will take place—rendering the therapy ineffective in children over time as the liver grows.

To get around the aforementioned dilutional effect, researchers are working on ways to bypass the limitations of a single dose administration and repeatedly administer the non-integrating vectors to keep the proteins levels at a therapeutic level. However, with a solution to one problem comes an entirely new problem—unwanted immune responses [21].

18.1.4 Immunogenicity

Both innate and adaptive immune responses can affect the safety and efficacy of AAV vector-mediated gene transfer in humans [23, 24]. Immune responses directed towards gene vectors, transgene product, or both limit the efficacy and safety of gene therapy [25, 26]. After administration of the vector or vector-transduced cells, a primary immune response against the vector envelopes or capsid proteins can occur [27]; in this case, it can limit re-administration of the same vector or cell product, but it should not affect the efficacy and safety of the procedure, as vector-derived antigens (Ags) are not maintained in the recipient. Indeed, viral vectors often lack viral genes, thus viral proteins are not actively produced by virally transduced cells. On the contrary, immune reactivity against vector components pre-existing to vector administration (such as following exposure to the virus that is being transposed) may inactivate the vector, inhibiting transduction, and/or attack transduced cells while still exposing vector-derived Ags, as described in some studies using adeno-associated virus (AAV) derived vectors [21, 28, 29]. Going back to our initial example of transferring a gene that codes for factor VIII using an AAV vector in people with hemophilia A, we see the potential for reduced efficacy due to either a dilutional effect or a significant immunogenetic response. Adenoviruses are common culprits of mild viral illness, therefore many already have pre-formed antibodies against adenoviruses [21, 30].

Recent discoveries have been made by A. Li et al. [31], which could alleviate many of the problems outlined above. Their research focused on the need for only transient need of CRISPR-

Cas9 upon gene transfer. They report a self-deleting AAV-CRISPR system that introduces insertion and deletion mutations into AAV episomes. They demonstrate that this system dramatically reduces the level of *Staphylococcus aureus* Cas9 protein, often greater than 79%, while achieving high rates of on-target editing in the liver. Off-target mutagenesis was not observed for the self-deleting Cas9 guide RNA at any of the predicted potential off-target sites examined. This system is efficient and versatile, as demonstrated by robust knockdown of liver-expressed proteins in vivo. This self-deleting AAV-CRISPR system is an important proof of concept that will help enable translation of liver-directed genome editing in humans [31]. Table 18.2 shows the properties of non-integrating gene therapy vectors [21]. Table 18.2 shows the properties of non-integrating gene therapy vectors (adapted from [21]).

18.1.5 History of Gene Therapy in Hemophilia

The evolution of hemophilia treatment has undergone a massive shift over the past 60+ years. In the 1960s, with the discovery of fractionation of plasma came the first uses of factor VIII and factor IX as replacement therapies. The next major development was the genetic cloning of the F8 and F9 genes. By utilizing recombinant DNA technology, scientists were able to develop a therapeutic approach where factor VIII and IX were injected into people. The major drawback with this therapeutic approach has been the short half-lives of these molecules in circulation. Fortunately, by adding IgG, albumin, or PEG, we have seen extended half-lives of these factors in circulation [32]. Next came the development of a unique therapy using the monoclonal antibody, emicizumab, which effectively binds to factors IXa and X at the same time, which in turn functions as an activated factor VIIIa does by activating factor X [33–35]. Although extending half-lives of factor therapy and monoclonal antibody therapy have proved to be an improvement when compared to treatment before their time, people with hemophilia (PWH) and families throughout the global community are looking for a permanent solution. Current hemophilia treatments are far from perfect and carry a stigma and risk of chronic disease; with factor levels peaks and troughs risking major joint disease from acute bleeds or chronic subclinical microdamage. Current therapies have made an impact on the disease process of hemophilia, but all treatments still tether a patient (and their family) to a lifetime of monitoring, medications and need to have emergency plans for even the simplest of activities. These are certain to impact life choices and quality of life. Genetic therapies as the technology have the potential to mature as a viable treatment option and change the global morbidity and mortality of hemophilia, much like how factor VIII and IX were initially used with the discovery of fractionation of plasma.

When considering gene therapy in hemophilia there are two guiding principles: (1) clotting factors are almost exclusively synthesized in the liver, making it the desired target for genetic manipulation. (2) Even a mild increase in circulating factor levels can drastically improve a patient's disease severity. Below, we examine the specific studies highlighting the evolution of genetic therapy in both hemophilia A and hemophilia B.

18.2 Genetic Therapy in Hemophilia A

In a recent 2020 study, 15 adult men with severe hemophilia A were treated with the factor VIII construct valoctocogene roxaparvovec (valrox). This study showed phenotypical improvements in terms of bleeding rates and increases in factor VIII activity [36]. Interestingly, the efficacy of this treatment proved to be dose-dependent. Increased vector dose showed both an increase in factor levels and decreased bleeding events (median of 0/year). With these encouraging results also came an awareness of risks and limitations, including one participant with increased liver function tests and fever, myalgia, and headache. There were no deaths, thromboses, inhibitor development, or persistent

Table 18.2 Properties of non-integrating gene therapy vectors

Vector	Carrying capacity (kb)	Features	Advantages	Disadvantages	Initial applications
Adenovirus	8–30	Nuclear episome	Efficient delivery to dividing and non-dividing cells. High, but transient expression	High immunogenicity	Cancer therapeutics vaccination
AAV	4.5	Episomal concatemers	Efficient delivery of dividing and non-dividing cells. Relatively low immunogenicity	Possible long-term persistence of capsids in vivo. Potential for encapsidation of prokaryotic sequences	Efficient and persistent in vivo delivery to post-mitotic tissues. Delivery of gene editing components
IDLV	7.5	Mutations of integrase gene in packaging plasmid	Efficient delivery to dividing and non-dividing cells. Transient expression in proliferating cells and sustained expression in post-mitotic tissues. Relatively low immunogenicity	Low expression in proliferating cells	Vaccination. Delivery of gene editing templates
Poxvirus	>25	Poxviral RNS pol-based	Large capacity delivery of substantial cassettes of heterologous antigens. Activates innate immune mediators	Potential for adverse events, particularly in immunocompromised patients	Transient expression of immunologically relevant proteins. Vaccination
Non-viral	Potentially unlimited	Chemical formulation	Inexpensive to manufacture. Can achieve stable expression with replication and segregation capacity. Relatively low immunogenicity	Relatively inefficient delivery	Gene delivery to muscle

elevations in liver function tests [36]. This study utilized the genetic transfer method using an AAV virus and a non-integrating vector which keeps the genetic carrier in an episomal form in the hepatocyte cytoplasm as outlined [37].

Studies that led up to this study included limited numbers of subjects who were treated with other gene therapy. These studies utilized retroviral and non-viral genetic vectors. Overall, these methods were also effective and encouraging. No serious adverse reactions were reported. Viral shedding was monitored closely and one patient who was treated with the retroviral vector had transient detection of the retrovirus in his semen (detected by PCR) [38, 39].

18.3 Genetic Therapy in Hemophilia B

A series of genetic transfer studies have been used for increase in factor IX activity. Research took advantage of a missense mutation in the *F9* gene which allowed for around 8–12× increase in factor IX activity [40–46].

One study selected 10 men with hemophilia B and a baseline factor IX activity level of less than 2% (severe disease). All participants were treated with a single-stranded AAV construct with liver tropism and liver-specific regulatory elements (AAV SPK-9001) expressing factor IX. These PWH displayed a mean steady-state factor IX expression level of 33.7% (range, 14–81%) and a reduction in mean annualized bleeding rate from 11.1 to 0.4 events per year [45, 47]. A hallmark of this study was that low doses of vector were given relative to studies that took place in the past, in hopes to limit a host immunogenic response. Fortunately for this study, there were no serious adverse events and no evidence of inhibitor development. Two individuals who had transient increases in liver function tests were treated with a course of glucocorticoids.

Results from a subsequent study showed reduced bleeding and increased factor IX activity levels (mean factor IX activity of 31% at 6 weeks and 47% at 26 weeks) via utilization of etranacogene dezaparvovec (AMT-061) as the gene therapy. This study was limited to three men with severe hemophilia B [48]. No transaminase elevations were observed in this study.

Interestingly enough, a prior study with similar approach to genetic therapy (codon-optimized factor IX in the same AAV5 vector) in ten men with hemophilia B displayed similar effects and had no concerning adverse effects [46].

Earlier studies demonstrated effectiveness of other methods, such as an AAV8 vector expressing a codon-optimized factor IX that produced dose-dependent decreases in dependence on factor IX concentrate and decreases in bleeding episodes [43, 44].

The genetic therapy trials listed above provide another chance to highlight the benefits of decreased genotoxicity utilizing the gene transfer method. Once again, the fact that the AAV-based therapies do not integrate into the host genome and stay in episomal form, dramatically reduces the direct integration into the host genome [49].

As genetic therapies for hemophilia A and hemophilia B surely will continue to evolve, there are other therapies on the horizon worth mentioning. First, we have cellular therapy. Cellular therapy focuses on introducing intact cells into the omentum of people with hemophilia. Dermal fibroblasts that have been transported autologously and sinusoidal endothelial cells from healthy animal donors have both resulted in increased factor levels and decreased bleeding episodes. An important upside of cellular therapy is focusing on the fact that cells capable of surviving in the host may be enclosed in immuno-protective devices before implantation to prevent rejection [39, 50].

Multiple studies [51–54] have also demonstrated effective therapy with the monoclonal antibody, Concizumab, which functions by inhibiting the tissue factor pathway inhibitor (TFPI), which normally blocks the function of factor Xa and factor VIIa. Inhibiting the inhibitor allows for increased concentrations of factor Xa and thrombin, conveniently avoiding factors VIII and IX entirely.

Hope was on the horizon when scientists noticed a decrease in bleeding episodes in patients with mild hemophilia with co-existent prothrombotic mutations like factor V Leiden and antithrombin deficiency. From this observation, scientists began targeting intrinsic anticoagulant proteins. Initially, this approach yielded encouraging results. Tragically, a patient in a study focusing on introducing anticoagulant proteins died of a direct thrombotic event attributable to the therapy, reminding the scientific community that we must approach these novel therapies with utmost humility and caution [55].

18.4 Risks to Genetic Therapy

Although the preceding section focuses mostly on the scientific breakthroughs of genetic therapy, we must carefully examine the risks to this evolving technology. We have touched on the principles of geno- and immunoreactivity, the dilutional effect, and some possible unintended genetic mutations resulting from genetic therapy. We will summarize the major risks below:

- Immunoreactivity: Because viral vectors are utilized in genetic therapy so heavily, some patients are capable of mounting profound immune responses, which can manifest as significant inflammatory reactions.
- Genotoxicity: Insertional mutagenesis (the creation of mutations of DNA by addition of one or more base pairs) can result in the unintentional creation of oncogenic proteins located near the desired location for genetic therapy. Sadly, some early genetic therapy trials of patients with immunodeficiencies, such as SCID, resulted in patients developing ALL and other T-cell lymphoproliferative disorders in 25% of patients [56–58]. Moreover, other trials resulted in patients with Wiskott–Aldrich Syndrome and chronic Granulomatous disease who received genetic therapy developed myelodysplasia and myeloid leukemias [59, 60]. From these horrendous side effects of genetic treatment, self-inactivating (SIN) viral vectors were developed which manipulate a different biochemical pathway to avoid oncogenic protein fusion altogether [61–63]. While this is encouraging for limiting the potential for genotoxicity, the scientific community remains hawkish when monitoring for genotoxic effects.

18.5 Ethics in Gene Therapy

Entire texts have been devoted to the ethical quandaries that have been brought to light with the development and implementation of genetic therapy.

18.5.1 Expecting the Unexpected

With new therapies come problems that you know you will have to face and problems you cannot even begin to prepare for. Take the infamous case of Jesse Gelsinger, for example. Jesse was an 18-year-old with Ornithine Trans Carbamylase (OTC) deficiency who was enrolled in a gene therapy trial at the University of Pennsylvania. Ultimately, Jesse had a profound systemic inflammatory response which resulted in multi-organ failure. Although the response to therapy was unexpected, it eventually proved to be fatal 98 hours/hrs after receiving the therapy. Jesse's family was obviously devastated and researchers were dumfounded. Why did Jesse react so differently than other participants in his cohort? Two main questions remain to this day: (1) was there a genetic predisposition to enhanced innate immunity for Jesse or (2) did Jesse have previous exposure to adenoviruses in the setting of natural infections that enhances the response of the host to a second exposure to the virus/vector?

Eventually, the Washington Post published a series of investigative reports alleging noncompliance in several aspects of the trial management. The Office for Human Research Protections, the NIH, the FDA, Committees from the US Senate and House of Representatives were just some of the regulatory agencies that came out with a number of allegations which included evaluating the safety of the pre-clinical models and the conduct of the clinical trial [64]. Because of the Jesse Gelsinger case, there have been substantial reforms across many institutions in the USA in terms of oversight of human subject research [64].

18.5.2 Cost/Genomic Justice

Suppose a highly efficacious genetic therapy with negligible side effects becomes available for clinical use. Imagine the headline: *A cure for hemophilia discovered.* How is this therapy distributed to societies across the globe? Developing new genetic the rapies over the past decades has brought the term *genomic justice* to the forefront. With cost already becoming an insurmountable barrier to therapy, the question must be asked: is it just to develop such a therapy if those who need it the most desperately cannot access it? In some cases, AAV-based gene therapy was priced at $ one million USD, which was cited as a reason for the eventual reason not to pursue further approval for the therapy [65]. Conversely, gene therapy for hemophilia B has been estimated to save over USD $200,000 annually for those who no longer need routine factor prophylaxis [47].

Central to the genomic justice conversation is the reality that most clinical research, at least in the USA, is primarily conducted on those of European descent with under representation of racial and ethnic minorities barriers, despite efforts to address recruitment and retention [66, 67]. Although the effects of gene therapy may be thought to be generalizable, conclusive efficacy of therapies or potential risks may not be applied to all racial and ethnic minorities—this drastic inequity in medicine proves to be a relatively new stain on the already tattered history of racial and ethnic inequities in medicine.

Genomic exploitation in developing countries [68]: with the discoveries and mass production of genetic therapies, troublesome concerns for exploitation of developing nations have garnered a lot of attention in the scientific community. Over the recent years, a trend of large scientific companies who pioneer genomic therapy has started to relocate in nations where mass production of therapies is much cheaper than if they were stationed in more developed nations. With this shift, ethical concerns such as ownership of genetic samples, data, and capacity to analyze genomic data must be addressed for any genomic research taking place in developed nations to be deemed successful. As you might imagine, a one size fits all approach, which tackling these ethical concerns will not be successful. Solutions must be tailored to specific research sites with the ethical principles of justice, ownership, and fair distribution of resources the highest priority. There is a need to dramatically reduce the disease burden for individuals living in developing nations. By globalization of genomic research, there is an opportunity to alleviate global injustices and inequities.

18.6 CRISPR + Somatic vs. Germline Mutations

With the advancement of CRISPR-Cas9 technology, came the inevitable discussion surrounding the safe and ethical deployment of this new therapeutic method. Originally, CRISPR-Cas9 experiments were performed on non-viable triploid zygotes [69, 70] However, eventually scientist moved to editing human embryos to evaluate the specificity and accuracy of the new technology [71], which ultimately led to the conversation of how to responsibly use gene editing methods [72]. In 2018, the Second International Summit on Human Genome Editing was held.

Over 500 researchers, policymakers, ethicists, representatives from medical and scientific academies, patient groups' representatives, and others attended the summit.

During the event, the potential benefits and risks of editing the human genome, cultural and ethical perspectives, regulatory and policy issues, and public outreach were debated. There was a special focus on ethical rules concerning both somatic (non-heritable) and germline (heritable) human genome editing. From this summit, the general acceptance of modifying single person's somatic DNA was thought to be more tolerable than a germline, which could be passed to offspring.

Somatic modification is significantly beneficial in treatment of monogenic diseases like hemophilia [73]. However, germline gene modification lacks societal consensus, and some countries even outlaw this practice. Moreover, from this summit, it was decided that genome editing of germline cells that could be passed on to the next generations as a part of the human gene pool seems outright irresponsible until the safety concerns are resolved and ethical concerns reach a consensus. The ethical debate on germline editing is easier to examine when broken down into three potential therapeutic scenarios:

1. The first scenario considers parents who want to decrease the probability of diseases developing in offspring. This would give parents another option instead of passing on known genetic diseases with deadly outcomes (Huntington's, SCD, Brugada, etc.).
2. The second scenario considers parents who want to inactivate particular genes that are known to predispose one to hypertension or hypercholesterolemia.
3. Lastly, the third scenario, and most controversial, considers parents who desire offspring with increased strength or certain cosmetic features or advantageous traits [74].

At the Second International Summit on Human Genome Editing, it was determined that germline genome editing could be *morally* permitted in certain circumstances, but there are no such circumstances in the world. Additionally, it was determined that risks and benefits of germline cells are still not clear enough to allow germline genome editing to continue [75, 76]. The following is a specific summary of why germline genome editing raises ethical concerns [77–81]:

- Lack of ability to consent before birth
- Lack of differentiation between research and clinical applications
- Equitable access and allocation of resources
- Exploitation for non-therapeutic modifications (e.g. "enhancement" of a feature rather than treatment/prevention of a disease)
- Potential unanticipated adverse effects
- Potential effects on future generations, including need for monitoring and lack of consent

18.7 Conclusions

In this chapter, we first took a brief dive into the history of the research and development that led to the development of gene therapy. Next, we examined the intricacies of each of the different methods of genetic therapy: gene editing and gene transfer. Next, we examine the possible adverse effects and overall risks of genetic therapy. Specifically, we break down how and why the dilutional effect and immunogenicity are limiting factors to broader implementation of genetic therapy. We focus on the history of therapy for hemophilia A and B and how genetic therapy has come to the center stage as a potential cure for the disease. Lastly, we examine the ethical concerns that surround genetic therapy in medicine. Ultimately, we urge the reader to heavily weigh the ethical concerns that surround the expanding conversations over genetic therapies, especially as they pertain to germline mutations, genetic therapy for advantageous traits, and genomic justice.

References

1. Alnasser SM. Review on mechanistic strategy of gene therapy in the treatment of disease. Gene. 2021;769:145246.
2. Wirth T, Parker N, Yla-Herttuala S. History of gene therapy. Gene. 2013;525(2):162–9.
3. High KA, Roncarolo MG. Gene therapy. N Engl J Med. 2019;381(5):455–64.
4. Richardson CD, et al. Enhancing homology-directed genome editing by catalytically active and inactive CRISPR-Cas9 using asymmetric donor DNA. Nat Biotechnol. 2016;34(3):339–44.
5. Haapaniemi E, et al. CRISPR-Cas9 genome editing induces a p53-mediated DNA damage response. Nat Med. 2018;24(7):927–30.
6. Shivram H, et al. Controlling and enhancing CRISPR systems. Nat Chem Biol. 2021;17(1):10–9.
7. Zhang M, et al. CRISPR technology: the engine that drives cancer therapy. Biomed Pharmacother. 2021;133:111007.
8. Mojica FJ, Juez G, Rodriguez-Valera F. Transcription at different salinities of Haloferax mediterranei sequences adjacent to partially modified PstI sites. Mol Microbiol. 1993;9(3):613–21.
9. Jansen R, et al. Identification of genes that are associated with DNA repeats in prokaryotes. Mol Microbiol. 2002;43(6):1565–75.
10. Gasiunas G, et al. Cas9–crRNA ribonucleoprotein complex mediates specific DNA cleavage for adaptive immunity in bacteria. Proc Natl Acad Sci. 2012;109(39):E2579–86.
11. Jinek M, et al. A programmable dual-RNA–guided DNA endonuclease in adaptive bacterial immunity. Science. 2012;337(6096):816–21.

12. Janik E, et al. Various aspects of a gene editing system-CRISPR-Cas9. Int J Mol Sci. 2020;21(24):9604.
13. Maeder ML, et al. Development of a gene-editing approach to restore vision loss in Leber congenital amaurosis type 10. Nat Med. 2019;25(2):229–33.
14. Nelson CE, et al. In vivo genome editing improves muscle function in a mouse model of Duchenne muscular dystrophy. Science. 2016;351(6271):403–7.
15. Wu Y, et al. Highly efficient therapeutic gene editing of human hematopoietic stem cells. Nat Med. 2019;25(5):776–83.
16. György B, et al. Allele-specific gene editing prevents deafness in a model of dominant progressive hearing loss. Nat Med. 2019;25(7):1123–30.
17. Makarova KS, et al. An updated evolutionary classification of CRISPR-Cas systems. Nat Rev Microbiol. 2015;13(11):722–36.
18. Mohanraju P, et al. Diverse evolutionary roots and mechanistic variations of the CRISPR-Cas systems. Science. 2016;353(6299):aad5147.
19. Wang F, et al. Advances in CRISPR-Cas systems for RNA targeting, tracking and editing. Biotechnol Adv. 2019;37(5):708–29.
20. Liu Z, et al. Application of different types of CRISPR/Cas-based systems in bacteria. Microb Cell Factories. 2020;19(1):172.
21. Athanasopoulos T, Munye MM, Yanez-Munoz RJ. Nonintegrating gene therapy vectors. Hematol Oncol Clin North Am. 2017;31(5):753–70.
22. Nowakowski A, et al. Genetic engineering of stem cells for enhanced therapy. Acta Neurobiol Exp. 2013;73:1–18.
23. Verdera HC, Kuranda K, Mingozzi F. AAV vector immunogenicity in humans: a long journey to successful gene transfer. Mol Ther. 2020;28(3):723–46.
24. Monahan PE, et al. Emerging immunogenicity and genotoxicity considerations of adeno-associated virus vector gene therapy for hemophilia. J Clin Med. 2021;10(11)
25. Nayak S, Herzog RW. Progress and prospects: immune responses to viral vectors. Gene Ther. 2010;17(3):295–304.
26. Herzog RW. Complexity of immune responses to AAV transgene products–example of factor IX. Cell Immunol. 2019;342:103658.
27. Abordo-Adesida E, et al. Stability of lentiviral vector-mediated transgene expression in the brain in the presence of systemic antivector immune responses. Hum Gene Ther. 2005;16(6):741–51.
28. Mingozzi F, et al. CD8+ T-cell responses to adeno-associated virus capsid in humans. Nat Med. 2007;13(4):419–22.
29. Ertl HC, High KA. Impact of AAV capsid-specific T-cell responses on design and outcome of clinical gene transfer trials with recombinant adeno-associated viral vectors: an evolving controversy. Hum Gene Ther. 2017;28(4):328–37.
30. Annoni A, et al. Modulation of immune responses in lentiviral vector-mediated gene transfer. Cell Immunol. 2019;342:103802.
31. Li A, et al. A self-deleting AAV-CRISPR system for in vivo genome editing. Mol Ther Methods Clin Dev. 2019;12:111–22.
32. Marchesini E, Morfini M, Valentino L. Recent advances in the treatment of hemophilia: a review. Biologics. 2021;15:221–35.
33. Kitazawa T, et al. A bispecific antibody to factors IXa and X restores factor VIII hemostatic activity in a hemophilia A model. Nat Med. 2012;18(10):1570–4.
34. Muto A, et al. Anti-factor IXa/X bispecific antibody (ACE910): hemostatic potency against ongoing bleeds in a hemophilia A model and the possibility of routine supplementation. J Thromb Haemost. 2014;12(2):206–13.
35. Muto A, et al. Anti-factor IXa/X bispecific antibody ACE910 prevents joint bleeds in a long-term primate model of acquired hemophilia A. Blood. 2014;124(20):3165–71.
36. Pasi KJ, et al. Multiyear follow-up of AAV5-hFVIII-SQ gene therapy for hemophilia A. N Engl J Med. 2020;382(1):29–40.
37. Rangarajan S, et al. AAV5-factor VIII gene transfer in severe hemophilia A. N Engl J Med. 2017;377(26):2519–30.
38. Powell JS, et al. Phase 1 trial of FVIII gene transfer for severe hemophilia A using a retroviral construct administered by peripheral intravenous infusion. Blood. 2003;102(6):2038–45.
39. Roth DA, et al. Nonviral transfer of the gene encoding coagulation factor VIII in patients with severe hemophilia A. N Engl J Med. 2001;344(23):1735–42.
40. Manno CS, et al. Successful transduction of liver in hemophilia by AAV-factor IX and limitations imposed by the host immune response. Nat Med. 2006;12(3):342–7.
41. Kay MA, et al. Evidence for gene transfer and expression of factor IX in haemophilia B patients treated with an AAV vector. Nat Genet. 2000;24(3):257–61.
42. Manno CS, et al. AAV-mediated factor IX gene transfer to skeletal muscle in patients with severe hemophilia B. Blood. 2003;101(8):2963–72.
43. Nathwani AC, et al. Adenovirus-associated virus vector-mediated gene transfer in hemophilia B. N Engl J Med. 2011;365(25):2357–65.
44. Nathwani AC, et al. Long-term safety and efficacy of factor IX gene therapy in hemophilia B. N Engl J Med. 2014;371(21):1994–2004.
45. George LA, et al. Hemophilia B gene therapy with a High-specific-activity factor IX variant. N Engl J Med. 2017;377(23):2215–27.
46. Miesbach W, et al. Gene therapy with adeno-associated virus vector 5-human factor IX in adults with hemophilia B. Blood. 2018;131(9):1022–31.
47. Porteus M. Closing in on treatment for hemophilia B. N Engl J Med. 2017;377(23):2274–5.
48. Von Drygalski A, et al. Etranacogene dezaparvovec (AMT-061 phase 2b): normal/near normal FIX activity and bleed cessation in hemophilia B. Blood Adv. 2019;3(21):3241–7.

49. George LA. Hemophilia gene therapy comes of age. Hematology Am Soc Hematol Educ Program. 2017;2017(1):587–94.
50. Follenzi A, et al. Transplanted endothelial cells repopulate the liver endothelium and correct the phenotype of hemophilia A mice. J Clin Invest. 2008;118(3):935–45.
51. Shapiro AD, et al. Subcutaneous concizumab prophylaxis in hemophilia A and hemophilia A/B with inhibitors: phase 2 trial results. Blood. 2019;134(22):1973–82.
52. Chowdary P, et al. Safety and pharmacokinetics of anti-TFPI antibody (concizumab) in healthy volunteers and patients with hemophilia: a randomized first human dose trial. J Thromb Haemost. 2015;13(5):743–54.
53. Agersø H, et al. Pharmacokinetics of an anti-TFPI monoclonal antibody (concizumab) blocking the TFPI interaction with the active site of FXa in Cynomolgus monkeys after iv and sc administration. Eur J Pharm Sci. 2014;56:65–9.
54. Eichler H, et al. A randomized trial of safety, pharmacokinetics and pharmacodynamics of concizumab in people with hemophilia A. J Thromb Haemost. 2018;16(11):2184–95.
55. Pasi KJ, et al. Targeting of antithrombin in hemophilia A or B with RNAi therapy. N Engl J Med. 2017;377(9):819–28.
56. Kohn DB. Historical perspective on the current renaissance for hematopoietic stem cell gene therapy. Hematol Oncol Clin North Am. 2017;31(5):721–35.
57. Howe SJ, et al. Insertional mutagenesis combined with acquired somatic mutations causes leukemogenesis following gene therapy of SCID-X1 patients. J Clin Invest. 2008;118(9):3143–50.
58. Hacein-Bey-Abina S, et al. Insertional oncogenesis in 4 patients after retrovirus-mediated gene therapy of SCID-X1. J Clin Invest. 2008;118(9):3132–42.
59. Stein S, et al. Genomic instability and myelodysplasia with monosomy 7 consequent to EVI1 activation after gene therapy for chronic granulomatous disease. Nat Med. 2010;16(2):198–204.
60. Braun CJ, et al. Gene therapy for Wiskott-Aldrich syndrome--long-term efficacy and genotoxicity. Sci Transl Med. 2014;6(227):227ra33.
61. Browning DL, et al. Evidence for the in vivo safety of insulated foamy viral vectors. Gene Ther. 2017;24(3):187–98.
62. El Ashkar S, et al. Engineering next-generation BET-independent MLV vectors for safer gene therapy. Mol Ther Nucleic Acids. 2017;7:231–45.
63. Mukherjee S, Thrasher AJ. Gene therapy for PIDs: progress, pitfalls and prospects. Gene. 2013;525(2):174–81.
64. Wilson JM. Lessons learned from the gene therapy trial for ornithine transcarbamylase deficiency. Mol Genet Metab. 2009;96(4):151–7.
65. Naldini L. Gene therapy returns to Centre stage. Nature. 2015;526(7573):351–60.
66. Niranjan SJ, et al. Bias and stereotyping among research and clinical professionals: perspectives on minority recruitment for oncology clinical trials. Cancer. 2020;126(9):1958–68.
67. Heller C, et al. Strategies addressing barriers to clinical trial enrollment of underrepresented populations: a systematic review. Contemp Clin Trials. 2014;39(2):169–82.
68. de Vries J, et al. Ethical issues in human genomics research in developing countries. BMC Med Ethics. 2011;12:5.
69. Kang X, et al. Introducing precise genetic modifications into human 3PN embryos by CRISPR/Cas-mediated genome editing. J Assist Reprod Genet. 2016;33(5):581–8.
70. Tang L, et al. CRISPR/Cas9-mediated gene editing in human zygotes using Cas9 protein. Mol Gen Genomics. 2017;292(3):525–33.
71. Liang P, et al. CRISPR/Cas9-mediated gene editing in human tripronuclear zygotes. Protein Cell. 2015;6(5):363–72.
72. Kaiser J, Normile D. Bioethics. Embryo engineering study splits scientific community. Science. 2015;348(6234):486–7.
73. Brokowski C, Adli M. CRISPR ethics: moral considerations for applications of a powerful tool. J Mol Biol. 2019;431(1):88–101.
74. Coller BS. Ethics of human genome editing. Annu Rev Med. 2019;70:289–305.
75. OlsonS, National Academies of Sciences, Engineering, and Medicine. International summit on human gene editing: a global discussion. International Summit on Human Gene Editing: A Global Discussion; 2016.
76. The U.S. National Academies of Sciences, Engineering, and Medicine. Second international summit on human genome editing: continuing the global discussion. In: Proceedings of a workshop—in brief. 2019.
77. Howard HC, et al. One small edit for humans, one giant edit for humankind? Points and questions to consider for a responsible way forward for gene editing in humans. Eur J Hum Genet. 2018;26(1):1–11.
78. Cwik B. Designing ethical trials of germline gene editing. N Engl J Med. 2017;377(20):1911–3.
79. Lanphier E, et al. Don't edit the human germ line. Nature. 2015;519(7544):410–1.
80. Benston S. Everything in moderation, even hype: learning from vaccine controversies to strike a balance with CRISPR. J Med Ethics. 2017;43(12):819–23.
81. Ormond KE, et al. Human germline genome editing. Am J Hum Genet. 2017;101(2):167–76.

A Summary of the Recent Recommendations of the World Federation of Hemophilia

19

E. Carlos Rodríguez-Merchán

19.1 Introduction

Hemophilia A is much more frequent than hemophilia B. Hemophilia A is calculated to comprise 80–85% of all hemophilia cases; hemophilia B is calculated to comprise 15%–20% of all hemophilia cases. Calculated frequency at birth is 24.6 cases per 100,000 males for all severities of hemophilia A (9.5 cases for severe hemophilia A) and 5 cases per 100,000 males for all severities of hemophilia B (1.5 cases for severe hemophilia B).

Hemophilia is commonly inherited via an X chromosome with an F8 or F9 gene mutation. Nonetheless, both the F8 and F9 genes are predisposed to novel mutations, and approximately 30% of all cases arise from spontaneous genetic variants. It has been published that more than 50% of people newly diagnosed with severe hemophilia have no previous family history of hemophilia.

Over the last few years enormous improvements have been achieved in a number of facets regarding the treatment of people with hemophilia (PWH). These cover genetic evaluation and management with numerous new therapeutic drugs including extended half-life factor VIII (FVIII) and factor IX (FIX) drugs and a bispecific antibody (subcutaneous factor substitution therapy with emicizumab). All of these permit for more efficacious hemostasis than was feasible in past times. Prophylaxis is established as the solely method to alter the natural history of bleeding. Besides, there are very efficacious treatments for PWH with inhibitors. All these advancements are included in the last edition of the WFH guidelines and are summarized in this chapter [1].

E. C. Rodríguez-Merchán (✉)
Department of Orthopedic Surgery, La Paz University Hospital, Madrid, Spain

19.2 Fundamentals of Management

For PWH prophylaxis is the gold standard of management. Episodic clotting factor concentrates (CFCs) replacement must not be considered a long-run alternative. PWH should have access to secure and efficacious management with optimal effectiveness in the prevention and treatment of bleeding. Treatment centers have to be based on a multidisciplinary team of specialists. All kind of clinical specialties and adequate laboratory services are required. Laboratory diagnosis and monitoring are required. Use of correct equipment and reagents is paramount. Gene therapy and genetic diagnosis of hemophilia must be available. Table 19.1 shows the main goals of treatment.

E. C. Rodríguez-Merchán (ed.), *Advances in Hemophilia Treatment*,
https://doi.org/10.1007/978-3-030-93990-8_19

Table 19.1 Main goals of treatment of hemophilia

Main goals
Rapid treatment of bleeding episodes including follow-up PRM
Adequate emergency management
Adequate pain treatment
Management of musculoskeletal adverse events and inhibitor formation
Treatment of comorbidities
Constant psychosocial evaluation and support as required
Continuous education on treatment and self-care for PWH and their families

PRM physical and rehabilitation medicine, *PWH* people with hemophilia

Table 19.2 Hemostatic products for the treatment of people with hemophilia (PWH)

Hemostatic products
Clotting factor concentrates (CFCs) • *FVIII CFCs* • *FIX CFCs* • *Extended half-life products*
Bypassing agents • *Recombinant activated factor VIIa (rFVIIa)* • *Activated prothrombin complex concentrate (aPCC)*
Other plasma products • *Cryoprecipitate* • *Fresh frozen plasma (FFP)*
Other pharmacological options • *Desmopressin (DDAVP)* • *Tranexamic acid* • *Epsilon aminocaproic acid (EACA)*
Non-factor replacement therapies • *Substitution therapy (emicizumab)*
Hemostatic rebalancing agents • *Fitusiran* • *Anti-TFPI (tissue factor pathway inhibitor) antibodies*

19.3 Hemostatic Products

CFCs are the management of choice for PWH as they are very secure and efficacious for treating and preventing bleeds. There are two principal types of CFCs: virally inactivated plasma-derived agents produced from plasma donated by human blood donors and recombinant agents made utilizing genetically engineered cells and recombinant technology. Table 19.2 summarizes the main hemostatic products available for the treatment of hemophilia.

19.4 Acute and Emergency Management of Bleeds

Treatment centers must create standards for emergency management of PWH, covering those with inhibitors, that embrace treatment of important acute side events such as intracranial hemorrhage and other kinds of significant internal hemorrhage and trauma.

Adjunctive treatments are essential in the management of bleeds, especially where coagulation therapies and hemostatic products are scarce (or unavailable) and may reduce the quantity of treatment product needed. They include: (a) The PRICE fundamentals (protection, rest, ice, compression, and elevation); (b) Physical and Rehabilitation Medicine; (c) Antifibrinolytic products are efficacious as adjunctive management for mucosal bleeds and invasive dental operations. (d) Some COX-2 inhibitors might be utilized for articular swelling following an acute bleed and for chronic joint degeneration (hemophilic arthropathy). (e) Supplementary methods for pain treatment (pain killers, distraction, mindfulness, or music therapy) might also be beneficial for PWH suffering from chronic hemophilic arthropathy.

19.5 Prophylaxis (Regular Replacement Therapy)

The standard of treatment for PWH with severe disease is regular replacement therapy (prophylaxis) with CFCs, or other hemostasis drugs to avert bleeding, initiated early in life (before age 3) to avert musculoskeletal side events from repetitive articular and muscle bleeds. Table 19.3 shows prevalent factor prophylaxis for hemophilia A and B established according to when prophylaxis is started. Table 19.4 shows prevalent factor prophylaxis with standard half-life clotting factor established according to its intensity. Table 19.5 shows essential prerequisites for efficacious prophylaxis.

Table 19.3 Prevalent factor prophylaxis for hemophilia A and B established according to when prophylaxis is started

Primary prophylaxis	Regular continuous prophylaxis initiated in the absence of documented joint illness, determined by physical examination and/or imaging studies, and prior to the second clinically evident joint bleed and 3 years of age
Secondary prophylaxis	Regular continuous prophylaxis started after 2 or more articular bleeds but prior to the onset of joint illness; this is commonly at 3 or more years of age
Tertiary prophylaxis	Regular continuous prophylaxis started after the onset of documented articular illness. Tertiary prophylaxis typically applies to prophylaxis initiated in adulthood

Table 19.4 Prevalent factor prophylaxis with standard half-life clotting factor established according to its intensity

Prophylaxis intensity	Hemophilia A	Hemophilia B
High-dose prophylaxis	25–40 IU FVIII/kg every 2 days (>4000 IU/kg per year)	40–60 IU FIX/kg twice per week (>4000 IU/kg per year)
Intermediate-dose prophylaxis	15–25 IU FVIII/kg 3 days per week (1500–4000 IU/kg per year)	20–40 IU FIX/kg twice per week (2000–4000 IU/kg per year)
Low-dose prophylaxis (with escalation of dose intensity, as required)[a]	10–15 IU FVIII/kg 2–3 days per week (1000–1500 IU/kg per year)	10–15 IU FIX/kg 2 days per week (1000–1500 IU/kg per year)

FIX factor IX, *FVIII* factor VIII, *IU* international unit, *kg* kilogram

[a]Should only be taken as the starting point of replacement therapy to be tailored, as possible, to prevent bleeding

Adherence to prophylaxis has been encountered to be poor in many teenagers (13–17 years of age) and young adults (18–30 years of age) with hemophilia. The crucial self-management abilities needed for PWH are summarized in Table 19.6.

Table 19.5 Essential prerequisites for efficacious prophylaxis

Dependable, constant supply of prophylactic treatments (clotting factor concentrates and/or non-factor therapies)
Consistent, expert monitoring (clinical and laboratory) of prophylaxis and its efficacy
Home therapy, by preference given by the patient/caregiver
Good patient understanding of the benefit of prophylaxis
Good patient adherence to prophylaxis

Table 19.6 Crucial self-management abilities needed for people with hemophilia (PWH)

Bleed identification
Self-infusion/self-management abilities
Self-care (i.e., nutrition and physical fitness) and drugs treatment (i.e., record-keeping, treatment habits, preservation of appropriate treatment provision, abilities in conservation, reconstitution, and administration of treatment drugs)
Pain treatment
Risk treatment and forming a concept of preventive therapy
Knowledge of adequate adjunctive therapies (antifibrinolytics, pain killers) and adjunctive management (the PRICE principles)

PRICE protection, rest, ice, compression, and elevation

19.6 Management of PWH with Inhibitors

Methodical monitoring for inhibitors and comprehensive treatment of inhibitors must be carried out for PWH A, especially when patients are at maximum peril during their first 20 exposures to CFCs (with one exposure established as all CFCs given within a 24-h period) and afterwards up to 75 exposures.

Elimination of inhibitors is currently best accomplished via immune tolerance induction (ITI) therapy. In severe hemophilia A, inhibitor elimination by ITI therapy is successful in 70–80% of PWH. In moderate/mild hemophilia A, response to ITI may be less positive.

PWH with inhibitors must have access to ITI and to appropriate hemostatic products for control of bleeding as well as surgical procedures, if required, at specialized centers with significant knowledge.

Bypassing agents and other adequate management drugs must be available for PWH who do not respond to enhanced factor dosages or ITI.

19.7 Treatment of Musculoskeletal Adverse Events

PWH must also have access to musculoskeletal specialists (orthopedic surgeon, physical medicine/rehabilitation specialist, physical therapist) with knowledge in hemophilia, with yearly musculoskeletal evaluations and continuous control of their musculoskeletal results and preventive or corrective techniques as required. Orthopedic surgeons must have specific training in surgical treatment of PWH.

Hemophilia is characterized by acute bleeds, over 80% of which happen in specific articulation (most usually the ankle, knee, and elbow joints, and often the hip, shoulder, and wrist joints) and in certain muscles (iliopsoas and gastrocnemius). Spontaneous bleeding might happen depending on the severity of the illness. In children with severe hemophilia, the first articulation and muscle bleeds commonly happen when they start to crawl and walk, normally between 1 and 2 years of age, but occasionally in later toddler years. Repetitive articular bleeds produce progressive articular damage due to blood collection in the articular cavity and synovial swelling. This causes adverse events such as chronic synovitis and hemophilic arthropathy. Insufficient management of intramuscular bleeds can produce muscle contractures, especially in bi-articular muscles (e.g., calf and iliopsoas muscles), frequently within the first decades of life. Other more severe side events such as compartment syndrome and pseudotumors might also occur.

For PWH, the WFH advises regular physical evaluation of the synovium following every bleed, preferably utilizing appropriate imaging techniques such as ultrasound (when possible) until the circumstance is controlled, as clinical evaluation alone is insufficient to detect early synovitis. For PWH who have unsolved chronic synovitis, the WFH advises nonsurgical synovectomy as a first-line treatment alternative utilizing radioisotope synovectomy with a pure beta emitter (phosphorus-32, yttrium-90, rhenium-186, or rhenium-188). One dose of CFC per dose of isotope must be utilized.

For PWH with chronic hemophilic arthropathy for whom nonsurgical therapies have been unsuccessful to produce satisfactory pain alleviation and ameliorated function, the WFH advises consultation with an orthopedic specialist on surgical procedure alternatives.

19.8 Management of Specific Problems and Comorbidities

19.8.1 Carriers of Hemophilia

A portion of carriers have little factor VIII (FVIII) or factor IX (FIX) activity because of lyonization (the unexpected suppression of one of the two X chromosomes, also called X inactivation), which may cause mild, moderate, or even severe hemophilia in unusual occasions. Symptomatic women must be designated as having hemophilia of a specified intensity, like men with hemophilia.

19.8.2 Surgery and Other Invasive Techniques

Neuraxial anesthesia needs factor levels over 50 IU/dL to avert bleeding and resulting in neurological adverse events. Surgery must be programmed early in the week and early in the day for optimal laboratory and blood bank support, if required. Appropriate amounts of CFCs (or bypassing agents for PWH with inhibitors) must be available for the surgery itself and to maintain appropriate coverage in the postoperative period for the duration needed for healing and/or rehabilitation.

19.8.3 Treatment of Comorbidities

Cardiovascular sickness, hypertension, and other cardiovascular risk factors are progressively occurring in adults with hemophilia.

19.8.4 Medical Problems with Aging

Elderly PWH must be treated in identical way as their equals in the general population, except for the required supplementary correction of deficient hemostasis with CFCs.

19.8.5 Management of Transfusion-Transmitted Infections

Anti-viral therapies must be accessible to all PWH who suffer from human immunodeficiency virus (HIV) and hepatitis C virus (HCV).

19.9 Central Venous Access Devices

For providing prophylaxis or ITI therapy in young children with difficult venous access, central venous access devices (CVADs) can facilitate steady, durable venous access to perform infusions easier. Possible adverse events of CVADS cover hospitalization, bleeding, catheter infection, thrombosis, breakage, and/or malfunction.

19.10 Pain Management

For PWH with acute pain secondary to a joint or muscle bleed, the WFH advises prompt administration of clotting factor concentrates to halt bleeding, pain killers, and adjunctive means such as immobilization, compression, and splinting to reduce pain, if adequate.

For children and adults with hemophilia with pain secondary to chronic hemophilic arthropathy, the WFH advises the utilization of paracetamol/acetaminophen, selective COX-2 inhibitors, tramadol, or morphine, and abstention of other NSAIDs. Codeine may be utilized for children over 12 years of age but is contraindicated in younger children.

Extended utilization of these drugs may have risks of dependence or addiction, as well as organ damage, and has to be meticulously monitored. PWH with constant pain must be referred to a specialized pain treatment team.

19.11 Dental Care

Preserving good oral health and averting dental complications is of great significance in PWH to preclude oral illnesses and conditions such as gingivitis, dental caries, and periodontal sicknesses which might produce severe gum bleeding, especially in those with severe/moderate hemophilia, and to elude the need for major dental surgery.

Since extended bleeding following dental management may produce severe or even life-threatening adverse events, PWH are a preference group for preventive dental and oral health care.

It is paramount to make sure that PWH have access to dental management and regular preventive dental care at a designated dental care center with experience in the treatment of PWH according to evidence-based dental protocols.

19.12 Genetic Counseling

Genetic counseling is a paramount but difficult component of comprehensive treatment for PWH and their families with a diagnosis of hemophilia and for those at risk. The principal purpose of genetic counselors is to educate PWH on the natural history of hemophilia, determine their family tree/pedigree, carry out risk evaluations related to the inheritance of hemophilia, promote genetic testing, assist them process and incorporate genetic knowledge, and debate important reproductive alternatives.

19.13 Circumcision

Circumcision is a vastly practiced surgical intervention; up to 30% of men in the world are circumcised. In PWH, circumcision is associated with several adverse events including prolonged bleeding, infection, delayed skin healing/augmented morbidity, gangrene, HIV and hepatitis infection acquired via contaminated blood agents to manage bleeding, risk of neonatal inhibitor appearance, psychosocial scarring, and risk of mortality. The crucial factors for circumcision in PWH include individual patient problems such as inhibitor appearance, venous access, and wound management, as well as the experience and means at the treatment center. PWH will always bleed when stitches are taken off, and this must be treated with clotting factor replacement.

19.14 Vaccination

Children and adults with hemophilia must receive the same routine vaccines as the general population; nevertheless, they must preferably get the vaccines subcutaneously rather than intramuscularly or intradermally, as it is as secure and efficacious as the latter and does not need clotting factor infusion. If intramuscular injection has to be the way of administration, a dose of clotting factor concentrate must be administered, and the smallest gauge needle available (25–27 gauge) has to be utilized. Besides, an ice pack must be applied to the injection area for 5 minutes prior to injection of the vaccine, and pressure has to be applied to the area for at least 10 min to diminish bleeding and inflammation.

19.15 Psychosocial Matters

Severe hemophilia is associated with significant psychological and economic troubles for PWH and their caregivers. As hemophilia can influence many facets of daily living and family life, psychological and social assistance are relevant elements of complete treatment for hemophilia. Psychosocial management is an important facet of healthcare services for PWH and their families.

19.16 Outcome Evaluation

In spite of the availability of many evaluation tools, a core set of means for result evaluation in PWH continues to be determined. Outcome evaluation in PWH should include two facets: illness-related and therapy-related results. Illness-related results concern to the efficacy of hemostatic therapy and are reflected in results such as: incidence of bleeding, and influence of bleeding on the musculoskeletal apparatus and other systems in the short and long run, including the psychosocial influence of hemophilia. Therapy-related results have to be monitored utilizing a prospective and systematic plan and must cover screening and testing of PWH treated with CFCs for inhibitor development. Other less common side events of CFC replacement therapy include thrombosis and allergic/anaphylactic reactions. Table 19.7 summarizes the main aspects of outcome assessment in PWH.

19.17 Conclusions

For PWH prophylaxis is the gold standard of management (regular replacement therapy with CFCs). Episodic CFCs replacement must not be

Table 19.7 Main aspects of outcome assessment in people with hemophilia (PWH)

Frequency of bleeding
Assessment of the impact of bleeding on the musculoskeletal apparatus and other systems
Pain evaluation
Body structure and function
Activities and participation
Environmental and personal factors
Economic factors
Health-related quality of life
Patient-reported results
Measures for utilization in the clinic or research setting

considered a long-run alternative. PWH should have access to secure and efficacious management with optimal effectiveness in the prevention and treatment of bleeding. Treatment hospitals must be based on a multidisciplinary team of specialists. PWH must have access to musculoskeletal specialists (orthopedic surgeon, physical medicine/rehabilitation specialist, physical therapist) with knowledge in hemophilia, with yearly musculoskeletal evaluations and continuous control of their musculoskeletal results and preventive or corrective techniques as required. Orthopedic surgeons must have specific training in surgical treatment of PWH.

Reference

1. Srivastava A, Santagostino E, Dougall A, Kitchen S, Sutherland M, Pipe SW, et al. WFH guidelines for the management of hemophilia, 3rd edition. Haemophilia. 2020;26(Suppl 6):1–158.

GPSR Compliance

The European Union's (EU) General Product Safety Regulation (GPSR) is a set of rules that requires consumer products to be safe and our obligations to ensure this.

If you have any concerns about our products, you can contact us on ProductSafety@springernature.com

In case Publisher is established outside the EU, the EU authorized representative is:

Springer Nature Customer Service Center GmbH
Europaplatz 3
69115 Heidelberg, Germany

Batch number: 10406427

Printed by Printforce, the Netherlands